THE WASHINGTON MANUAL™

Endocrinology Subspecialty Consult

Second Edition

Editors

Katherine E. Henderson, MD

Instructor in Medicine
Department of Internal Medicine
Division of Medical Education
Washington University School of
  Medicine
Barnes-Jewish Hospital
St. Louis, Missouri

Thomas J. Baranski, MD, PhD

Associate Professor
Department of Internal Medicine
Division of Endocrinology, Metabolism,
  and Lipid Research
Washington University School of
  Medicine
St. Louis, Missouri

Perry E. Bickel, MD

Associate Professor and Director
Center for Obesity and Diabetes
  Research
Brown Foundation Institute of Molecular
  Medicine
University of Texas Health Science Center
  at Houston
Houston, Texas

William E. Clutter, MD

Associate Professor of Medicine
Department of Internal Medicine
Division of Endocrinology, Metabolism,
  and Lipid Research
Washington University School of Medicine
St. Louis, Missouri

Janet B. McGill, MD

Associate Professor of Medicine
Department of Internal Medicine
Division of Endocrinology, Metabolism, and
  Lipid Research
Washington University School of Medicine
St. Louis, Missouri

Series Editors

Katherine E. Henderson, MD

Instructor in Medicine
Department of Internal Medicine
Division of Medical Education
Washington University School of Medicine
Barnes-Jewish Hospital
St. Louis, Missouri

Thomas M. De Fer, MD

Associate Professor of Internal Medicine
Washington University School of Medicine
St. Louis, Missouri

Wolters Kluwer | Lippincott Williams & Wilkins
Health
Philadelphia · Baltimore · New York · London
Buenos Aires · Hong Kong · Sydney · Tokyo

Acquisitions Editor: Ave McCracken
Managing Editor: Michelle LaPlante
Project Manager: Bridgett Dougherty
Marketing Manager: Kimberly Schonberger
Manufacturing Manager: Kathleen Brown
Design Coordinator: Risa Clow
Cover Designer: Joseph DePinho
Production Service: Aptara®

Second Edition

9 8 7 6 5 4 3 2

Library of Congress Cataloging-in-Publication Data

The Washington manual endocrinology subspecialty consult / editors, Katherine E. Henderson . . . [et al.]. — 2nd ed.
    p. ; cm. — (Washington manual subspecialty consult series)
  Includes bibliographical references and index.
  ISBN 978-0-7817-9154-0 (pbk. : alk. paper) 1. Endocrinology—Handbooks, manuals, etc. 2. Endocrine glands—Diseases—Handbooks, manuals, etc. I. Henderson, Katherine E. II. Washington University (Saint Louis, Mo.). School of Medicine. III. Title: Endocrinology subspecialty consult. IV. Series.
  [DNLM: 1. Endocrine System Diseases—Handbooks. 2. Metabolic Diseases—Handbooks. WK 39 W319 2009]
  RC649.W28 2009
  616.4—dc22

                                                                                        2008020985

The Washington Manual™ is an intent-to-use mark belonging to Washington University in St. Louis to which international legal protection applies. The mark is used in this publication by LWW under license from Washington University.

Care has been taken to confirm the accuracy of the information present and to describe generally accepted practices. However, the authors, editors, and publisher are not responsible for errors or omissions or for any consequences from application of the information in this book and make no warranty, expressed or implied, with respect to the currency, completeness, or accuracy of the contents of the publication. Application of this information in a particular situation remains the professional responsibility of the practitioner; the clinical treatments described and recommended may not be considered absolute and universal recommendations.

The authors, editors, and publisher have exerted every effort to ensure that drug selection and dosage set forth in this text are in accordance with current recommendations and practice at the time of publication. However, in view of ongoing research, changes in government regulations, and the constant flow of information relating to drug therapy and drug reactions, the reader is urged to check the package insert for each drug for any change in indications and dosage and for added warnings and precautions. This is particularly important when the recommended agent is a new or infrequently employed drug.

Some drugs and medical devices presented in this publication have Food and Drug Administration (FDA) clearance for limited use in restricted research settings. It is the responsibility of health care providers to ascertain the FDA status of each drug or device planned for use in their clinical practice.

To purchase additional copies of this book, call our customer service department at **(800) 638-3030** or fax orders to **(301) 223-2320**. International customers should call **(301) 223-2300**.

Visit Lippincott Williams & Wilkins on the Internet: http://www.lww.com. Lippincott Williams & Wilkins customer service representatives are available from 8:30 am to 6:00 pm, EST

RRS0904

Table of Contents

PART I. HYPOTHALAMIC AND PITUITARY DISORDERS

PART II. THYROID DISORDERS

PART III. ADRENAL DISORDERS

PART IV. GONADAL DISORDERS

PART V. DISORDERS OF BONE AND MINERAL METABOLISM

PART VIII. OTHER ENDOCRINE DISORDERS

Contributing Authors

Ana Maria Arbelaez, MD
Assistant Professor of Pediatrics
Washington University School of Medicine
St. Louis Children's Hospital
St. Louis, Missouri

Carlos Bernal-Mizrachi, MD
Assistant Professor of Medicine
Division of Endocrinology, Metabolism and
    Lipid Research
Washington University School of Medicine
Barnes-Jewish Hospital
St. Louis, Missouri

Sweety Bhandare, MD
Attending Physician
Hamilton Community Health Network
Flint, Michigan

Manu V. Chakravarthy, MD, PhD
Instructor in Medicine
Division of Endocrinology, Metabolism and
    Lipid Research
Washington University School of Medicine
Barnes-Jewish Hospital
St. Louis, Missouri

William E. Clutter, MD
Associate Professor of Medicine
Division of Medical Education and Division
    of Endocrinology, Metabolism and Lipid
    Research
Washington University School of Medicine
St. Louis, Missouri

Benjamin Cooperberg, MD
Fellow in Endocrinology
Division of Endocrinology, Metabolism and
    Lipid Research
Washington University School of Medicine
St. Louis, Missouri

Pascual De Santis, MD
Attending Physician
Cleveland Clinic Foundation
Weston, Florida

Shaili K. Felton, MD
Fellow in Endocrinology
Division of Endocrinology, Metabolism and
    Lipid Research
Washington University School of Medicine
St. Louis, Missouri

Anne C. Goldberg, MD
Associate Professor of Medicine
Division of Endocrinology, Metabolism and
    Lipid Research
Washington University School of Medicine
St. Louis, Missouri

Jason S. Goldfeder, MD
Assistant Professor of Medicine
Division of Medical Education
Washington University School of Medicine
Barnes-Jewish Hospital
St. Louis, Missouri

Joan M. Heins, MA, RD, LD
Clinical Coordinator
Division of Geriatrics and Nutritional Sciences
Washington University School of Medicine
St. Louis, Missouri

James N. Heins, MD
Professor of Clinical Medicine
Division of Endocrinology, Metabolism and
    Lipid Research
Washington University School of Medicine
St. Louis, Missouri

Katherine E. Henderson, MD
Instructor in Medicine
Department of Internal Medicine
Division of Medical Education
Washington University School of
    Medicine
Barnes-Jewish Hospital
St. Louis, Missouri

Runhua Hou, MD
Fellow in Endocrinology
Division of Endocrinology, Metabolism and
   Lipid Research
Washington University School of Medicine
St. Louis, Missouri

Paul Hruz, MD, PhD
Assistant Professor of Pediatrics
Division of Pediatric Endocrinology and
   Diabetes
Washington University School of Medicine
St. Louis Children's Hospital
St. Louis, Missouri

Kent Ishihara, MD
Atttending Physician
Hellman and Rosen Endocrine Associates
North Kansas City Hospital
North Kansas City, Missouri

Matteo Levisetti, MD
Assistant Professor of Medicine
Division of Endocrinology, Metabolism and
   Lipid Research
Washington University School of Medicine
Barnes-Jewish Hospital
St. Louis, Missouri

Janet B. McGill, MD
Associate Professor of Medicine
Division of Endocrinology, Metabolism and
   Lipid Research
Washington University School of Medicine
Barnes-Jewish Hospital
St. Louis, Missouri

Paraskevi Mentzelopoulos, MD
Instructor in Medicine
Department of Medicine
Beth Israel-Deaconess Hospital
Harvard Medical School
Joslin Diabetes Center
Boston, Massachusetts

Sheri Nishimoto, MD
Fellow in Endocrinology
Division of Endocrinology, Metabolism and
   Lipid Research
Washington University School of Medicine
Barnes-Jewish Hospital
St. Louis, Missouri

Parvin F. Peddi, MD
Resident Physician
Division of Medical Education
Washington University School of Medicine
Barnes-Jewish Hospital
St. Louis, Missouri

Dominic N. Reeds, MD
Assistant Professor of Medicine
Division of Geriatrics and Nutritional Science
Washington University School of Medicine
Barnes-Jewish Hospital
St. Louis, Missouri

Richard I. Stein, PhD
Research Assistant Professor of Medicine
Division of Geriatrics and Nutritional Science
Washington University School of Medicine
St. Louis, Missouri

Kevin E. Yarasheski, PhD
Professor of Medicine, Cell Biology &
   Physiology, and Physical Therapy
Division of Endocrinology, Metabolism and
   Lipid Research
Washington University School of Medicine
St. Louis, Missouri

Chairman's Note

Medical knowledge is increasing at an exponential rate, and physicians are being bombarded with new facts at a pace that many find overwhelming. The Washington Manual™ Subspecialty Consult Series was developed in this context for interns, residents, medical students, and other practitioners in need of readily accessible practical clinical information. They, therefore, meet an important unmet need in an era of information overload.

I would like to acknowledge the authors who have contributed to these books. In particular, the series editors, Katherine E. Henderson, MD and Thomas M. De Fer, MD, for their oversight of the project. I'd also like to recognize Melvin Blanchard, MD, Chief of the Division of Medical Education in the Department of Medicine at Washington University for his guidance and advice. The efforts and outstanding skill of the lead authors are evident in the quality of the final product. I am confident that this series will meet its desired goal of providing practical knowledge that can be directly applied to improving patient care.

Kenneth S. Polonsky, MD
Adolphus Busch Professor
Chairman, Department of Medicine
Washington University School of Medicine
St. Louis, Missouri

Preface

T his second edition of *The Washington Manual™ Endocrinology Subspecialty Consult* was written by Washington University house staff, fellows, and endocrine faculty. The manual is designed to serve as a guide for students, house staff, and fellows involved in inpatient and outpatient endocrinology consults. It is not meant to serve as a comprehensive review of the field of endocrinology. Rather, it focuses on practical approaches to endocrine disorders commonly seen in consultation, with emphasis on key components of evaluation and treatment.

Several changes in content were made with the second edition. All chapters have been updated to provide the latest information on the pathophysiology and treatment of endocrine disorders. New chapters have been added that cover obesity, vitamin D deficiency, autoimmune polyendocrine syndromes, and endocrine disorders in HIV/AIDS. Drug dosing information was also reviewed and updated in each chapter. Bulleted key points highlight the salient features of each chapter. Clinical pearls are highlighted in bold-faced text within the chapters.

We are indebted to the remarkable efforts of the house staff, fellows, and attending physicians who contributed to the current edition and worked enthusiastically to provide high-quality, contemporary, concise chapters. We would also like to acknowledge and thank the authors of the first edition for the interest and effort they put into this project.

We would like to thank the following faculty for their expert editorial advice: Dr. Samuel Klein for the Obesity chapter and Dr. Philip E. Cryer for the Hypoglycemia chapter.

—K.E.H.
—T.J.B.
—P.E.B.
—W.E.C
—J.B.M

Pituitary Adenomas

Pascual De Santis

INTRODUCTION

Pituitary tumors constitute 10% of intracranial tumors. They can be benign or malignant, hormone-producing, or functionally inactive. According to their size, they are classified as microadenomas (<10 mm in greatest diameter) or macroadenomas (≥10 mm in greatest diameter). The most frequent primary tumors are pituitary adenomas, which are benign neoplasms arising in the adenohypophysial cells. They can be divided into:

- Somatotroph adenomas: Growth hormone (GH)–producing tumors clinically associated with acromegaly or gigantism. They account for approximately 15% of tumors.
- Lactotroph adenomas: Prolactinomas account for approximately 25% of symptomatic pituitary tumors.
- Thyrotroph adenomas (<1% of pituitary tumors): Associated with hyperthyroidism, or they can be silent, depending on whether the thyroid-stimulating hormone (TSH) subunits are processed correctly.
- Corticotroph adenomas (~15% of pituitary tumors): Contain adrenocorticotropic hormone (ACTH) and related peptides. Clinically they are associated with Cushing's disease or Nelson's syndrome (after bilateral adrenalectomy).
- Gonadotroph adenomas (~10% of pituitary tumors): Result in elevated serum alpha subunit, follicle-stimulating hormone (FSH) and, rarely, luteinizing hormone (LH) levels.
- Plurihormonal adenomas (~15% of pituitary tumors): Produce more than one type of hormone. Apart from the frequent occurrence of elevated GH and prolactin levels, the most common association of combined endocrine disorders is acromegaly and hyperthyroidism.
- Null cell adenomas (~20% of pituitary tumors): No histologic, immunocytologic, or electron microscopic markers of hormone excess.

Any type of tumor may be clinically nonfunctioning and present with symptoms of sellar and extrasellar mass effect and hypopituitarism. The majority of these tumors are gonadotroph or null cell adenomas.

CAUSES

Pituitary adenomas arise as a result of monoclonal pituitary cell proliferation. Oncogenes and tumor suppressor genes commonly found to be mutated in most malignancies are encountered infrequently in pituitary adenomas. Several different mutations have been associated with pituitary adenomas. Activating *gsp* mutations are present in 40% of GH-secreting adenomas. These are point mutations of the G protein alpha subunit (Gs alpha) gene, which activate Gs alpha protein and increase cyclic adenosine monophosphate (cAMP) levels, leading to GH hypersecretion and cell proliferation. H-ras gene mutations were identified in metastatic pituitary carcinomas. Pituitary tumor transforming gene (PTTG) is abundant in all pituitary tumor types, especially prolactinomas. In addition to somatic mutations, hypothalamic factors may promote and maintain growth of trans-formed pituitary adenomatous cells. There are emerging data for the importance of fibro-blast growth factor system, dysregulation of cell-cycle control proteins, and loss of reticulin network in pituitary tumor formation.

PRESENTATION

If the adenoma secretes functional hormones, the patient usually presents with symptoms caused by the hormone excess (see Disorders of the Pituitary Hormone Axis in this chap-ter). Some patients present with symptoms secondary to mass effects of the adenoma. Most pituitary masses are benign neoplasms, but they may aggressively invade locally into con-tiguous structures. Large infarcts may lead to partially or totally empty pituitary sella. Most masses arising from within the sella are benign, hormonally functional, or nonfunctional, with a relatively good prognosis, and their invasiveness is relatively limited. In contrast, parasellar masses are often malignant or invasive and have a less favorable prognosis. It is important to differentiate pituitary adenomas from other pituitary lesions.

Differential Diagnosis of Pituitary Tumors

Sellar/Parasellar Cysts

The most common cysts are **craniopharyngiomas**. They are calcified, cystic, suprasellar tumors derived from embryonic squamous cell rests of Rathke's cleft. They have a bimodal peak of incidence, occurring predominantly in children between the ages of 5 and 10 years; a second peak occurs in late middle age. There is a female preponderance, and most cysts present as calcified sellar/suprasellar masses. Children present with headache, vomiting, visual field deficits, and growth failure. Adults may present with bitemporal hemianopsia, cranial nerve abnormalities (cranial nerves III, IV, VI, and V1), anterior pituitary hormone deficits, and diabetes insipidus (DI). **Rathke's cleft cysts** are benign, uncalcified lesions that mimic endocrinologically inactive adenomas or craniopharyngiomas, but that have a par-ticularly low recurrence rate after partial excision.

Chordomas

Chordomas are rare tumors that arise from notochordal remnants within the clivus. They produce bony destruction with local infiltration, and they tend to recur. They are more common in men ages 30 to 50 years. They produce cranial neuropathy and diplopia. Endocrine dysfunction is unusual. Calcification is seen in 50% of cases.

Germinomas

Germinomas arise in sellar/suprasellar regions and involve the hypothalamus, chiasm, optic nerves, and pineal region. Patients present with hypopituitarism or pituitary hyperfunction, precocious puberty, DI, visual field defects, and signs of increased intracranial pressure. They metastasize within the central nervous system (CNS) in 10% of cases.

Dermoid Tumors

Dermoid tumors are rare developmental tumors in childhood that produce recurrent meningitis from leakage of tumor contents.

Pituitary Metastases

Pituitary metastases occur most commonly in elderly patients and usually arise from breast carcinomas (women) and lung carcinomas. Other sites of primary malignancies that metastasize to the pituitary include gastrointestinal tract, kidney, prostate, and skin (melanoma). Patients present with anterior pituitary dysfunction, visual field abnormalities, DI, and cranial nerve palsies. A rapidly enlarging mass is highly suggestive of a metastatic lesion.

Aneurysms

Aneurysms can arise from the cavernous sinus, or from the infraclinoid or supraclinoid internal carotid arteries. They may compress the optic nerve or chiasm and produce bitemporal deficits, ocular motor palsies, intense headache, and supraorbital pain. They may extend into the sella and cause direct pituitary compression, producing hypopituitarism and hyperprolactinemia. They are identified by magnetic resonance imaging (MRI) and MR angiography (MRA) and need to be excluded before transsphenoidal biopsy.

Pituitary Granulomas

- Tuberculous meningitis can involve the sellar and parasellar regions. A tuberculoma may be sellar or suprasellar and is associated with hypopituitarism, visual field changes, and DI.
- Sarcoidosis of the hypothalamic–pituitary region occurs in most patients with CNS involvement and can cause hypopituitarism with or without symptoms of an intrasellar mass. Sarcoidosis has a predilection for the hypothalamus, posterior pituitary, and cranial nerves. The most common hormonal abnormalities are hypogonadotropic hypogonadism, mild hyperprolactinemia, and DI.
- Giant cell granuloma (granulomatous hypophysitis) is a rare noncaseating giant cell granulomata that partially or completely replaces the pituitary gland in the absence of involvement of other organs. It is most common in middle-aged to older women. The cause is unknown. It produces hypopituitarism and hyperprolactinemia.
- Histiocytosis X (HX): It can be a unifocal or multifocal eosinophilic granuloma (Hand-Schüller-Christian [HSC] disease or the more malignant form, Letterer-Siwe disease). HX has predilection for the hypothalamus, and one half of patients present with DI. Children can present with growth retardation and anterior pituitary hormone deficits. HSC disease includes the triad of DI, exophthalmos, and lytic bone disease (only 25% of patients present with this triad). Other features of the disease include axillary skin rash and a history of recurrent pneumothorax.

Lymphocytic Hypophysitis

Lymphocytic hypophysitis affects mostly women, and in 60% to 70% of cases presents in late pregnancy or during the postpartum period. Other autoimmune diseases (autoimmune thyroiditis) are present in 20% to 25%. It can present as an enlarging intrasellar/suprasellar mass, hypopituitarism, DI, and/or visual impairment (56%–70%). Partial recovery of pituitary function and resolution of the sellar mass can occur spontaneously or with use of corticosteroids and hormone replacement. The diagnosis is confirmed by histology or resolution of the mass over time. Surgery is needed if visual or compressive symptoms develop.

Pituitary Abscesses

Pituitary abscesses are rare, and they occur from direct extension of adjacent infection in the sphenoid sinuses and other CNS infections. Most abscesses arise in previously healthy pituitary glands, but one-third are associated with pituitary adenomas or craniopharyngiomas. Gram-positive streptococci or staphylococci may be isolated, or, rarely, *Aspergillus*, *Candida albicans*, or *Entamoeba histolytica*. Patients present with visual compromise, hypopituitarism, and DI (50%). MRI shows ring enhancement and a central isointense cavity with contrast.

Intrapituitary Hemorrhage and Infarction

Intrapituitary hemorrhage and infarction are caused by ischemic damage to the hypophyseal-portal system, and pituitary insufficiency is clinically apparent when 75% of the gland is damaged. The damage is limited to the anterior lobe, and the posterior pituitary function remains intact. In pregnancy, the pituitary gland enlarges in response to estrogen stimulation, making it vulnerable to arterial pressure changes. Sheehan's syndrome, described after severe postpartum hemorrhage, is less commonly seen.

Pituitary Carcinomas

Pituitary carcinomas are rare tumors and may produce GH, ACTH, or prolactin, or they may be clinically nonfunctioning. The diagnosis can only be established when the lesion metastasizes.

Pituitary Hyperplasia

Generalized enlargement of the pituitary can occur in thyrotroph hyperplasia owing to long-standing primary hypothyroidism, gonadotroph hyperplasia in long-standing primary hypogonadism, lactotroph hyperplasia during pregnancy and, very rarely, somatotroph hyperplasia in ectopic secretion of growth hormone-releasing hormone (GHRH).

Primary Central Nervous System Lymphoma

Primary CNS lymphoma may involve the pituitary and the hypothalamus, causing neurologic symptoms sometimes associated with anterior and/or posterior pituitary hormone insufficiencies.

Disorders of the Pituitary Hormone Axis

Prolactinomas

Hyperprolactinemia produces amenorrhea and galactorrhea in women and decreased libido and impotence in men. Macroadenomas also produce visual symptoms, secondary to compression of the optic chiasm, cranial neuropathies, and hypopituitarism (see Chapter 2, Prolactinoma).

Growth Hormone–Secreting Tumors

- **Acromegaly:** The insidious progression over years often results in a delay in diagnosis (6–10 years). Symptomatic cardiac disease is present in 20% (hypertension occurs in 50%, left ventricular hypertrophy, arrhythmias, cardiac failure) and accounts for 60% of deaths. Diabetes mellitus can develop in 10% to 25% of patients. There is a two- to threefold increased rate of developing colon cancer and premalignant polyps (see Chapter 3, Acromegaly).
- **Gigantism:** It should be considered in children >3 SD (standard deviations) above the normal mean height for age or >2 SD above normal mean parental height. It is caused by excess of GH secretion before the epiphyses close.

Adrenocorticotropic Hormone–Secreting Tumors (Cushing's Disease)

(See also Chapter 14, Cushing's Syndrome.)

The classic features of centripetal obesity, hirsutism, and plethora are not always present. Children can present with generalized obesity and poor linear growth. Patients develop fat depots over the thoracocervical spine (buffalo hump), supraclavicular region, cheeks, and temporal regions (moon facies). Gonadal dysfunction is common, with menstrual irregularities in women and loss of libido in men and women. Hirsutism (vellus hypertrichosis of face) and acne are common. Psychiatric abnormalities occur in 50% of patients (depression, lethargy, paranoia, and psychosis). Long-standing Cushing's disease can produce osteoporotic vertebral collapse, rib fractures, and aseptic necrosis of the femoral head and the humeral head. Hypercortisolism produces skin thinning, bruising with minimal trauma, red-purple striae >1 cm in diameter (usually found on the abdomen, upper thighs, and arms), and proximal muscle weakness of the lower limb and shoulder girdle (inability to climb stairs or rise from a deep chair). Hypertension occurs in 75% of patients. Infections are more common (poor wound healing, reactivation of tuberculosis, and onychomycosis). Glucose intolerance occurs, and overt diabetes mellitus is present in more than one third of patients.

Thyroid Stimulating Hormone–Secreting Tumors

TSH-secreting tumors are usually large macroadenomas, and >60% are locally invasive. Patients present with visual field abnormalities, cranial nerve palsies, headache, hyperthyroidism (palpitations, arrhythmias, weight loss, and tremors), and goiter.

Gonadotropin-producing Pituitary Tumors (Clinically Nonfunctioning Tumors)

Gonadotropin-producing pituitary tumors are usually macroadenomas, and patients present with visual disturbance, symptoms of hypopituitarism, or headache. Some tumors produce elevated FSH, LH, or alpha subunit concentration, and patients present with hypogonadism related to gonadal downregulation.

Pituitary Apoplexy

An endocrine emergency, pituitary apoplexy results from spontaneous hemorrhage into a pituitary adenoma, or after head trauma. It evolves over 1 to 2 days, with severe headache, neck stiffness, and progressive cranial nerve damage, cardiovascular collapse, change in consciousness, bilateral visual disturbances, hyperglycemia, fever, CNS hemorrhage, and coma. Acute adrenal insufficiency may also be superimposed. Pituitary imaging reveals intra-adenomal hemorrhage and stalk deviation. Most patients recover spontaneously but experience long-term pituitary insufficiency. Ophthalmoplegia may resolve spontaneously, but signs of reduced visual acuity and altered mental status are indications for transsphenoidal surgical decompression.

Hypopituitarism

In congenital forms of hypopituitarism, an earlier age of onset will result in greater severity of thyroid, gonadal, adrenal, growth, or water disturbances. The corticotrophs and thyrotrophs are most resistant to mass effects and the last to lose function. ACTH deficiency produces hypotension, shock, hypoglycemia, nausea, vomiting, fatigue, and dilutional hyponatremia. Serum cortisol and ACTH levels can be determined before glucocorticoid administration. A cosyntropin stimulation test can be done several weeks after the onset of ACTH deficiency (see Chapter 11, Adrenal Insufficiency, for further details about this test). Hypothyroidism becomes apparent weeks after pituitary insufficiency. TSH is not elevated in secondary hypothyroidism, and free thyroxine (T_4) is used for follow-up. Patients develop coarse and cold skin and delayed ankle reflex relaxation. Even in the absence of symptoms, T_4 should be administered (glucocorticoids should be replaced first). Sexual dysfunction related to gonadotropin deficiency is common: Women present with abnormal menses or amenorrhea with no elevation of LH or FSH levels, and men present with sexual dysfunction and low testosterone. Sex hormone replacement is important to prevent osteoporosis, although sexual function may not be normalized. GH deficiency is present when two or more hormones are deficient. Prolactin deficiency is rare and occurs when the anterior pituitary is completely destroyed, as in apoplexy.

Local Effects of Sellar Masses

Headaches are common, and they do not correlate with the size of the adenoma. Upward compression and pressure on the optic chiasm may result in bitemporal hemianopsia, loss of red perception, scotomas, and blindness. Lateral invasion may impinge on the cavernous sinus, leading to lesions of the III, IV, VI, and V1 cranial nerves, producing diplopia, ptosis, ophthalmoplegia, and facial numbness. Uncinate seizures, personality disorders, and anosmia occur if temporal and frontal brain lobes are invaded by the expanding parasellar mass. Direct hypothalamic involvement produces recurrent vomiting with or without extrapyramidal or pyramidal tract involvement, precocious puberty, hypogonadism, DI (partial or complete) and/or adipsia, or essential hypernatremia owing to an impaired thirst mechanism, syndrome of inappropriate secretion of antidiuretic hormone (SIADH), sleep disturbances, dysthermia, and appetite disorders (obesity, hyperphagia, anorexia, adipsia, and compulsive drinking).

MANAGEMENT

Diagnostic Evaluation

The screening tests for functional pituitary adenomas include the following.

Prolactinomas

Elevated serum prolactin levels (although a mild elevation should be confirmed on serial samples). Mild hyperprolactinemia raises the possibilities of "hook effect," medication induced hyperprolactinemia or stalk compression (see Chapter 2, Prolactinoma).

Acromegaly

Elevated insulin-like growth factor 1 (IGF-1) levels, GH nadir >1 mcg/L during an oral glucose tolerance test are consistent with acromegaly (see Chapter 3, Acromegaly).

Cushing's Disease

High 24-hour urine free cortisol or failed dexamethasone suppression tests (cortisol levels are not suppressed with the low dose but are suppressed with the high dose), high normal ACTH levels (but they are inappropriately elevated for the plasma cortisol), elevated late-night plasma, and salivary cortisol levels are diagnostic of Cushing's disease. Corticotropin-releasing hormone (CRH) testing produces a rise in plasma ACTH and cortisol levels in contrast to ectopic ACTH secretion. The most reliable way to differentiate pituitary from ectopic ACTH secretion is by inferior petrosal sinus sampling (measuring ACTH levels in the venous blood draining the pituitary). (The reader is referred to Chapter 14, Cushing's Syndrome, for further details.)

Thyroid-Stimulating Hormone–Secreting Tumors

High T_4, triiodothyronine (T_3), and alpha subunit with high or inappropriately normal TSH and a pituitary tumor seen in MRI confirm the diagnosis. Thyrotropin-releasing hormone (TRH) stimulation distinguishes between TSH overproduction by a TSH-secreting tumor (TSH response to TRH is blunted) and thyroid hormone insensitivity (TSH rises in response to TRH). The molar ratio of alpha subunit to TRH is high (>1) in 85% of patients. Genetic testing for thyroid hormone receptor mutations are also available.

Incidentalomas

The term refers to a pituitary lesion that was previously unsuspected and discovered in the course of evaluation for an unrelated problem. They are thought to be present in ~10% of the general, unselected population based on autopsy and MRI studies. The evaluation and management of these lesions are controversial, and their natural history is only partially known. Microadenomas are less likely to grow, especially when <5 mm. The cost-effective approach depends on the radiologic characteristics of a pituitary MRI, the size of the lesion, and the clinical findings of possible hormonal hypersecretion. There is precedent in measuring serum prolactin levels as the sole hormonal evaluation in a patient without any clinical findings consistent with any hormonal abnormalities. However, if the patient has features of the metabolic syndrome, most physicians would agree to screen for Cushing's syndrome. Macroadenomas require formal visual field testing, and may require investigation for decreased anterior pituitary function. Follow-up imaging studies may be required, but the frequency is not established. Microadenomas may not require additional imaging when they are <5 mm. Microadenomas measuring 5 to 9 mm may need follow-up imaging for 1 or 2 years. If hormonal abnormalities, visual field defects, or size changes are detected during the evaluation of these lesions, appropriate management according to the specific circumstances is warranted.

Hypopituitarism

- To evaluate adrenal insufficiency, check 8 AM cortisol, ACTH levels, and cosyntropin stimulation test (if it is inconclusive, the insulin tolerance test can be done).
- To evaluate hypothyroidism, check serum free T_4.
- For GH deficiency, perform insulin-induced hypoglycemia and arginine–GHRH tests.
- For gonadotropin deficiency, obtain LH, FSH, testosterone in men, and prolactin (hyperprolactinemia is associated with hypogonadism). The GRH stimulation test rarely differentiates causes of gonadotropin deficiency and is usually not indicated.

Imaging Studies

Tumors of the pituitary gland are best diagnosed with MRI focused on the pituitary (contiguous sections detect lesions of 1–3 mm). MRI detects tumor effect on soft tissue structures, cavernous sinus or optic chiasm, sphenoid sinus, and hypothalamus. T1-weighted sections with gadolinium distinguish most pituitary masses. T2-weighted images are important for diagnosing high-signal hemorrhage. During pregnancy, the gland should not exceed 10 to 12 mm. A thickened stalk may indicate the presence of hypophysitis, granuloma, or atypical chordomas. Microadenomas enlarge the sella turcica and can grow upward toward the optic chiasm. MRI can distinguish pituitary adenomas from other masses. Pituitary computed tomography (CT) allows visualization of bony structures, including the sellar floor and clinoid bones. CT recognizes calcifications of craniopharyngiomas that are not evident on MRI. There is a 5% risk of developing nephrogenic systemic fibrosis after the administration of gadolinium in patients with a glomerular filtration rate (GFR) of <30 mL/minute.

Treatment and Follow-Up

Nonfunctioning Pituitary Adenomas

The risk of significant tumor enlargement is low for microadenomas. MRI may be repeated at yearly intervals for 2 years, and if there is no evidence of growth of the lesion, the interval between scans may subsequently be lengthened. Surgery is not indicated unless growth is demonstrated. Macroadenomas have already indicated a propensity for growth, and if the lesion is asymptomatic, MRI can be repeated at 6 and 12 months and then yearly, and surgery may be deferred unless there is evidence of growth. If the macroadenoma is accompanied by compression of the optic chiasm, cavernous sinus invasion, or pituitary hormone deficiencies, surgery should be performed and irradiation of the mass considered (especially gamma-knife, external beam radiation therapy). Ten percent of these tumors respond to bromocriptine with tumor size reduction.

Prolactinomas

Treat with dopamine receptor agonists such as bromocriptine (see Chapter 2, Prolactinoma).

Acromegaly

Transsphenoidal surgery is the treatment of choice, and 70% of patients achieve GH levels <5 ng/mL and have normal IGF-1 levels, but recurrence rate is 5% to 10%. After use of conventional radiation, GH levels of <5 ng/mL are achieved in 40% of patients by 5 years and 60% to 70% of patients by 10 years (see Chapter 3, Acromegaly).

Cushing's Disease

Transsphenoidal surgery is the mainstay of treatment, and cure is expected in 80% to 90% of patients, with a 5% to 10% recurrence rate. The hypothalamus–pituitary–adrenal axis (HPA) may be suppressed for up to 1 year. Radiotherapy is used for patients not cured by surgery and those with bilateral adrenalectomy or with Nelson's syndrome. Sixty-one percent of patients are in remission by 12 months, and 70% by 24 months. At the time of surgery, patients should be treated with corticosteroids for any potential or confirmed HPA-axis deficit. On postoperative day 5, plasma cortisol should be measured at 9 AM, with the patient having omitted hydrocortisone for 24 hours: A nonsuppressed plasma cortisol postoperatively suggests residual tumor activity or an ectopic source of ACTH. Medical therapy can provide some benefit and includes:

- Ketoconazole (Nizoral) (200–1200 mg/day). It blocks cortisol synthesis, and 90% of patients normalize cortisol levels without a rise in ACTH levels.
- Other medications (less effective) are metyrapone, aminoglutethimide, and mitotane (see Chapter 14, Cushing's Syndrome).

TSH-Secreting Adenomas

Transsphenoidal surgery is the treatment of choice but rarely results in cure. Most cases respond well to octreotide acetate (Sandostatin, Sandostatin LAR) with tumor shrinkage, but in one third of patients tachyphylaxis may develop. Radiation therapy is adjunctive when surgery is not curative. For treatment of hyperthyroidism, propranolol, radioactive iodine thyroid ablation, thyroidectomy, methimazole, or propylthiouracil are used.

KEY POINTS TO REMEMBER

- Most pituitary masses are benign neoplasms but may aggressively invade contiguous structures.
- Pituitary adenomas can produce symptoms due to local effects (headache, visual disturbances, and cranial neuropathies of cranial nerves III, IV, VI, V1 if they impinge the cavernous sinus) or to hormone secretion (acromegaly, Cushing's disease, hyperthyroidism).
- Pituitary apoplexy is an endocrine emergency that results from hemorrhage into a pituitary adenoma.
- Pituitary masses most commonly are pituitary adenomas, but other etiologies need to be excluded.

REFERENCES AND SUGGESTED READINGS

Braunstein G. Hypothalamic syndromes. In: DeGroot LJ, Jameson JL, eds. *Endocrinology*, 5th ed. Philadelphia: WB Saunders; 2006:373–386.

Ezzat S, Asa S. Mechanisms of disease: The pathogenesis of pituitary tumors. *Nat Clin Pract Endocrinol Metab* 2006;2(4):220–230.

Freda P, Post KD. Differential diagnosis of sellar masses. *Endocrinol Metab Clin North Am* 1999;28:81–117.

Freda P, Wardlaw S. Diagnosis and treatment of pituitary tumors. *J Clin Endocrinol Metab* 1999;84:3859–3866.

Katsnelson L, Alexander JM, Klibanski A. Clinically nonfunctioning pituitary adenomas. *J Clin Endocrinol Metab* 1993;76:1089–1094.

Krikorian A, Aron D. Evaluation and management of pituitary incidentalomas—revisiting an acquaintance. *Nat Clin Pract Endocrinol Metab* 2006;2(3):138–148.

Maccagnan P, Macedo CL, Kayath MJ, et al. Conservative management of pituitary apoplexy: A perspective study. *J Clin Endocrinol Metab* 1995;80:2190–2197.

Melmed S, Kleinberg D. Anterior pituitary. In: Larsen PR, Kronenberg HM, Melmed S, et al., eds. *Williams textbook of endocrinology*, 10th ed. Philadelphia: WB Saunders; 2003:177–179.

Melmed S. Evaluation of pituitary masses. In: DeGroot LJ, Jameson JL, eds. *Endocrinology*, 5th ed. Philadelphia: WB Saunders; 2006:387–393.

Melmed S. Functional pituitary anatomy and histology. In: DeGroot LJ, Jameson JL, eds. *Endocrinology*, 5th ed. Philadelphia: WB Saunders; 2006:167–182.

Molitch M. Evaluation and treatment of the patient with a pituitary incidentaloma. *J Clin Endocrinol Metab* 1995;80:3–6.

Rennert J, Doerfler A. Imaging of sellar and parasellar lesions. *Clin Neurol Neurosurg* 2007;09:111–124.

Rivera J. Lymphocytic hypophysitis: Disease spectrum and approach to diagnosis and therapy. *Pituitary* 2006;9:35–45.

Saeger W, Lüdecke DK, Buchfelder M, et al. Pathohistological classification or pituitary tumors: 10 years of experience with the German Pituitary Tumor Registry. *Eur J Endocrinol* 2007;156:203–216.

Sonabend A, Musleh W, Lesniak M. Oncogenesis and mutagenesis of pituitary tumors. *Expert Rev Anticancer Ther* 2006;6[Suppl 9]:S3–S14.

Prolactinoma

2

Shaili K. Felton

INTRODUCTION

Prolactinomas are the most frequent secretory pituitary tumors, occurring with an annual incidence of 6 in 100,000. Autopsy studies found prolactin-staining microadenoma in ~10% of individuals. Prolactinomas account for 40% to 50% of pituitary adenomas. The female-to-male ratio for microprolactinomas (tumors <10 mm in greatest diameter) is 20:1 and for macroprolactinomas (>10 mm in greatest diameter) is 1:1. Tumor size correlates with serum prolactin levels. Prolactin levels >200 ng/mL are indicative of a macroprolactinoma. The risk of progression from prolactin-secreting microadenoma to macroadenoma is less than 30%. Prolactinoma is the most frequent pituitary tumor occurring in the multiple endocrine neoplasia syndrome. 10% of prolactinomas also secrete other hormones. The most frequent mixed tumors are growth hormone (GH)/prolactin-secreting adenomas.

Malignant prolactinomas are extremely rare and are defined by the presence of metastases. Of the 140 cases of pituitary carcinomas reported in the literature as of 2006, one-third were malignant prolactinomas. These neoplasms can invade the sphenoidal and cavernous sinuses and give rise to distant metastases to the bone, lymph nodes, lung, liver, or spinal cord.

CAUSES

The **hypothalamus** exerts a predominantly inhibitory influence on prolactin secretion through inhibitory factors (e.g., dopamine). Alterations of D2 dopamine receptors seem to occur in prolactinomas. An alteration in the neuroendocrine mechanisms regulating prolactin secretion results in modestly elevated prolactin levels (25–150 ng/mL; normal values, 5–20 ng/mL).

Differential Diagnosis for Hyperprolactinemia

Medications

Drugs that are D2 dopamine receptor antagonists may increase serum prolactin concentrations by an unknown mechanism. Examples include antipsychotics (risperidone [Risperdal], phenothiazines, haloperidol), metoclopramide, and antihypertensives (methyldopa [Aldomet], reserpine, verapamil). Other drugs that can raise prolactin levels include tricyclic antidepressants, serotonin reuptake inhibitors, estrogens, opiates, and cocaine.

Physiologic Causes

Physiologic causes of increased prolactin levels include pregnancy and nipple stimulation.

Lactotroph Adenomas (Prolactinomas)

Lactotroph adenomas arise from monoclonal expansion of a cell that has undergone somatic mutations.

Lactotroph Hyperplasia

Lactotroph hyperplasia is due to stalk compression that reduces inhibition of the lactotroph cells by prolactin inhibitory factors (i.e., dopamine). This may occur because of tumors of the hypothalamus (craniopharyngiomas or metastatic breast carcinoma), infiltrative diseases (sarcoidosis), disruption of the hypothalamic-pituitary stalk in head trauma, or pituitary adenomas.

Hypothyroidism

Most patients with hypothyroidism have normal prolactin levels. Rarely patients with hypothyroidism present with elevated prolactin values. Thyroid hormone replacement typically restores normal prolactin values.

Chest Wall Injury and Spinal Cord Lesions

Chest wall injuries or irritating lesions (e.g., herpes zoster) activate neural reflexes similar to nipple stimulation and, therefore, can increase prolactin levels.

Chronic Renal Failure

Patients with chronic renal failure may have a threefold increase in prolactin values, owing to decreased clearance. In the setting of renal failure, medications (e.g., metoclopramide) can cause markedly elevated prolactin levels (>500 ng/mL). Levels should return to normal after renal transplantation.

Cirrhosis

Basal prolactin levels are increased in 5% to 20% of patients with cirrhosis, possibly because of alterations in hypothalamic dopamine generation.

Adrenal Insufficiency

Glucocorticoids have a suppressive effect on prolactin gene transcription and release.

Idiopathic Hyperprolactinemia

In some patients with prolactin concentrations between 20 and 100 ng/mL, no cause can be found. Many of these patients have undetectable lactotroph microadenomas. Long-term follow-up revealed that in one third of these patients, prolactin levels returned to normal; in 10% to 15% of these patients, prolactin levels rose to 50% over baseline; and in the remaining patients, prolactin levels remained stable and mildly elevated.

Macroprolactinemia ("Big Prolactin")

A small amount of a 25-kDa glycosylated form of prolactin (instead of the normal 23-kDa nonglycosylated prolactin) can circulate in aggregates. These aggregates of macroprolactin can be distinguished from hyperprolactinemia by gel filtration or polyethylene glycol precipitation. In a series of such patients, none had a history of amenorrhea, few had oligomenorrhea or galactorrhea, and none had adenomas seen on magnetic resonance imaging (MRI).

Hook Effect (Prozone Effect)

Measurement of serum prolactin levels is important in the differentiation of prolactinomas from nonfunctioning adenomas. Immunoradiometric assay is frequently used for measurement of serum prolactin levels. The sensitivity and the precision of the assay is good, with a short incubation time. Falsely low values have been reported with this technique when a large amount of prolactin is present that saturates the antibodies. This is known as the hook effect. In the setting of a pituitary macroadenoma, prolactin concentrations between 20 and 200 ng/mL might lead the clinician to conclude that the adenoma is non-functioning because macroadenomas can increase prolactin levels to this range due to stalk compression. Hook effect (prozone effect) artifact should be considered and excluded by performing an additional determination of a 1:10 dilution of serum. If the diluted specimen yields the same value (or even a higher value) then the diagnosis of macroprolactinoma can be made.

PRESENTATION

Clinical Manifestations

Signs and symptoms of an expanding pituitary lesion include headache (common in patients with macroadenoma and ameliorates after tumor shrinkage), diminished visual acuity, and visual field defects. Ophthalmoplegia may occur when tumors expand laterally and invade the cavernous sinus. Rhinorrhea may occur if the tumor invades the sphenoid or ethmoid sinuses, or after rapid drug-induced tumor shrinkage.

The history should focus on a search for medications, symptoms of hypothyroidism, renal disease or cirrhosis, headache, and visual symptoms. The physical examination should evaluate for bitemporal field loss and signs of hypothyroidism or hypogonadism. Prolactin is secreted periodically. The finding of a mildly elevated prolactin level requires confirmation in several samples. A careful history of drug ingestion is recommended. Routine blood tests such as a thyroid-stimulating hormone (TSH) and blood chemistry panel can exclude hypothyroidism, chronic renal failure, and liver cirrhosis. Serum prolactin levels <100 ng/mL that progressively drop to within normal limits during multiple samplings exclude the diagnosis of hyperprolactinemia. Serum prolactin levels >200 ng/mL are highly indicative of a macroprolactinoma. When there is no obvious cause of hyperprolactinemia, MRI with gadolinium enhancement provides the best anatomic detail of the hypothalamic-pituitary area. Large nonsecreting tumors can cause modest elevations in prolactin due to stalk compression (prolactin elevation, <150 ng/mL), whereas prolactin-secreting macroadenomas have much higher levels of prolactin (>250 ng/mL). Visual field testing (Goldmann's perimetry) should be obtained in patients with tumors that are adjacent to or compressing the optic chiasm.

Premenopausal Women

Premenopausal women present with secondary hypogonadism (infertility, oligomenorrhea, or amenorrhea), and galactorrhea is present in 30% to 80%. Hyperprolactinemia accounts for 10% to 20% of cases of amenorrhea (excluding pregnancy) in this group of women. A serum prolactin >100 ng/mL is associated with overt hypogonadism and can cause hot flashes and vaginal dryness. Mild hyperprolactinemia (20–50 ng/mL) can cause infertility, even if there is no abnormality of the menstrual cycle. Women who are amenorrheic for longer periods are at risk for osteopenia and osteoporosis and are less likely to present with galactorrhea.

Postmenopausal Women

Postmenopausal women rarely present with galactorrhea, since they have very low estrogen levels. Hyperprolactinemia in these women is recognized after a prolactinoma is sufficiently large to produce mass effect, for example, headaches or visual impairment. Seborrhea and moderate hirsutism may be present. These symptoms may be accompanied by elevations of androstenedione and dehydroepiandrosterone sulfate, suggesting a stimulatory effect of prolactin on adrenocortical androgen secretion.

Men

Men present with hypogonadotropic hypogonadism and symptoms of decreased libido, impotence, infertility, gynecomastia, and, rarely, galactorrhea. Hyperprolactinemia results in decreased testosterone secretion, which in turn produces decreased energy, libido, muscle mass, and body hair, and promotes osteoporosis.

MANAGEMENT

Indications for therapy depend on tumor size and effects of hyperprolactinemia. Invasion or compression of the stalk or optic chiasm, or symptoms caused by hyperprolactinemia are indications for initiating therapy. In 95% of patients, microprolactinomas did not enlarge over a 6-year period of observation. It is unlikely that a prolactinoma will grow significantly without a concomitant increase in serum prolactin levels; therefore, most patients with microadenomas can be monitored safely with serial prolactin levels. If prolactin levels rise significantly, repeat imaging is indicated.

Medical Therapy

The mainstays of management for prolactinomas are the dopaminergic agonists (bromocriptine and cabergoline). Most patients will respond to therapy within weeks of initiation, as evidenced by symptoms and prolactin levels. The majority of patients will also have a greater than 50% decrease in the size of the adenoma. Several recent studies demonstrate that cabergoline or bromocriptine can be withdrawn safely and that 40% to 70% of individuals will have a long-lasting remission.

Bromocriptine
Bromocriptine is an ergot derivative D2 receptor agonist. It can be administered orally once or twice a day at doses of 2.5 to 20 mg/day and produces reduction in prolactin levels to the normal range in 60% to 100% of cases. Women resume regular ovulatory menses, and galactorrhea should resolve after 2 to 3 months of therapy. For macroprolactinomas, the reduction in tumor size is usually associated with improved visual fields, reduction of hyperprolactinemia, and improvement in other pituitary function (owing to reduced mass effect). Most series suggest that bromocriptine therapy has little or no effect on later surgical results for microadenomas; however, in patients with macroadenomas, bromocriptine treatment lasting >6 to 12 weeks has been associated with perivascular fibrosis of the tumor, which can complicate complete tumor resection. The most common side effects of bromocriptine are nausea and vomiting. Orthostatic hypotension may occur when initiating therapy. Between 5% and 10% of patients either do not respond to bromocriptine or have only minimal responses. To overcome resistance to treatment, other dopamine agonists have been developed.

Cabergoline
Cabergoline is a nonergot D2 receptor agonist with a long half-life, and can be given orally at 0.25 to 1 mg twice a week. Several noninferiority studies have shown that cabergoline is at least as effective as bromocriptine in lowering prolactin levels and reducing tumor size, and some studies have shown success rates superior to that of bromocriptine. Side effects are much less frequent and less severe than with bromocriptine. Recent studies have shown that cabergoline can cause valvular fibrosis at higher doses (used for off-label treatment of Parkinson's disease). For hyperprolactinemic disorders, a considerably lower dose of cabergoline is used. At these lower doses, there appears to be little chance of valvular abnormalities.

Other Dopamine Agonists
Pergolide, a dopamine agonist that was recently taken off the market, was approved only for Parkinson's disease and not for treatment of hyperprolactinemia. It was taken off the market when two new studies showed that patients with Parkinson's disease who were treated with pergolide had an increased chance of serious damage to their heart valves when compared to patients who did not receive the drug.

Quinagolide, which can be given once daily, is another potential therapy. Fifty percent of patients with resistance to bromocriptine respond to quinagolide, but it is not yet approved for use in the United States.

Surgery

Pituitary surgery is recommended for patients with microprolactinomas or macroprolactinomas who are refractory to or intolerant of dopamine agonists, for those in whom medical treatment is unable to shrink the adenoma, or for patients with cystic or rapidly expanding tumors. Pituitary surgery aimed at debulking the tumor mass and preventing tumor expansion is indicated for women with macroprolactinoma who wish to become pregnant. Transsphenoidal surgery is the preferred technique for treating microadenomas in patients who do not wish to receive lifelong medical therapy.

Radiotherapy

Radiotherapy is limited to patients with macroprolactinomas that are refractory to medical treatment and surgery. It is occasionally used in conjunction with medical treatment. Approximately 30% of patients achieve normal serum prolactin levels gradually over a period of years.

Prolactinomas and Pregnancy

Patients with prolactinomas wishing to become pregnant should be referred to specialists in high-risk obstetrics and endocrinology because they may need to be pretreated with bromocriptine to achieve fertility. Pregnancy rates of 37% to 81% have been reported in patients with prolactinoma. Bromocriptine should be discontinued once pregnancy is achieved. No teratogenic effects of bromocriptine have been reported when it is discontinued within a few weeks of conception.

In women with **microprolactinomas,** pregnancy and delivery are usually uneventful. Women with **macroprolactinomas** who desire pregnancy should be pretreated with bromocriptine for a sufficient period to cause substantial tumor shrinkage. Once this has occurred and pregnancy is achieved, the drug should be discontinued.

During pregnancy, the normal pituitary increases in size, owing to marked lactotroph hyperplasia due to the effect of estrogen on prolactin synthesis. The risk of tumor expansion is <5.5% for microprolactinomas and 15.5% to 35.7% for macroprolactinomas. Prepregnancy transsphenoidal surgical debulking of a large macroadenoma reduces the risk of serious tumor enlargement. Monitoring periodic prolactin levels in pregnant patients is of no benefit, as prolactin levels do not always rise during pregnancy and may not rise with tumor enlargement. Visual field testing should be limited to those patients who become symptomatic. Repeat scanning is reserved for patients with symptoms of tumor enlargement. Reinstitution of bromocriptine therapy at the lowest effective dose during pregnancy is the treatment of choice for patients with symptomatic tumor enlargement, as any type of surgery during pregnancy results in 1.5-fold increase in fetal loss in the first trimester and a fivefold increase in the second trimester. Transsphenoidal surgery or delivery (if pregnancy is far enough advanced) should be performed if there is no response to bromocriptine and vision is progressively worsening.

KEY POINTS TO REMEMBER

- Prolactin levels >200 ng/mL are indicative of a macroprolactinoma.
- The most common clinical manifestations of prolactinomas are infertility, oligomenorrhea, amenorrhea, and galactorrhea. Macroadenomas can also produce headaches and visual field defects.

KEY POINTS TO REMEMBER *(Continued)*

- A careful history should be taken of medications that elevate prolactin levels. A physical exam should be performed to test for signs of hypothyroidism, hypogonadism, and bitemporal field loss. Routine blood tests should be checked to exclude hypothyroidism, chronic renal failure and liver cirrhosis as a cause of hyperprolactinemia.
- The initial treatment for patients with microprolactinomas and macroprolactinomas is medical therapy with either bromocriptine or cabergoline. Cabergoline produces less frequent side effects, but it is more expensive.
- In women with large macroadenomas who desire pregnancy, prepregnancy transsphenoidal surgery to debulk the tumor reduces the risk for serious tumor enlargement. Bromocriptine given for a sufficient period to shrink the tumor can also reduce the chance of clinically important enlargement during pregnancy.

REFERENCES AND SUGGESTED READINGS

Abrahamson MJ, Snyder PJ. Causes of hyperprolactinemia. In: Rose BD, ed. *UpToDate*. Wellesley, MA: UpToDate; 2004.

Bevan J, Webster J, Burke CW, et al. Dopamine agonists and pituitary tumor shrinkage. *Endocr Rev* 1992;13(2):220–240.

Faglia G. Prolactinomas and hyperprolactinemic syndrome. In: De Groot L, Jameson JL, eds. *Endocrinology*, 4th ed. Philadelphia: WB Saunders; 2001:329–342.

Kars M, Roelfsema F, Romijn JA, et al. Malignant prolactinoma: case report and review of literature. *Eur J Endocrinol* 2006;155:523–534.

Melmed S, Kleinberg D. Anterior pituitary. In: Larsen PR, et al., eds. *Williams Textbook of Endocrinology*, 10th ed. Philadelphia: WB Saunders; 2003:177–279.

Molitch M. Medical treatment of prolactinomas. *Endocrinol Metab Clin North Am* 1999;28:143–169.

Molitch ME, Thorner MO, Wilson C, et al. Therapeutic controversy: management of prolactinomas. *J Clin Endocrinol Metab* 1997;82(4):996–1000.

Petakov MS, Damjanovic SS, Nikolić-Durović MM, et al. Pituitary adenomas secreting large amounts of prolactin may give false low values in immunoradiometric assays: the hook effect. *J Endocrinol Invest* 1998;21:184–188.

Schade R, Andersohn F, Suissa S, et al. Dopamine agonists and the risk of cardiac-valve regurgitation. *N Engl J Med* 2007;356(1):29–38.

Snyder PJ. Clinical manifestations and diagnosis of hyperprolactinemia. In: Rose BD, ed. *UpToDate*. Wellesley, MA: UpToDate; 2004.

Zanettini R, et al. Valvular heart disease and the use of dopamine agonists for Parkinson's disease. *N Engl J Med* 2007;356(1):39–46.

Acromegaly

Dominic N. Reeds

3

INTRODUCTION

Acromegaly is a disorder characterized by overproduction of growth hormone (GH), most commonly as a result of a pituitary adenoma. When these tumors occur before puberty, they may cause hypogonadism with failure of growth-plate closure, resulting in gigantism. Acromegaly, when occurring postpubertally, is insidious, with an average lag time of almost 10 years from disease onset to diagnosis. The incidence of acromegaly is low—three cases per million people per year. Recently, abuse of GH by athletes and patients seeking "the fountain of youth" has led to an increase in the incidence of drug-induced acromegaly.

CAUSES

Acromegaly is usually a result of a benign, monoclonal adenoma derived from somatotroph cells in the anterior pituitary gland. These cells normally secrete GH, stimulated by GH-releasing hormone (GHRH) from the hypothalamus and inhibited by both somatostatin from the hypothalamus and insulin-like growth factor 1 (IGF-1) from peripheral tissue. Most of the effects of GH are mediated through IGF-1, a growth and differentiation factor made in the liver. GH and IGF-1 cause growth of bone and cartilage and lead to impaired glucose tolerance and changes in protein and fat metabolism. Overproduction of GH, and the consequent increased synthesis of IGF-1, results in the clinical findings outlined in this chapter.

Differential Diagnosis

The differential diagnosis of acromegaly includes other causes of elevated GH levels. Exogenous use of GH should be considered in adolescent patients and body builders. Nonpituitary GH-secreting tumors are extremely rare. Familial forms of acromegaly include multiple endocrine neoplasia, McCune-Albright's syndrome, and Carney's syndrome.

PRESENTATION

Patients present with skeletal overgrowth and soft tissue enlargement. Tumor growth is often more rapid in younger patients. Endocrine symptoms arise from compression of the remaining pituitary gland by the enlarging mass. The most frequent signs and symptoms are:

- Dermatologic: Excessive sweating, oily skin, more or enlarging skin tags
- Musculoskeletal: Arthralgias; osteoarthritis of large weight-bearing joints; larger hat, ring, or shoe size; enlarged gaps between the teeth; kyphoscoliosis

- Endocrine: Hypothyroidism, including cold intolerance, weight gain, and fatigue; hypogonadism, including menstrual irregularities, reduced libido, and infertility; diabetes mellitus, galactorrhea
- Neurologic: Headache, carpal tunnel syndrome, peripheral paresthesias, visual disturbances
- Pulmonary: Obstructive sleep apnea
- Cardiac: Increased left ventricular mass, hypertension
- Gastrointestinal: Organomegaly, polyps
- Renal: Hypercalciuria

MANAGEMENT

Diagnostic Evaluation

The initial laboratory tests to be ordered in a patient suspected of having acromegaly should be IGF-1 and GH levels. A GH level <0.4 mcg/L and IGF-1 level within the normal range (adjusted for age and gender) exclude the diagnosis of acromegaly. If either of these tests is abnormal, a 2-hour oral glucose tolerance test should be performed as follows:

- Draw blood for baseline serum glucose and GH levels
- Patient consumes 75 g of oral glucose
- Draw blood for GH and glucose levels every 30 minutes for 2 hours

If the GH level falls to <1 mcg/L during the oral glucose tolerance test, acromegaly is excluded. False positives may occur in patients with diabetes, chronic hepatitis, renal failure, and anorexia.

The initial imaging study should be magnetic resonance imaging (MRI) of the head, with and without gadolinium contrast to evaluate for pituitary adenoma.

Treatment

Patients with acromegaly have premature mortality (relative risk, ~1.5-fold), with an increased incidence of insulin resistance, left ventricular hypertrophy, hypertension, and death due to cardiovascular disease. Acromegaly appears to be associated with an increased risk for development of colonic carcinoma, and it is recommended that colonoscopy be performed in all patients. Studies have shown that reducing GH levels improves survival in patients with acromegaly. The goal of therapy is a GH level <2 mcg/L or an IGF-1 level in the age- and sex-adjusted normal range. A reduction in GH can be achieved with surgery, medical therapy, and/or radiotherapy.

Surgery

Surgery results in the most rapid reduction in GH levels; however, its efficacy depends on (a) the size of the adenoma and (b) the experience of the surgeon. Surgery is the treatment of choice for microadenomas, which are cured surgically in 90% of cases. Results for macroadenomas are more disappointing, with <50% of individuals cured by surgery alone.

Medical Therapy

Somatostatin analogs, including octreotide (Sandostatin) and lanreotide (Somatuline), are more effective agents for treatment of acromegaly. They act as agonists on somatostatin receptors on the tumor and achieve adequate IGF-1 suppression in up to 50% of patients. Dosing is titrated based on the patient's GH and IGF-1 levels. These drugs may be administered as monthly depot injections. Dopamine agonists, bromocriptine (Parlodel) and cabergoline (Dostinex), inhibit secretion of GH by stimulating dopaminergic receptors on the adenoma. Bromocriptine is effective in <20% of patients with acromegaly; however, cabergoline appears to be more efficacious. These drugs should be used at low doses initially to prevent nausea. Pegvisomant (Somavert) blocks GH action in peripheral tissues by antagonizing the GH receptor. This results in normalization of IGF-1 levels in 89% of patients; however, a significant rise in GH levels is seen. This increase in GH levels has not been shown to increase tumor size; however, two patients have required surgery for rapidly enlarging pituitary tumors while receiving pegvisomant. Liver function tests should be followed every 6 months because elevated liver enzymes have been reported.

Radiotherapy

Both conventional fractionated radiotherapy and stereotactic radiotherapy (gamma-knife) have been used to treat pituitary adenomas, including GH-secreting adenomas. Full response to treatment with fractionated therapy may not be seen for up to 15 years. Treatment with gamma-knife therapy appears to provide faster normalization of GH levels, with less damage to surrounding brain tissue. Use of gamma-knife therapy is limited by tumor size and proximity to the optic nerves. Up to 60% of patients develop hypopituitarism after radiotherapy. Radiation therapy should not be used as primary therapy for acromegaly unless the patient is unwilling or unable to undergo surgery.

KEY POINTS TO REMEMBER

- Acromegaly is a rare condition with a long lag time between disease onset and diagnosis.
- Abuse of GH may result in similar clinical features.
- Ask about an increase in shoe size and ring size.
- Surgery is the initial treatment of choice when the tumor appears resectable.
- Radiotherapy and medical therapy provide adjunctive support and can achieve normalization of IGF-1 levels in up to 90% of patients.

REFERENCES AND SUGGESTED READINGS

Abosch A, Tyrrell JB, Lamborn KR, et al. Transsphenoidal microsurgery for growth hormone secreting pituitary adenomas: initial outcome and long-term results. *J Clin Endocrinol Metab* 1998;83: 3411–3418.

Abs R, Verhelst J, Maiter D, et al. Cabergoline in the treatment of acromegaly: a study in 64 patients. *J Clin Endocrinol Metab* 1998;83:374–378.

Bates AS. An audit of outcome of treatment in acromegaly. *QJM* 1993;86:293–299.

Jaffe CA, Barkan AL. Treatment of acromegaly with dopamine agonists. *Endocrinol Metab Clin North Am* 1992;21:713–735.

Landolt AM, Haller D, Lomax N, et al. Stereotactic radiosurgery for recurrent surgically treated acromegaly: comparison with fractionated radiotherapy. *J Neurosurg* 1998;88:1002–1008.

Melmed S. Acromegaly. *N Engl J Med* 2006;355:2558–2573.

Molitch ME. Clinical manifestations of acromegaly. *Endocrinol Metab Clin North Am* 1992;21:597–615.

Newman CB, Melmed S, Snyder PJ, et al. Safety and efficacy of long-term octreotide therapy of acromegaly: results of a multicenter trial in 103 patients—a clinical research center study. *J Clin Endocrinol Metab* 1995;80:2768–2775.

Orme SM, McNally RJ, Cartwright RA, et al., for the United Kingdom Acromegaly Study Group. Mortality and cancer incidence in acromegaly: a retrospective cohort study. *J Clin Endocrinol Metab* 1998;83:2730–2734.

Sheppard MC. Primary medical therapy for acromegaly. *Clin Endocrinol* 2003;58: 387–399.

Trainer PJ, Drake WM, Katznelson L, et al. Treatment of acromegaly with the growth-hormone receptor antagonist pegvisomant. *N Engl J Med* 2000;342:1171–1177.

Diabetes Insipidus

4

Kent Ishihara

INTRODUCTION

Diabetes insipidus (DI) is a disorder of water balance caused by nonosmotic renal losses of water. DI is caused by either deficient arginine vasopressin (AVP) secretion from the posterior pituitary gland (central DI) or end-organ unresponsiveness of the kidneys to AVP (nephrogenic DI). AVP is also commonly referred to as antidiuretic hormone (ADH), and for the purposes of this discussion about water balance and DI, ADH will be the preferred term to help remember the important physiologic role of this hormone. Loss of the antidiuretic action of ADH in patients with DI leads to polyuria, and eventually to dehydration and hypernatremia if water intake is not able to keep up with water loss.

ADH is synthesized in the supraoptic and paraventricular nuclei of the hypothalamus and transported to the posterior pituitary gland for storage and secretion. Osmoreceptors in the hypothalamus are very sensitive to changes in plasma osmolality, which is primarily determined by the sodium concentration. The release of ADH is inhibited until the osmolality rises above a threshold level, after which ADH secretion rises rapidly in proportion to the plasma osmolality.

ADH primarily acts upon the kidneys at the level of the distal tubule and collecting duct to increase water permeability and reabsorption. The effects of ADH are mediated via a G protein–coupled V2 receptor that signals the translocation of aquaporin-2 channels into the apical membrane of the principal cells in the collecting duct. In conjunction with aquaporin-3 and aquaporin-4 channels on the basal–lateral surface of these cells, water is then allowed to flow freely down the osmotic gradient from the relatively dilute tubular fluid to the highly concentrated renal medulla. Therefore, decreased production or activity of ADH results in impaired water resorption in the nephron, leading to a dilute urine and loss of free water.

Other stimuli of ADH release include nausea, decreased intravascular volume, acute hypoglycemia, glucocorticoid deficiency, manipulation of abdominal contents during surgery, physiologic and pathophysiologic stressors, and cigarette smoking.

CAUSES

The causes of DI are summarized in Table 4-1.

Pathophysiology

There are two basic abnormalities that lead to DI:

- **Central DI**—Destruction of the ADH-producing cells in the posterior pituitary gland results in decreased circulating levels of ADH. Central DI may result from a

TABLE 4-1	CAUSES OF DIABETES INSIPIDUS
Central DI	Head trauma (may remit after 6 months)
	Postsurgical (develops 1–6 days after surgery and often disappears, recurs, or becomes chronic)
	Tumors—Craniopharyngioma, pinealoma, meningioma, germinoma, glioma, benign cysts, leukemia, lymphoma, metastatic breast or lung
	Infections—TB, syphilis, mycoses, toxoplasmosis, encephalitis, meningitis
	Granulomatous disease—Sarcoidosis, histiocytosis X, Wegener's granulomatosis
	Cerebrovascular disease—Aneurysms, thrombosis, Sheehan's syndrome, cerebrovascular accident
	Idiopathic—Sporadic or familial (rare autosomal dominant trait)
Nephrogenic DI	Congenital—Rare inherited disorder caused by inherited mutations in the AVP receptor (X-linked recessive) or in the water channel of the renal tubule (autosomal recessive)
	Acquired—Much more common and less severe
	Medications (lithium, amphotericin B, demeclocycline, cisplatin, aminoglycosides, rifampin, foscarnet, methoxyflurane, vincristine)
	Electrolyte disorders (hypercalcemia, hypercalciuria, hypokalemia)
	Chronic tubulointerstitial diseases (polycystic kidney disease, medullary sponge kidney, obstructive uropathy, papillary necrosis)
	Sickle cell disease and trait
	Multiple myeloma, amyloidosis
	Sarcoidosis

AVP, arginine vasopressin; DI, diabetes insipidus; TB, tuberculosis.
From Fried LF, Palevsky PM. Hyponatremia and hypernatremia. *Med Clin North Am* 1997;81: 585–609, with permission.

complete lack of ADH, but is more commonly *partial*, so that ADH levels will submaximally rise in response to a strong osmotic stimulus such as fluid deprivation.
- **Nephrogenic DI**—Nephrogenic DI is caused by impaired renal responsiveness to ADH, usually owing to an abnormality in the collecting ducts. Nephrogenic DI may be *complete*, in which case the renal tubule does not respond to any concentration of ADH, or *partial*, so that increased circulating levels of ADH will produce a submaximal renal response.

In both central and nephrogenic DI, plasma sodium and osmolality increase because the kidney is not able to appropriately concentrate urine. Increased plasma osmolality triggers the thirst mechanism, and water intake increases to compensate for urinary water losses. However, if the thirst mechanism is impaired, or if access to water is restricted, severe hypernatremia and hyperosmolality can develop.

Differential Diagnosis

The main symptom or sign of DI is polyuria, which must be differentiated from other causes of polyuria. Polyuria can be either *hypotonic* (water diuresis) or *nonhypotonic* (solute diuresis). Hypotonic polyuria is defined by a urine osmolality of <300 mOsm/kg, and can be either *physiologic* or *pathologic*. Physiologic hypotonic polyuria occurs in the setting of an increased free water intake leading to an appropriate suppression of ADH, free water diuresis, and a normal serum osmolality. For example, with primary polydipsia, excessive free water intake leads to a large volume of dilute urine that is appropriate to maintain a normal plasma sodium and osmolality. Primary polydipsia may lead to hyponatremia, but does not cause hypernatremia. On the other hand, DI results in a pathologic hypotonic polyuria that leads to an increase in thirst and free water intake to maintain a normal plasma sodium and osmolality. If free water intake does not match output, DI may lead to hypernatremia.

Nonhypotonic polyuria is commonly caused by diuretic medications or hyperglycemia, and can be distinguished from hypotonic polyuria by the presence of a relatively high urine osmolality in the appropriate clinical setting.

When hypernatremia is present, the differential diagnosis includes other causes of free water loss—for example, insensible losses from the skin or respiratory tract, vomiting, diarrhea, or diuretic use. As with DI, hypernatremia develops when the patient does not drink enough water to compensate for the water loss.

PRESENTATION

The primary symptoms of DI are thirst and polyuria, with a daily urine volume typically exceeding 3 L. Symptoms of hypernatremia (e.g. weakness, altered mental status, coma, or seizures) may develop with significant or rapid dehydration. The physical examination is usually normal unless significant dehydration has developed.

MANAGEMENT

Diagnosis

- **Is polyuria present?** Polyuria is usually defined as a 24-hour urine output >30 to 50 mL/kg in adults or >100 mL/kg in children. A good history and physical examination can be very helpful. Age, onset, duration, and degree of polyuria may provide important clues. Intermittent, transient, or frequent urination with low urine volumes are not suggestive of DI. Nocturia is often present in DI, since the polyuria is not entirely dependent on fluid intake. Dietary habits, fluid intake, thirst, and medication use may be important factors. Headaches, vision changes, recent head trauma or surgery, and any underlying psychiatric illnesses may also provide additional clues. Orthostatic hypotension and skin tenting may be signs of volume depletion. Urine color may be a clue to the kidney's ability to concentrate urine. In the hospital setting, an accurate review of the patient's intake and output is essential. A plasma glucose measurement is a quick way to rule out diabetes as the cause of polyuria—typically a glucose level >200 to 300 mg/dL is required to cause glucose to spill over into the urine and induce an osmotic diuresis.
- **Are hypernatremia and hyperosmolality present?** Simultaneous measurements of urine and plasma for sodium and osmolality are essential. In DI, plasma sodium may be normal or elevated. If hyponatremia is present, primary polydipsia is the most likely cause of hypotonic polyuria.
- **Is the urine osmolality inappropriately low for the plasma osmolality?** In DI, urine osmolality is typically low (<300 mOsm/kg, specific gravity <1.010) and inappropriate for any elevation of plasma osmolality that may be present; however, urine osmolality can be >300 mOsm/kg if there is only partial DI, or in complete DI

complicated by volume depletion. Urine sodium can be variable, but is often inappropriately low for the degree of hypernatremia that may be present. On the other hand, a fully concentrated urine (urine osmolality, 800–1200 mOsm/kg) essentially rules out DI as the cause of hypernatremia, and other causes should be considered (e.g., insensible water losses from skin, lungs, and gastrointestinal tract; salt loading from feedings, medications, and/or intravenous fluids).

- **Are any other biochemical abnormalities present?** Measurements of serum calcium, potassium, blood urea nitrogen (BUN), and creatinine may be helpful. Chronic hypokalemia and hypercalcemia can cause partial nephrogenic DI. On the other hand, hypokalemia can also be a consequence of DI, and hypercalcemia could be caused by volume depletion. Patients with chronic kidney disease may also develop partial DI owing to defects in the renal concentrating capacity of diseased nephrons.

- **Fluid Deprivation Test.** A fluid deprivation test may be helpful in deciding whether hypotonic polyuria is caused by DI or primary polydipsia when the plasma sodium and osmolality are normal. The test is not necessary, and could be dangerous, in the setting of hypertonic hypernatremia, in which primary polydipsia is not a consideration. Likewise, if the patient has hypotonic hyponatremia, DI is not a consideration. Therefore, *a fluid deprivation test should be done only in a patient with hypotonic polyuria and a normal plasma sodium/osmolality.*

  - Drugs that influence ADH secretion or action should be discontinued if possible. Caffeine, alcohol, and tobacco should be avoided for at least 24 hours. Other stimuli of ADH secretion (e.g., nausea and hypotension) should also be monitored to aid in the interpretation of the results.

  - The test should begin in the morning, and body weight, plasma osmolality, serum sodium concentration, urine osmolality, and urine volume should be followed hourly.

  - Fluids are withheld until body weight decreases by 5%, plasma sodium and osmolality reach the upper limits of normal (sodium >145 mEq/L and osmolality >295 mOsm/kg), or a stable hourly urinary osmolality (variation of $<5\%$ over 3 hours) is established. If urine osmolality does not reach 300 mOsm/kg before these parameters are achieved, primary polydipsia is excluded. In patients with partial DI, urine osmolality will be greater than plasma osmolality, but the urine will remain submaximally concentrated. In patients with complete DI, the urine osmolality will remain less than the plasma osmolality.

  - If a diagnosis of complete DI is established with a lower urine osmolality than plasma osmolality when the goals of the test are met, ADH can be given to help differentiate between central and nephrogenic DI. DDAVP (desmopressin) 0.03 mcg/kg can be given subcutaneously and urine osmolality measured at 30, 60, and 120 minutes. In central DI, the urine osmolality should increase more than 50% from the level achieved during dehydration. In nephrogenic DI, the urine osmolality may increase, but usually not by more than 50%.

  - ADH levels drawn before and during fluid deprivation can be plotted on a nomogram and can help differentiate between partial central DI, partial nephrogenic DI, and primary polydipsia.

- **Hypertonic Saline Test.** The fluid deprivation test may not be able to distinguish between patients who are able to submaximally concentrate their urine during fluid deprivation. In these patients, the target plasma sodium and osmolality required to maximally stimulate ADH secretion may not be reached with fluid deprivation alone, and the administration of hypertonic saline may be necessary to reach those goals. Patients with partial DI (central or nephrogenic) may be able to partially concentrate their urine in proportion to the defect in ADH secretion or action. Patients with primary polydipsia may also develop an impaired ability to concentrate their urine. ADH secretion and action should be normal in patients with primary polydipsia, but chronic polyuria can lead to washout of the medullary interstitium, resulting in loss of the transtubular osmolar gradient that is required to maintain the maximum urinary concentrating ability of the kidneys. Therefore, patients with primary polydipsia may be difficult to distinguish from those with partial DI. In these patients, the administration of hypertonic saline and measurement of ADH levels will almost always be able to differentiate between primary polydipsia, partial central DI, and partial nephrogenic DI.

- Hypertonic (3%) saline is infused at 0.05–0.1 mL/kg/minute for 1 to 2 hours, and plasma osmolality and sodium are measured every 30 minutes.
- ADH is measured once the serum sodium and osmolality are above the upper limits of normal (sodium >145 mEq/L and osmolality >295 mOsm/kg).
- Nomograms have been established that can then be used to distinguish among primary polydipsia, partial central DI, and partial nephrogenic DI.
- Of note, this test may be contraindicated in patients at risk for complications of volume overload (e.g., those with underlying heart disease or congestive heart failure).

Treatment

The treatment of DI has two goals: (a) replace the water deficit and (b) treat the underlying abnormality in water balance.

Managing the Water Deficit

The water deficit should be calculated (see subsequent text) and replaced orally with water whenever possible; otherwise, a hypotonic fluid (usually D5W or 0.2% NaCl) can be given intravenously. If the hypernatremia has developed rapidly over a period of hours, the water deficit can be corrected to decrease the plasma sodium at a rate up to 1 mEq/L/hour. If the hypernatremia has developed more slowly, the rate should be no more than 0.5 mEq/L/hour, up to a maximum of 8 to 10 mEq/L/day, using the smallest volume of fluid possible to avoid cerebral edema. If the patient is hypotensive due to volume contraction, normal saline should be used initially until the blood pressure is restored. As the hypernatremia is being corrected, serum sodium concentration and urine output should be followed closely.

The water deficit can be calculated from the plasma sodium ($[Na+]_{plasma}$) using the following formula:

$$\text{Water deficit (L)} = [0.6 \text{ (men) or } 0.5 \text{ (women)}] \times \text{body weight (kg)} \times ([Na+]_{plasma} - 140) \div 140$$

For example, if an asymptomatic 70-kg man has a plasma sodium of 150 mEq/L, the calculated water deficit is 3 L [$0.6 \times 70 \times (150 - 140) \div 140$]. To decrease the sodium at a rate of 0.5 mEq/L/hour, 3 L of D5W can be administered over 20 hours [($150 - 140$ mEq/L) $\div$ 0.5 mEq/L/hour] at a rate of 150 mL/hour (3 L $\div$ 20 hours).

Alternatively, the change in $[Na+]_{plasma}$ in mEq/L for each liter of fluid given can be approximated from the following equation:

$$\text{Change in } [Na+]_{plasma} = ([Na+]_{infusate} + [K+]_{infusate} - [Na+]_{plasma}) \div (\text{total body water} + 1),$$

where $[Na+]_{infusate}$ = mEq/L of sodium in the infusate (e.g., 0 mEq/L of D5W or 34 mEq/L of 0.2% NaCl), $[K+]_{infusate}$ = mEq/L of potassium in the infusate, and total body water = body weight (kg) $\times$ (0.6 for men, 0.5 for women).

Therefore, if the same 70-kg man has a plasma sodium of 150 mEq/L, the calculated decrease in sodium per liter of D5W would be ($0 + 0 - 150$) $\div$ ($0.6 \times 70 + 1$) = -3.5

mEq/L. To decrease the sodium at an initial rate of 0.5 mEq/L/hour, D5W should be infused at ~143 mL/hour (0.5 mEq/L/hour ÷ 3.5 mEq/L × 1000 mL). This formula is particularly useful when choosing a hypotonic fluid other than D5W, or when potassium is added to the fluid to replace any concomitant potassium deficits.

It should be recognized that both of these strategies offer only approximations of the expected change in sodium. If there are other ongoing free water losses, the rate of infusion will need to be increased accordingly. When DDAVP is used to treat DI, reducing free water losses, the rate of infusion may need to be decreased. Therefore, plasma sodium and volume status should be assessed frequently (initially every 2 hours, and reduced to every 4 hours when the correction rate is stable) to monitor and make adjustments to therapy.

Correcting Chronic Water Loss

- **Central DI.** The agent most commonly used to treat central DI is the ADH-analog DDAVP. Compared to ADH (vasopressin), DDAVP has a longer half-life, almost no pressor activity, and few side effects. It may be administered parentally, intranasally, or orally. DDAVP given intravenously or subcutaneously has a rapid onset of action and is usually given at a dose of 1 to 2 mcg once or twice daily. The intranasal route has a rapid onset of action and can be given at a dose of 1 to 4 sprays per day (10 mcg per spray) divided one to three times daily. Oral DDAVP has an onset of action of 30 to 60 minutes and can be given at a dose of 0.1 to 0.4 mg one to four times daily, up to a maximum dose of 1.2 mg/day. The use of oral DDAVP has been shown to be very effective, but may be limited in some patients owing to variable gut absorption and reduced bioavailability. In addition, converting from nasal to parenteral administration is easily accomplished by reducing the dose by a factor of ten; whereas, because of the variable bioavailability with oral administration, a dose titration may be required when converting to or from oral dosing.

For stable patients who are tolerating PO and who have an intact thirst response, a simple and safe method for dosing DDAVP is to start with 0.1 mg PO and assess for a response (decreased urine output, increased urine osmolality, and decreased thirst). If there is no response, or a suboptimal response, within a few hours, the dose should be increased by 0.1 mg every few hours until there is an appropriate response. Once an effective dose is found, the patient should be monitored for breakthrough hypotonic polyuria (typically >200–250 mL/hour with osmolality <300 mOsm/kg or specific gravity <1.010). If the polyuria is persistent for at least a couple of hours, the effective dose of DDAVP should then be retitrated. If breakthrough consistently occurs before 6 to 8 hours, the dose can be increased up to a maximum dose of 0.4 mg, since higher doses may prolong the duration of action, even though they usually do not have a greater effect on urinary concentrating ability. The patient should continue to receive the DDAVP on an as needed (PRN) basis until a stable regimen is found in which the patient is taking a maximum of 1.2 mg daily divided in up to three or four doses. Throughout this dose titration, the patients should be given free access to water and told to drink *only* when thirsty, thereby avoiding the possibility of water intoxication and hyponatremia. Likewise, patients should be encouraged to drink water liberally whenever they are thirsty to protect against hypernatremia and volume depletion during times when the DDAVP has worn off. This regimen can be used in any stable patient with an intact thirst mechanism, and is particularly effective in those who may have transient DI (e.g., after pituitary surgery or head trauma), since the DDAVP will only be dosed if the patient has continued evidence of DI. Similar PRN regimens can be devised using parenterally or nasally administered DDAVP, including in those patients who are less stable or who have a defective thirst mechanism, as long as they are monitored closely for water balance and breakthrough polyuria.

In patients with an intact thirst mechanism who have chronic DI, a fixed dosing regimen of DDAVP may be used. The lowest dose that reduces the symptoms of DI to tolerable levels with minimal risk of hyponatremia should be used, since patients should be able to compensate for hypernatremia by increasing fluid intake whenever they are thirsty, but do not have a similar means to detect hyponatremia if they increase their fluid intake for other reasons. For some patients, dosing once at bedtime to reduce nocturia may be all that is needed. In others, more frequent dosing may be necessary.

In adipsic patients with DI, management can be extremely difficult. In general, these patients are given a fixed dose of DDAVP and instructed to carefully maintain adequate hydration and adjust their fluid intake based on other indirect indicators of water balance (e.g., daily weight measurements).

Several other medications have also been shown to be effective in the treatment of central DI. Chlorpropamide (Diabinese) is an oral hypoglycemic agent that may also be useful in the treatment of partial central DI, since it can potentiate ADH-mediated water reabsorption. The usual dose is 125 to 500 mg PO once daily, but may take up to 4 days for maximum effect. Carbamazepine at doses of 100 to 300 mg twice daily may improve polyuria by enhancing the response to ADH. Clofibrate at doses of 500 mg q6h can improve polyuria by increasing ADH release. A low-salt diet combined with a thiazide diuretic can be an effective treatment for central DI by inducing mild volume depletion and increased proximal tubular resorption of sodium and water, but it is probably more effective for treating nephrogenic DI. Indomethacin is an nonsteroidal anti-inflammatory drug (NSAID) that can increase the concentrating ability of the kidney by inhibiting renal prostaglandin synthesis, decreasing the glomerular filtration rate, and increasing the renal response to ADH.

- **Nephrogenic DI.** Because the kidney is unresponsive to ADH, DDAVP is not an effective treatment for nephrogenic DI. If nephrogenic DI is acquired, the concentration defect usually improves quickly with discontinuation of the offending drug or correction of the electrolyte disorder. Otherwise, nephrogenic DI is usually controlled with a sodium-restricted diet and a thiazide diuretic (e.g., hydrochlorothiazide, 25 mg once or twice daily). Thiazides cause an overall reduction in electrolyte-free water excretion by stimulating proximal tubular sodium resorption and diminishing sodium delivery to more distal sites. Patients on this therapy should be monitored for hypovolemia and hypokalemia. Amiloride may enhance the effect of the thiazide diuretic by increasing sodium excretion and the resulting antipolyuric response to volume depletion, while reducing potassium excretion. Amiloride may also be the treatment of choice for lithium-induced DI, since it blocks the sodium channels in the collecting duct through which lithium enters and interferes with the tubular response to ADH. NSAIDs can also be a useful adjunct to treatment because they may decrease glomerular filtration rate as well as decrease the synthesis of prostaglandins that normally antagonize the action of ADH. Finally, because some cases of nephrogenic DI are only partial, DDAVP may be effective in some patients.
- **Follow-up.** Patients with central DI who are treated with DDAVP on a fixed dosing schedule should be followed for the development of hyponatremia. Occasional withdrawal of the DDAVP should be performed to confirm recurrence of polyuria, and serum sodium concentration should be checked periodically. All patients with central DI should wear or carry a medical alert tag or card. When a patient with DI loses access to water, as may occur during a medical emergency or surgery, he or she is at high risk of dehydration. Under these circumstances, urine output and serum sodium concentration should be followed closely, and DDAVP should be administered on a PRN basis until the patient is stable.

KEY POINTS TO REMEMBER

- DI results from either deficient ADH secretion (Central DI) or end-organ unresponsiveness to ADH (Nephrogenic DI).
- To establish a diagnosis of DI, the urine should be inappropriately dilute for the serum osmolality.
- Treatment of DI should be aimed at replacing the patient's water deficit and treating the underlying cause.
- Central DI is most commonly treated with DDAVP.
- DDAVP is usually not an effective treatment for nephrogenic DI, which is typically controlled with a sodium-restricted diet and a thiazide diuretic.

REFERENCES AND SUGGESTED READINGS

Adrogue HJ, Madias NE. Hypernatremia. *N Engl J Med* 2000;342:1493–1499.

Ball SG, Baylis PH. Vasopressin, diabetes insipidus, and syndrome of inappropriate antidiuresis. In: DeGroot LJ, Jameson JL, eds. *Endocrinology*, 5th ed. Philadelphia: Elsevier; 2006:537–556.

Bichet DG. Diagnosis of polyuria and diabetes insipidus. *UpToDate* 2007;15.1.

Bichet DG. Treatment of central diabetes insipidus. *UpToDate* 2007;15.1.

Bichet DG. Treatment of nephrogenic diabetes insipidus. *UpToDate* 2007;15.1.

Chlorpropamide in diabetes insipidus. *Br Med J* 1971;1:302–303.

Hockaday TDR. Diabetes insipidus. *Br Med J* 1972;2:210–213.

Loh JA, Verbalis JG. Diabetes insipidus as a complication after pituitary surgery. *Nat Clin Pract Endocrinol Metab* 2007;3:489–494.

Makaryus AN, McFarlane SI. Diabetes insipidus: diagnosis and treatment of a complex disease. *Cleve Clin J Med* 2006;73:65–71.

Mohn A, Acerini CL, Cheetham TD, et al. Hypertonic saline test for the investigation of posterior pituitary function. *Arch Dis Child* 1998;79:431–434.

Pomerleau OF. Nicotine and the central nervous system: biobehavioral effects of cigarette smoking. *Am J Med* 1992;93[Suppl 1A]:2S-7S.

Robertson GL. Antidiuretic hormone. Normal and disordered function. *Endocrinol Metab Clin North Am* 2001;30:671–694.

Robertson GL. Disorders of the neurohypophysis. In: Jameson JL, ed. *Harrison's Endocrinology*. New York: McGraw-Hill; 2006:57–69.

Verbalis JG. Disorders of body water homeostasis. *Best Pract Res Clin Endocrinol Metab* 2003;17:471–503.

Victorina WM, Rydstedt LL, Sowers JR. Clinical disorders of vasopressin. In: Lavin N, ed. *Manual of Endocrinology and Metabolism*, 3rd ed. Philadelphia: Lippincott Williams & Wilkins; 2002:68–82.

Syndrome of Inappropriate Antidiuretic Hormone

5

Kent Ishihara

INTRODUCTION

Hyponatremia is the most common electrolyte abnormality in hospitalized patients, with a prevalence estimated to be as high as 30% in some series. The syndrome of inappropriate antidiuretic hormone (SIADH) is the most common cause of hyponatremia, and is typically caused by the inappropriate secretion of antidiuretic hormone (ADH) from the pituitary gland or from an ectopic source. However, a recently recognized genetic disorder caused by mutations in the vasopressin receptor also causes a syndrome that meets the criteria for SIADH, but with low or undetectable levels of ADH. Therefore, some are now referring to the syndrome as the "syndrome of inappropriate antidiuresis" (SIAD). Nevertheless, because the latter entity seems to be rare at this point, the more commonly recognized term SIADH will be used in this discussion to avoid any confusion.

ADH, also known as arginine vasopressin (AVP), is a key component of the homeostatic mechanisms that regulate water balance (see also Chapter 4, Diabetes Insipidus). ADH is released from cells in the neurohypophysis in response to increased serum osmolality or decreased intravascular volume. In the kidneys, ADH acts through the vasopressin V2 receptor to increase water permeability at the distal tubule and collecting duct of the nephron, enhancing water reabsorption at these sites. With excess ADH, dilutional hyponatremia develops because water cannot be excreted normally. SIADH can also occur with ectopic production of ADH from a malignancy or inflamed tissue.

The hallmark of SIADH is an inappropriately elevated urine osmolality in the setting of a low plasma osmolality. More specifically, hypotonic hyponatremia and a relatively concentrated urine are found in the setting of euvolemia and normal renal, thyroid, and adrenal function.

CAUSES

The causes of SIADH are summarized in Table 5-1.

Differential Diagnosis

Unlike hypernatremia, which is always hypertonic, hyponatremia can be hypotonic, isotonic, or hypertonic. Hypertonic hyponatremia results from transcellular shifts of water out of cells owing to solutes confined to the extracellular space. For example, glucose lowers the serum sodium level by 1.6 mEq/L for each 100 mg/dL of plasma glucose >100 mg/dL, and by an additional 4.0 mEq/L for each 100 mg/dL of plasma glucose >400 mg/dL (an average value of 2.4 mEq/L for each 100 mg/dL >100 mg/dL can be used when the plasma glucose is >400 mg/dL). Similarly, isotonic hyponatremia results from the presence of large volumes of isotonic fluids in the extracellular space (e.g., isotonic

TABLE 5-1	CAUSES OF THE SYNDROME OF INAPPROPRIATE ANTIDIURETIC HORMONE

CNS (excess ADH release)

Acute intermittent porphyria

Bleeding (hematoma/hemorrhage)

CVA

Delirium tremens

Guillain-Barré syndrome

Head trauma

Hydrocephalus

Infections (meningitis/encephalitis/abscess)

Tumors

Medications

Bromocriptine mesylate (Bromocriptine)

Carbamazepine (Tegretol)

Chlorpropamide

Clofibrate

Cyclophosphamide

Desmopressin (DDAVP)

Ecstasy

Haloperidol (Haldol)

Nicotine

Opiates

Oxytocin

Phenothiazines

Selective serotonin reuptake inhibitors (SSRIs)

Tricyclic antidepressants (TCAs)

Vinblastine

Vincristine

Miscellaneous

HIV

Nausea

Neuropsychiatric disorders (increased thirst, ADH release at lower osmolality, increased renal sensitivity to ADH)

Pain

Postoperative state (excessive amounts of electrolyte-free water)

Neoplasms (ectopic ADH secretion)

Duodenal carcinoma

Lymphoma

Mesothelioma

TABLE 5-1	CAUSES OF THE SYNDROME OF INAPPROPRIATE ANTIDIURETIC HORMONE *(Continued)*

Olfactory neuroblastoma

Pancreatic carcinoma

Prostate carcinoma

Small cell carcinoma of lung

Thymoma

Pulmonary diseases

Bronchiectasis

COPD

Cystic fibrosis

Pneumonia (PCP, TB, aspergillosis)

Positive pressure ventilation

ADH, antidiuretic hormone; CNS, central nervous system; COPD, chronic obstructive pulmonary disease; CVA, cerebrovascular accident; PCP, *Pneumocystis carinii* pneumonia; TB, tuberculosis.

mannitol) that do not contain sodium. Both hypertonic and isotonic hyponatremias are usually easily identifiable by history and laboratory studies or both.

Pseudohyponatremia is a form of isotonic hyponatremia that is caused by spurious laboratory measurements of sodium in the setting of severe hypertriglyceridemia or paraproteinemia. In the past, this was a problem found when using only a few specific analytic chemistry techniques, but may not be as much of a problem with more modern chemistry analyzers. Nevertheless, in the appropriate clinical settings, consultation with the laboratory director may be helpful in determining if pseudohyponatremia may be a possibility.

The differential diagnosis of SIADH includes other causes of hypotonic hyponatremia. Hypotonic hyponatremias are caused by excess water intake and/or impaired renal excretion of water, and can be further categorized by the volume status of the patient.

Hypervolemic hypotonic hyponatremia is characterized by sodium retention and an increase in total body water. The usual causes include congestive heart failure, cirrhosis, nephrotic syndrome, acute and chronic renal failure, and pregnancy, all of which are usually identifiable clinically.

Hypovolemic hypotonic hyponatremia is characterized by sodium depletion and a loss of total body water. The usual causes include diuresis (medication-induced or osmotic), salt-wasting nephropathies, acute adrenal insufficiency, gastrointestinal losses, excessive sweating, blood loss, and third-spacing (e.g., with pancreatitis or severe burns). In patients with neurologic disease or injuries, cerebral salt wasting is another cause of hypovolemic hypotonic hyponatremia that is often mistaken for SIADH when volume status is difficult to determine. Patients with cerebral salt wasting may not have overt hypovolemia, but there is usually evidence of volume depletion when carefully examined (e.g., reviewing fluid intake vs. output during the development of hyponatremia). The mechanism by which this occurs is not fully known, but it is thought to be mediated either by decreased neural input to the kidney or increased release of a circulating natriuretic factor (e.g., atrial natriuretic peptide or brain natriuretic peptide) that leads to sodium loss and volume depletion.

Euvolemic hypotonic hyponatremia is characterized by a low to normal total body sodium and a normal to elevated total body water. The most common cause is SIADH, but it can also result from hypothyroidism, adrenal insufficiency, primary polydipsia, potomania, thiazide diuretics, extreme exercise, a reset osmostat, or the nephrogenic syndrome of inappropriate antidiuresis.

- Hypothyroidism rarely causes hyponatremia, and the mechanisms by which this occurs are not entirely understood. Proposed mechanisms include dysregulation of ADH release or clearance, or both, as well as effects on vascular tone, cardiac output, and renal blood flow.

- Adrenal insufficiency is also an unusual cause of hyponatremia. ADH is an adrenocorticotropic hormone (ACTH) secretagogue and is subject to negative feedback by glucocorticoids. Hyponatremia can occur in both primary and secondary adrenal insufficiency, and is thought to be caused by the loss of negative feedback on ADH secretion, in addition to any loss of mineralocorticoid effects in primary, but not secondary, adrenal insufficiency.

- Primary polydipsia may lead to hyponatremia if free water intake exceeds the capacity of the kidneys to excrete free water. Under normal circumstances, acute free water ingestion does not lead to hyponatremia because the average person is capable of excreting more than 20 L of urine per day. Hyponatremia develops in only a minority of patients with primary polydipsia, and the mechanisms by which this occurs is unclear. These patients appear to have abnormal osmoregulation of free water clearance that is not clearly dependent on altered ADH secretion or action.

- Potomania was classically described in binge beer drinkers, but is now found more commonly in people with unusual dietary habits or eating disorders (e.g., anorexia nervosa). These patients develop hypotonic hyponatremia in the setting of a dilute urine because of low solute intake and excretion. Free water clearance is dependent on solute excretion by the kidneys, and solute excretion is dependent on solute intake. Therefore, if solute intake is decreased because of a restricted diet, solute excretion will also be decreased, and the kidneys will not be able to clear as much free water. With a severe decrease in solute excretion, as little as 2 to 3 L of free water can be excreted per day, so any free water ingested that is more than 2 to 3 L per day will be retained by the body and contribute to hyponatremia.

- Thiazide diuretics typically cause hypotonic hyponatremia associated with hypovolemia, but patients can be euvolemic if free water intake is increased to compensate for thirst and volume depletion.

- Exercise-associated hyponatremia (EAH) is a recently defined entity that is now believed to be a form of SIADH. EAH is most often described in marathon runners, who can become severely hyponatremic resulting in severe neurologic symptoms, cerebral edema, and even death. In the past, this disorder was thought to be related to excessive free water intake in the setting of volume depletion and solute loss by prolonged sweating. However, these patients meet all of the criteria for SIADH, and have been found to have inappropriately detectable ADH levels in the setting of significant hyponatremia. Therefore, electrolyte-supplemented (but still hypotonic) sports drinks as compared to electrolyte-free drinking water may decrease the rate at which hyponatremia develops, but the sports drinks are not likely to prevent EAH, and may even exacerbate the hyponatremia if used to treat this disorder.

- Reset osmostat syndrome is a variant of SIADH in which there is a shift in the setpoint for ADH release to a lower plasma osmolality. Therefore, the patient may have an inappropriately concentrated urine in the setting of hypotonic hyponatremia, but will be able to dilute urine normally in response to a water load and concentrate urine in response to dehydration.

- **Nephrogenic syndrome of inappropriate antidiuresis** is a newly described genetic syndrome in which all of the criteria for SIADH are met, but in which ADH levels are undetectable. Mutations in the vasopressin V2 receptor were first identified as the cause of this syndrome in two male infants with symptomatic hyponatremia. Since then, more individuals have been identified with these mutations, including a family that showed variable phenotypic expression of this syndrome in both male and female adults.

PRESENTATION

As with other causes of hyponatremia, symptoms are dependent on the degree of hyponatremia and the rapidity at which it develops. It is rare to have symptoms with serum sodium levels of ≥ 125 mEq/L, but with acute hyponatremia (<48 hours) patients may complain of malaise and nausea. At levels of <125 mEq/L, patients may present with neuropsychiatric signs and symptoms, ranging from muscular weakness, headache, lethargy, ataxia, and psychosis to cerebral edema, increased intracranial pressure (ICP), seizures, and coma. Signs of either volume depletion or overload are not consistent with SIADH and should prompt an evaluation for other causes of hyponatremia.

MANAGEMENT

Diagnosis

SIADH is a diagnosis of exclusion, and therefore, other causes of hyponatremia must be ruled out.

Essential diagnostic criteria include:

- Low plasma osmolality: A plasma osmolality <275 mOsm/kg is consistent with SIADH, and will rule out hypertonic causes of hyponatremia.
- Inappropriately elevated urine osmolality and urine sodium concentration: A urine osmolality >100 mOsm/kg and urine sodium concentration >20 to 40 mEq/L are consistent with SIADH.
- Euvolemia: Volume depletion or overload should prompt an evaluation for an alternative diagnosis.
- Normal renal, adrenal, and thyroid function: Measurements of blood urea nitrogen (BUN) and creatinine, cortisol (30–60 minutes following intravenous or intramuscular administration of cosyntropin, 250 mcg), and thyroid-stimulating hormone (TSH) and free thyroxine (T_4) must be normal to establish the diagnosis of SIADH.
- No recent use of diuretic agents.

Supplemental diagnostic criteria include:

- Abnormal water load test, which is defined as the inability to excrete at least 80% of a water load (20 mL/kg water ingested in 10–20 minutes) after 4 hours and/or the failure to dilute urinary osmolality to <100 mOsm/kg. This test should be administered after the serum sodium level is >125 mEq/L through water restriction and/or saline administration.
- Plasma ADH level inappropriately elevated relative to plasma osmolality.
- Low to normal BUN and creatinine level, fractional excretion of sodium >1%, and uric acid <4 mg/dL, all suggesting that the patient is not hypovolemic.
- No significant correction of plasma sodium with volume expansion, but improvement after fluid restriction. Likewise, if cerebral salt wasting is in the differential

diagnosis, and the hyponatremia does not improve or worsens with fluid restriction, a trial of volume expansion may be helpful in determining whether sodium and volume replacement will be the most appropriate treatment.

Treatment

SIADH is usually self-limited, and the primary management strategy is to correct the underlying etiology. However, immediate treatment strategies are based on the severity of the hyponatremia and any associated symptoms.

Symptomatic Hyponatremia

Acute symptomatic hyponatremia is a medical emergency and is managed primarily according to the severity of symptoms and secondarily according to the level of sodium. Severe neurologic symptoms (e.g., obtundation, seizures, and coma) should be treated promptly with hypertonic (3%) saline until symptoms have resolved. However, *overly aggressive correction of hyponatremia may result in the development of central pontine myelinolysis* (CPM), a potentially devastating neurologic condition; therefore, correction of hyponatremia should always be done with caution. If the rate of development of hyponatremia is rapid (<48 hours), an equally rapid rate of correction is felt to be safe. However, resolving the symptoms should be the primary goal, whereas correction to normonatremia should be performed more judiciously as if the development of hyponatremia were more chronic. In cases where the acuity or chronicity of the hyponatremia is not known, the rate of correction should be limited to 1 to 2 mEq/L/hour for the first 3 to 4 hours, and by no more than 0.5 mEq/L/hour thereafter, for a maximum correction of 8 to 10 mEq/L per 24 hours. Fortunately, symptoms will usually resolve when the serum sodium changes by as little as 5%, or 3 to 7 mEq/L.

Many strategies have been employed to calculate the initial rate of hypertonic saline. Two of the simplest strategies include the following:

- The change in plasma sodium ($[Na+]_{plasma}$) in mEq/L for each liter of fluid given can be approximated from the following equation:

$$\text{Change in } [Na+]_{plasma} = ([Na+]_{infusate} + [K+]_{infusate} - [Na+]_{plasma}) \div (\text{total body water} + 1)$$

where $[Na+]_{infusate}$ = mEq/L of sodium in the infusate (e.g., 513 mEq/L of 3% saline), $[K+]_{infusate}$ = mEq/L of potassium in the infusate, and total body water = body weight (kg) × (0.6 for men or 0.5 for women).

For example, if a 70-kg man is having seizures and has a plasma sodium of 110 mEq/L, the calculated increase in sodium per liter of 3% saline would be $(513 + 0 - 110) \div (0.6 \times 70 \div 1) = 9.4$ mEq/L. To increase the sodium at an initial rate of 2 mEq/L/hour, 3% NaCl should be infused at ~213 mL/hour (2 mEq/L/hour ÷ 9.4mEq/L × 1000 mL).

- Alternatively, 3% saline can be administered at a rate of 1–2 mL/kg of body weight per hour to increase the sodium level by 1 to 2 mEq/L/hour. In patients with coma or seizure, the initial rate can be doubled. In patients with mild symptoms, half the rate should be used.

Therefore, in the same 70-kg man with a plasma sodium of 110 mEq/L who is having seizures, the initial rate of 3% NaCl would be 210 to 280 mL/hour (3 to 4 mL/kg/hour × 70 kg).

It is important to note that both of these strategies offer only approximations of the expected change in sodium. If there are other ongoing free water losses or if a loop diuretic is used to increase free water excretion and prevent volume overload, the infusion rate should be decreased. With any strategy, plasma sodium and volume status should be assessed frequently (initially every 2 hours, and reduced to every 4 hours when the correction rate is stable) to monitor and make adjustments to therapy.

For mild to moderate symptoms, 3% saline can be used cautiously to raise plasma sodium and alleviate symptoms. Alternatively, normal saline plus a loop diuretic can be used in place of 3% saline, or a vasopressin receptor antagonist (see below) may be considered. It should be noted that the use of normal saline alone could worsen the hyponatremia if the kidney is unable to dilute the urine to less than the osmolality of normal saline (~300 mOsm/L). For example, if the concentration of the urine is fixed at 400 mOsm/L, and 1 L of normal saline is given, the 300 mOsm of NaCl will be excreted in 750 mL of water (urine concentration, 400 mOsm/L), and the remaining 250 mL of free water will be retained by the body and will lower the plasma sodium. Irrespective of the fluid strategy that is determined to be best for a particular patient, the initial rate of correction should not exceed 2 mEq/L/hour, and should be reduced quickly to no more than 0.5 mEq/L/hour (up to a maximum of 8–10 mEq/L/day). Plasma sodium and volume status should be measured frequently to monitor and adjust therapy.

Vasopressin receptor antagonists are a promising new treatment option for SIADH. Conivaptan (Vaprisol) is the first agent in this new class of medications and was approved by the U.S. Food and Drug Administration (FDA) in 2005 for the intravenous (IV) treatment of euvolemic hyponatremia (including SIADH), and in 2007 for hypervolemic hyponatremia. Conivaptan is a nonselective vasopressin (V1a and V2) receptor antagonist that is metabolized through the CYP3A4 pathway. It is contraindicated in hypovolemic hyponatremia and with potent CYP3A4 inhibitors, such as ketoconazole, itraconazole, clarithromycin, ritonavir, and indinavir. A loading dose of 20 mg IV is administered over 30 minutes, followed by a continuous infusion of 20 mg/day for an additional 1 to 3 days (up to a maximum of 4 days). The dose may be increased to 40 mg/day if the sodium level is not rising at the desired rate. Injection site reactions are usually mild, but they occur in up to 50% of patients, and it is recommended to rotate the infusion site every 24 hours. Hypotension is a concern because of the drug's V1a-receptor antagonism, but this has not been a significant side effect in early studies. Overall, the drug seems to be well-tolerated.

Asymptomatic Hyponatremia

Hyponatremia may be asymptomatic if the degree of hyponatremia is only mild or if the development of more profound hyponatremia has occurred gradually over time. Severe neurologic sequelae are rare when hyponatremia is chronic, but the risk of developing CPM with correction of the hyponatremia may be much greater in this context. Therefore, conservative management strategies are often utilized to gradually increase the sodium level in these patients.

The cornerstone of treatment for asymptomatic hyponatremia resulting from SIADH is fluid restriction, so that free water excretion in the urine exceeds dietary intake. An appropriate prescription for fluid restriction can be estimated by measuring plasma sodium and a spot urine sample for sodium and potassium. These values can then be used to determine the urine-to-plasma (U/P) electrolyte ratio:

$$\text{U/P ratio} = ([Na+]_{urine} + [K+]_{urine}) \div [Na+]_{plasma}$$

where $[Na+]_{urine}$ = mEq/L of sodium in the urine, $[K+]_{urine}$ = mEq/L of potassium in the urine, and $[Na+]_{plasma}$ = mEq/L of sodium in the plasma.

If the U/P ratio is ≥1.0, free water should be maximally restricted. If the ratio is 0.5–1.0, free water should be restricted to ≤500 mL/day, and if the ratio is ≤0.5, free water should be restricted to ≤1000 mL/day.

If more profound hyponatremia is present (usually <110 mEq/L), patients may be at increased risk of developing severe symptoms. Therefore, even if asymptomatic, it may be reasonable to correct the hyponatremia at a maximum rate of 0.5 mEq/L/hour, and no more than 8 to 10 mEq/L over 24 hours. Hypertonic saline or vasopressin receptor antagonists may be necessary to achieve this goal, but should be discontinued as soon as the sodium level is approximately 120 to 125 mEq/L, after which more conservative measures should be instituted.

Adequate intake of dietary protein and salt should be encouraged, since maximal free water clearance by the kidneys is dependent on the intake and excretion of solutes. Oral intake of urea (30 g/day) has been shown to be effective as well, but it is not well tolerated. Loop diuretics can also be added to increase free water excretion.

For cases of SIADH that are not self-limited or are refractory to fluid restriction, demeclocycline (Declomycin) may be administered. Demeclocycline (Declomycin) inhibits the renal effect of ADH (effectively producing nephrogenic diabetes insipidus) and can improve the serum sodium concentration without fluid restriction. Initial dosing is 600 mg daily in 2 to 3 divided doses, with an onset of action 3 to 6 days after treatment initiation. It should be given 1 to 2 hours after meals. The major side effect is nephrotoxicity, so renal function should be monitored closely.

Oral vasopressin receptor antagonists specific for the V2 receptor (tolvaptan, lixivaptan, stavaptan) are promising new agents for the long-term management of refractory SIADH, but are not yet clinically available.

Prognosis

Prognosis is dependent on the underlying etiology as well as the severity of the hyponatremia and associated symptoms. More profound or symptomatic hyponatremia has a much higher morbidity and mortality than mild or chronic asymptomatic hyponatremia. SIADH usually resolves with therapy for the underlying etiology.

KEY POINTS TO REMEMBER

- SIADH is a diagnosis of exclusion.
- A low serum osmolality in conjunction with an inappropriately elevated urine osmolality and urine sodium are consistent with SIADH.
- The cornerstone of treatment is fluid restriction.
- Hypertonic fluids can be administered in cases of acute symptomatic hyponatremia, but care should be taken not to correct the serum sodium level too rapidly.
- V2 receptor antagonists are now available for the treatment of SIADH.

REFERENCES AND SUGGESTED READINGS

Adrogue HJ, Madia NE. Hyponatremia. *N Engl J Med* 2000;342:1581–1589.

Ball SG, Baylis PH. Vasopressin, diabetes insipidus, and syndrome of inappropriate antidiuresis. In: DeGroot LJ, Jameson JL, eds. *Endocrinology*, 5th ed. Philadelphia: Elsevier; 2006:537–556.

Cawley MJ. Hyponatremia: current treatment strategies and the role of vasopressin antagonists. *Ann Pharmacother* 2007;41:840–850.

Decaux G, Vandergheynst F, Bouko Y, et al. Nephrogenic syndrome of inappropriate antidiuresis in adults: high phenotypic variability in men and women from a large pedigree. *J Am Soc Nephrol* 2007;18:606–612.

Ellison DH, Berl T. Clinical practice. The syndrome of inappropriate antidiuresis. *N Engl J Med* 2007;356:2064–2072.

Feldman BJ, Rosenthal SM, Vargas GA, et al. Nephrogenic syndrome of inappropriate antidiuresis. *N Engl J Med* 2005;352:1884–1890.

Furst H, Hallows KR, Post J, et al. The urine/plasma electrolyte ratio: a predictive guide to water restriction. *Am J Med Sci* 2000;319:240–244.

Goldman MB, Luchins DJ, Robertson GL. Mechanisms of altered water metabolism in psychotic patients with polydipsia and hyponatremia. *N Engl J Med* 1988;318:397–403.

Goldman MB, Robertson GL, Luchins DJ, et al. The influence of polydipsia on water excretion in hyponatremic, polydipsic, schizophrenic patients. *J Clin Endocrinol Metab* 1996;81:1465–1470.

Hillier TA, Abbott RD, Barrett EJ. Hyponatremia: evaluating the correction factor for hyperglycemia. *Am J Med* 1999;106:399–403.

Jacobi J, Titze J, Niewerth P, Lang R, et al. Severe hyponatraemia due to hypothalamic—pituitary adrenal insufficiency. *Nephrol Dial Transplant* 2001;16:1708–1710.

Palmer BF. Hyponatremia in patients with central nervous system disease: SIADH versus CSW. *Trends Endocrinol Metab* 2003;14:182–187.

Rose BD. Treatment of hyponatremia: SIADH and reset osmostat. *UpToDate* 2007:15.1.

Siegel AJ, Verbalis JG, Clement S, et al. Hyponatremia in marathon runners due to inappropriate arginine vasopressin secretion. *Am J Med* 2007;120:461.e11–e17.

Upadhyay A, Jaber BL, Madias NE. Incidence and prevalence of hyponatremia. *Am J Med* 2006;119[Suppl 1]:S30–35.

Weisberg LS. Pseudohyponatremia: a reappraisal. *Am J Med* 1989;86:315–318.

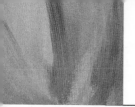

Evaluation of Thyroid Function

6

William E. Clutter

INTRODUCTION

The major hormone secreted by the thyroid is **thyroxine** (T_4), which is converted by deiodinases in many tissues to the more potent **triiodothyronine** (T_3). Both are reversibly bound to plasma proteins, primarily **thyroxine-binding globulin** (**TBG**), and also thyroxine-binding prealbumin (TBPA) and albumin. Only the free (unbound) fraction enters cells and produces biological effects.

T4 secretion is stimulated by **thyroid-stimulating hormone** (**TSH**). In turn, pituitary TSH secretion is inhibited by thyroid hormones, forming a sensitive negative-feedback loop that keeps free T_4 levels within a narrow normal range. TSH secretion is stimulated by hypothalamic thyrotropin-releasing hormone (TRH).

Diagnosis of thyroid disease is based on clinical findings, palpation of the thyroid, and measurement of plasma TSH and thyroid hormones.

CLINICAL EVALUATION

Thyroid palpation determines the size and consistency of the thyroid, and the presence of nodules, tenderness, or a thrill. Auscultation may detect a bruit over the gland in severe hyperthyroidism.

Examination of the eyes includes assessment for lid lag and proptosis in suspected hyperthyroidism and periorbital edema in suspected hypothyroidism. Skin examination may reveal warm, moist skin in hyperthyroidism and dry, cool skin or myxedema in hypothyroidism. Neurologic signs include brisk tendon reflex relaxation and fine tremor in hyperthyroidism and delayed reflex relaxation in hypothyroidism.

LABORATORY EVALUATION

Thyroid-Stimulating Hormone

Plasma TSH is the initial test of choice in most patients with suspected thyroid disease, except when thyroid function is not in a steady state or TSH secretion by the pituitary may be abnormal (Table 6-1).

TSH levels are elevated in even very mild primary hypothyroidism and are suppressed to <0.1 μU/mL in even very mild hyperthyroidism. Therefore, **a normal plasma TSH level excludes hyperthyroidism and primary hypothyroidism.** Because even slight changes in thyroid hormone levels affect TSH secretion, **abnormal TSH levels are not specific for clinically important thyroid disease.** Changes in plasma TSH lag behind changes in plasma T_4, and TSH levels may be misleading when plasma T_4 levels are changing rapidly, as during treatment of hyperthyroidism, or in the first few weeks after changes in the dose of thyroxine.

TABLE 6-1	PLASMA TSH MEASUREMENT

Appropriate Uses:

Diagnosis of suspected hyperthyroidism or primary hypothyroidism

Monitoring and adjustment of therapy for primary hypothyroidism

Monitoring TSH suppression therapy for thyroid cancer

Inappropriate Uses:

Evaluation of suspected secondary hypothyroidism

Monitoring and adjustment of therapy for secondary hypothyroidism

Within several weeks of a change in thyroxine dose

During early stages of treatment of hyperthyroidism

Plasma TSH is mildly elevated (<20 μU/mL) in some euthyroid patients recovering from **nonthyroidal illnesses** and in **mild (or subclinical) hypothyroidism.**

TSH levels may be suppressed to <0.1 μU/mL in severe nonthyroidal illness, in **mild (or subclinical) hyperthyroidism**, and during treatment with dopamine or high doses of glucocorticoids (Table 6-2). Also, TSH levels remain <0.1 μU/mL for some time **after hyperthyroidism is corrected.** TSH levels decrease in the first trimester of **pregnancy** (owing to thyroid stimulation by chorionic gonadotropin) and may fall to <0.1 μU/mL.

TSH levels are usually within the reference range in secondary hypothyroidism due to pituitary or hypothalamic disease, and are not useful for detection of this rare form of hypothyroidism.

Plasma Free T_4

Measurement of plasma free T_4 confirms the diagnosis and assesses the severity of **hyperthyroidism** when plasma TSH is <0.1 μU/mL (Table 6-3). It is also used to diagnose **secondary hypothyroidism** and adjust thyroxine therapy in patients with pituitary disease. Most laboratories measure free T_4 by one of several types of immunoassay.

Plasma Free T_4 Measured by Equilibrium Dialysis

Plasma free T_4 by equilibrium dialysis (ED) is the most reliable measure of clinical thyroid status, but results are seldom rapidly available. ED is needed only in rare cases in which the diagnosis is not clear from measurement of plasma TSH and free T_4 by immunoassay.

TABLE 6-2	CAUSES OF A SUPPRESSED PLASMA TSH

Clinical hyperthyroidism

Subclinical hyperthyroidism

Recently resolved hyperthyroidism

First trimester of pregnancy

Nonthyroidal illness

Dopamine therapy

High-dose glucocorticoid therapy

TABLE 6-3	APPROPRIATE USES OF PLASMA FREE T_4
Confirmation of the diagnosis and severity of hyperthyroidism	
Confirmation of the severity of primary hypothyroidism	
Diagnosis of suspected secondary hypothyroidism	
Monitoring and adjustment of therapy for secondary hypothyroidism	

Plasma Total T_4

Plasma total T_4 assays measure both bound and free hormone. Because altered levels of TBG cause abnormal total T_4 levels in euthyroid patients, total T_4 is less reliable than free T_4 and should not be used, except when free T_4 may be artifactually elevated by heparin treatment (see Effect of Drugs on Thyroid Function Tests in this chapter). Some common causes of increased TBG are estrogen treatment, including oral contraceptives, and pregnancy. Low TBG levels are common in cirrhosis, nephrotic syndrome, and many severe illnesses.

Plasma Total T_3

Although T_3 is the biologically active hormone, much of it is derived from deiodination of T_4 within target cells, making T_4 the major circulating thyroid hormone. Plasma T_3 level is affected by alterations in plasma TBG just as is plasma T_4. This test has very limited use in the evaluation of suspected thyroid disease, and **should only be measured in patients with suspected hyperthyroidism with suppressed plasma TSH but normal plasma free T_4**. Some of these patients have clinical hyperthyroidism with elevation of plasma T_3 alone (**T_3 toxicosis**). Plasma T_3 assays are not useful in the diagnosis of hypothyroidism. Many laboratories offer assays of plasma free T_3, but their reliability is unknown.

Plasma Thyroglobulin

Thyroglobulin (Tg), the precursor of thyroid hormones, is a glycoprotein synthesized only by thyroid follicular cells. Most thyroglobulin is broken down within the thyroid to release T_4 and T_3, but a small amount enters the circulation intact. Plasma thyroglobulin levels are increased in all thyroid diseases and are undetectable when all thyroid tissue has been removed. The only use of plasma thyroglobulin assays is **monitoring of patients with papillary or follicular thyroid carcinoma after total thyroidectomy** to detect persistent or recurrent disease.

An assay for **antithyroglobulin antibodies** should always be done in conjunction with the thyroglobulin assay, since the presence of such antibodies renders the thyroglobulin assay useless.

Antithyroid Antibodies

Patients with autoimmune thyroid diseases (Hashimoto's thyroiditis, painless thyroiditis, and Graves' disease) often have **autoantibodies against thyroid peroxidase**, **thyroglobulin**, or both. Measurement of these antibodies has a very limited role in thyroid diagnosis. They can be used to confirm that primary hypothyroidism or a euthyroid goiter is due to Hashimoto's thyroiditis, but this diagnosis can usually be made on clinical grounds.

Thyroid-Stimulating Immunoglobulins

Thyroid-stimulating immunoglobulins (TSIs) are **autoantibodies to the TSH receptor** that mimic the stimulatory effect of TSH on thyroid growth and hormone production, and cause hyperthyroidism in **Graves' disease**. Measurement of these antibodies is seldom needed to make this diagnosis, which is usually obvious on clinical grounds. Its primary use is in **pregnant women with a history of Graves' disease treated by radioactive iodine or thyroidectomy.** These patients may still have high levels of TSI, which can no longer produce hyperthyroidism in the mother, but can cross the placenta and cause neonatal hyperthyroidism. Assay of TSI in the third trimester has some value in predicting this rare complication.

Plasma Calcitonin

Calcitonin is the secretory product of thyroid parafollicular or C cells. Although it has no apparent physiologic role, it is a useful tumor marker for **medullary carcinoma of the thyroid** (MCT), which is derived from parafollicular cells. Mild elevations of plasma calcitonin are not specific for MCT.

Radioactive Iodine Uptake

Radioactive iodine uptake (RAIU) is the percentage of a small oral dose of iodine-131 (^{131}I) retained by the thyroid after 24 hours. It occasionally helps in **differential diagnosis of hyperthyroidism** (see Chapter 8), and is also used to calculate the dose for RAI therapy. Large doses of exogenous iodine in the form of x-ray contrast media or iodine-containing drugs suppress RAIU temporarily. The normal range of RAIU for dietary iodine intake in the United States is 10% to 30%. Note that RAIU is a number, not an image.

THYROID IMAGING

Although thyroid imaging tests are widely used, they have very limited value in the assessment of patients with suspected thyroid disease, since clinically important abnormalities of thyroid anatomy are readily assessed by palpation.

Radioisotope Thyroid Scan

Radioisotope thyroid scans use technetium-99m pertechnetate, which is taken up by the sodium-iodine symporter of thyroid cells. These scans can determine the functional activity of thyroid nodules: hypofunctioning ("cold"), isofunctioning ("warm"), or hyperfunctioning ("hot"). Almost all thyroid carcinomas are hypofunctioning, but unfortunately for the usefulness of this test, so are most benign nodules, resulting in a very low positive predictive value (PPV). This test has been supplanted in the evaluation of thyroid nodules by fine-needle aspiration cytology (FNAC). The only indication for radioisotope thyroid scanning is the presence of **a single palpable thyroid nodule in a patient with hyperthyroidism.** If the nodule is hyperfunctioning and causing hyperthyroidism, it is assuredly benign and does not require biopsy. On the other hand, a hypofunctioning nodule in a gland affected by Graves' disease should be evaluated by FNAC.

Ultrasonography

High-resolution ultrasonography (US) of the thyroid has become widely used, despite a lack of evidence that its use improves the clinical outcome in patients with thyroid disease. Its primary role is in the evaluation of thyroid nodules. It differentiates solid from cystic nodules and may be used to guide fine-needle biopsy, particularly of nonpalpable nodules. The critical limitation of US is the **high prevalence of incidental thyroid nodules, which are found in 20% to 60% of the population.** Most of these nodules are of no clinical importance, and their detection leads only to unnecessary anxiety, further testing, and even unnecessary surgery. **US has no role in the evaluation of diffuse goiters, or of patients with hypo- or hyperthyroidism.**

FINE-NEEDLE ASPIRATION CYTOLOGY (FNAC)

FNAC is the method of choice for evaluating thyroid nodules for the presence of malignancy. It is a safe and simple bedside procedure, and provides a definitive diagnosis in the great majority of patients. If the specimen obtained is inadequate for diagnosis, the procedure should be repeated. Complications are rare and consist mostly of transient painful swelling of the nodule due to bleeding within it.

SPECIAL TOPICS

Effect of Nonthyroidal Illness on Thyroid Function Tests

Many illnesses alter thyroid tests without causing true thyroid dysfunction (the nonthyroidal illness or euthyroid sick syndrome). These changes must be recognized to avoid mistaken diagnosis and therapy.

The **low T_3 syndrome** occurs in many illnesses, during starvation, and after trauma or surgery. Conversion of T_4 to T_3 by type 1 deiodinase is decreased, and plasma T_3 levels are low. Plasma free T_4 and TSH levels are normal. This may be an adaptive response to illness, and thyroid hormone therapy is not beneficial.

The **low T_4 syndrome** occurs in severe illness. Plasma total T_4 levels fall due to decreased levels of TBG and perhaps due to inhibition of T_4 binding to TBG. **Plasma free T_4 measured by equilibrium dialysis usually remains normal.** However, when measured by commonly available immunoassays, free T_4 may be low. **TSH levels decrease early in severe illness**, sometimes to <0.1 μU/mL. **During recovery they rise, sometimes to levels higher than the normal range** (although rarely >20 μU/mL).

Effect of Drugs on Thyroid Function Tests

A number of drugs affect thyroid function tests (Table 6-4). Iodine-containing drugs (**amiodarone** and **radiographic contrast media**) may cause hyperthyroidism or hypothyroidism in susceptible patients. Other drugs alter thyroid function tests, especially plasma total T_4, without causing true thyroid dysfunction. In general, plasma TSH levels are reliable in determining whether true hyperthyroidism or hypothyroidism is present.

Evaluation of Thyroid Function in Pregnancy

Thyroid hormone is critical for fetal brain development, and several changes occur in maternal thyroid function during pregnancy. **TBG and total T_4 levels** rise early in pregnancy. **Chorionic gonadotropin** is homologous to TSH, and very high levels in the first trimester stimulate the TSH receptor, causing a transient **fall in TSH levels** by stimulating T_4 secretion. The mother usually remains euthyroid, but rarely she develops a transient clinical hyperthyroidism, often associated with hyperemesis gravidarum.

The **placenta contains high levels of type 3 deiodinase (D3), which inactivates T_4** and severely limits T_4 transfer from mother to fetus. Nevertheless, some T_4 crosses the placenta and is important for early fetal brain development. **In mothers with preexisting hypothyroidism, increased T_4 metabolism by placental D3 means that their levothyroxine dose must usually be increased to maintain euthyroidism.** Urinary iodine excretion increases, and in areas of iodine deficiency, it becomes more difficult for the thyroid to maintain adequate hormone secretion, with development of a transient goiter. If the iodine deficiency is too severe, the fetus receives inadequate thyroid hormone, and endemic cretinism results.

Thyroid disorders and pregnancy often coincide (because of the frequency of thyroid disease in young women). Important interactions between the two include (a) the normal

TABLE 6-4   EFFECTS OF DRUGS ON THYROID FUNCTION TESTS

Effect	Drug
Decreased free and total T_4	
True hypothyroidism (TSH elevated)	Iodine (amiodarone, radiographic contrast) Others (see Chapter 9)
Inhibition of TSH secretion	Glucocorticoids Dopamine
Multiple mechanisms (TSH normal)	Phenytoin
Decreased total T_4 only	
Decreased TBG (TSH normal)	Androgens
Inhibition of T_4 binding to TBG (TSH normal)	Furosemide (high doses), salicylates
Increased free and total T_4	
True hyperthyroidism (TSH <0.1 μU/mL)	Iodine (amiodarone, radiographic contrast)
Inhibited T_4 to T_3 conversion (TSH normal)	Amiodarone
Increased free T_4 only	
Displacement of T4 from TBG in vitro (TSH normal)	Heparin, low-molecular-weight heparin
Increased total T_4 only	
Increased TBG (TSH normal)	Estrogens, tamoxifen

T_3, triiodothyronine; T_4, thyroxine; TBG, thyroxine-binding globulin; TSH, thyroid-stimulating hormone.

decrease in TSH in the first trimester, which may be mistaken for hyperthyroidism; (b) in hypothyroid women, the frequent need to increase levothyroxine dose in pregnancy; (c) the complexity of treating hyperthyroidism in pregnant women without adversely affecting the fetus; and (d) the occasional occurrence of a transient hyperthyroidism caused by painless thyroiditis in the months after delivery.

KEY POINTS TO REMEMBER

- Plasma TSH is the best initial test in most patients with suspected thyroid disease.
- Plasma free T_4 is used to diagnose secondary hypothyroidism.
- Nonthyroidal illness, pregnancy, and some drugs affect thyroid function tests and may cause diagnostic confusion.
- FNAC is the method of choice for evaluating thyroid nodules for malignancy.
- Plasma thyroglobulin is a useful tumor marker in patients who have undergone thyroidectomy for thyroid carcinoma, unless antithyroglobulin antibodies are present.
- Twenty percent to 60% of the population have incidental, clinically unimportant thyroid nodules detectable by ultrasonography.

REFERENCES AND SUGGESTED READINGS

Adler SM, Wartofsky L. The nonthyroidal illness syndrome. *Endocrinol Metab Clin North Am* 2007;36:657–672.

Dufour DR. Laboratory tests of thyroid function: uses and limitations. *Endocrinol Metab Clin North Am* 2007;36:579–594.

LeBeau SO, Mandel SJ. Thyroid disorders during pregnancy. *Endocrinol Metab Clin North Am* 2006;35:117–136.

Euthyroid Goiter and Thyroid Nodules

William E. Clutter

7

INTRODUCTION

Euthyroid goiter is defined as thyroid enlargement with normal thyroid function. There are three forms: **diffuse goiter, multinodular goiter,** and a **solitary thyroid nodule. The diagnosis of euthyroid goiter is based on palpation of the thyroid and evaluation of thyroid function.** If the thyroid is enlarged, the examiner should determine whether the enlargement is diffuse or multinodular, or whether a single nodule is palpable. **All three forms of euthyroid goiter are common, especially in women.** Imaging studies, such as thyroid scans or ultrasonography, provide no useful additional information about goiters that are diffuse or multinodular by palpation and should not be performed in these patients. Furthermore, **20% to 60% of people have nonpalpable thyroid nodules that are detectable by ultrasound.** These nodules rarely have any clinical importance, but their incidental discovery may lead to unnecessary diagnostic testing and treatment.

EUTHYROID DIFFUSE GOITER

Causes

Almost all euthyroid diffuse goiters in iodine-sufficient regions such as the United States are caused by **chronic lymphocytic thyroiditis (Hashimoto's thyroiditis). Iodine deficiency** also causes diffuse colloid goiter in much of the world. Because Hashimoto's thyroiditis may also cause hypothyroidism, **plasma thyroid-stimulating hormone (TSH)** should be measured even in patients who are clinically euthyroid. The presence of antithyroid antibodies confirms the diagnosis of Hashimoto's disease, but this test is seldom needed. Thyroid imaging should not be performed.

Clinical Presentation and Management

Small diffuse goiters usually are **asymptomatic**, and therapy is seldom required. Larger goiters may cause **compressive symptoms** such as **dysphagia, dyspnea,** or **neck fullness.** Symptomatic diffuse goiters may shrink with suppression of plasma TSH to the lower part of the normal range by levothyroxine therapy. If levothyroxine is not given, the patient should be monitored for the development of hypothyroidism. Patients should be followed annually with thyroid palpation and measurement of plasma TSH. Most diffuse goiters do not progressively enlarge, but in a few, thyroidectomy may be needed to relieve compressive symptoms or for cosmetic reasons.

MULTINODULAR GOITER

Clinical Presentation

Multinodular goiter (MNG) is caused by nodular hyperplasia of thyroid follicles. It occurs most commonly in iodine-deficient regions, but is also very common in iodine-sufficient areas such as the United States, primarily in **older patients and in women**. Most patients are asymptomatic and require no treatment. In a few patients, **hyperthyroidism (toxic MNG)** develops (see Chapter 8). In some patients, the goiter causes compressive symptoms, and treatment is required. The risk of malignancy in MNG is comparable to the frequency of incidental thyroid carcinoma in clinically normal glands. Evaluation for thyroid carcinoma with fine-needle aspiration cytology (FNAC) is warranted if there is a dominant nodule (a nodule that is disproportionately larger than the other nodules). Some centers have adopted a policy of performing thyroid ultrasonography (US) in all patients with MNG, and evaluating all nodules larger than 1 cm by FNAC. This policy dramatically increases the number of thyroid biopsies and the cost of managing this common condition. There is no evidence that routine thyroid US improves clinical outcomes in patients with MNG, and it is not recommended.

Management

Subtotal thyroidectomy is the treatment of choice for patients with compressive symptoms. If the patient is a poor candidate for surgery or refuses surgery, a high dose (about 50 mCi) of radioactive iodine will reduce gland size and improve symptoms in most patients. Thyroxine treatment has little if any effect on the size of MNGs and should not be used.

SINGLE THYROID NODULES

Single thyroid nodules are palpable in about 5% of women and 1% of men. They are usually due to benign nodular hyperplasia or thyroid adenomas, but about 5% are thyroid carcinomas, and the main diagnostic task is establishing or excluding this diagnosis.

Clinical Presentation

Most thyroid nodules present as a **painless lump in the neck** discovered by the patient or physician. **Clinical findings that increase the likelihood of carcinoma** include age <20 years, the presence of cervical lymphadenopathy, a history of radiation to the head or neck in childhood, and a family history of medullary thyroid carcinoma or multiple endocrine neoplasia (MEN) syndromes type 2A or 2B. A hard, fixed nodule; recent nodule growth; or hoarseness due to invasion of the recurrent laryngeal nerve also suggests malignancy. However, most patients with thyroid carcinomas have none of these risk factors, and their lesions cannot be distinguished clinically from benign nodules. Thus, **nearly all palpable single thyroid nodules should be evaluated with FNAC.**

A few solitary thyroid nodules are **adenomas producing hyperthyroidism** (see Chapter 8). Some thyroid nodules present with the sudden onset of pain and tenderness, indicating hemorrhage into a preexisting, usually benign, nodule. Solitary nodules rarely cause compressive symptoms.

Diagnostic Evaluation

Plasma TSH should be measured, since a nodule in a hyperthyroid patient is more likely to be benign. **If plasma TSH is suppressed**, a radioisotope thyroid scan should

TABLE 7-1	DIAGNOSTIC CATEGORIES OF FINE-NEEDLE ASPIRATION CYTOLOGY

Benign

Malignant

Indeterminate (also termed suspicious or follicular lesion)

Inadequate for diagnosis

be performed. If the nodule is hyperfunctioning and causing hyperthyroidism, it is assuredly benign and does not require biopsy. On the other hand, a hypofunctioning nodule in a gland affected by Graves' disease should be evaluated by FNAC. This is the only indication for radioisotope scanning in patients with a thyroid nodule.

Plasma calcitonin should be measured if there is a family history of medullary carcinoma or MEN 2A or 2B.

The key diagnostic evaluation is FNAC, the results of which are classified into four categories (Table 7-1):

- Nodules with **benign** cytology should be reevaluated periodically by palpation, since there is a low risk of false-negative cytology. Repeat biopsy should be considered if the nodule enlarges. Levothyroxine therapy has little or no effect on the size of single thyroid nodules, and is not indicated.
- If the specimen is **inadequate**, the biopsy should be repeated.
- Nodules with **malignant** cytology should be treated by total thyroidectomy followed by treatment described in the section Thyroid Carcinoma in this chapter.
- About 20% of nodules with indeterminate cytology are malignant, so these lesions should also be treated surgically. A lobectomy is often performed, with completion thyroidectomy if carcinoma is confirmed.

Some centers have adopted a policy of performing thyroid US in all patients with a single palpable nodule, and performing FNAC on all nodules larger than 1 cm. Some ultrasonographic features of thyroid nodules are suggestive of malignancy, but they are neither sensitive nor specific enough to establish or exclude the diagnosis. There is no evidence that routine thyroid US improves clinical outcomes in these patients, and it is not recommended.

THYROID CARCINOMA

Most thyroid malignancies are differentiated carcinomas arising from follicular cells (**papillary or follicular carcinomas**) (Table 7-2). These cancers retain many properties of normal thyroid cells: they **take up iodine** and **synthesize thyroglobulin**, although less efficiently than normal thyroid tissue. **Their growth and function is stimulated by TSH.** These three properties are used in treatment and follow-up of thyroid carcinoma.

The most common type of thyroid cancer is papillary carcinoma, which is a slow growing tumor that may remain localized for years. It characteristically metastasizes first to cervical lymph nodes. Microscopic foci of papillary carcinoma are common at autopsy. Thus, a small papillary carcinoma found incidentally in a thyroid removed for other reasons, is usually not clinically important. **Follicular carcinoma** is more aggressive, and may metastasize early to lung and bone. Many thyroid cancers have mixed papillary and

TABLE 7-2	MAJOR TYPES OF THYROID CANCER
Type	**Frequency**
Follicular cell origin:	
Papillary	80%
Follicular	15%
Anaplastic	Rare
C-cell (parafollicular cell) origin:	
Medullary carcinoma	5%
Thyroid lymphoma	Rare

follicular morphology; these behave like papillary carcinoma. **Anaplastic** carcinoma is a rare, rapidly progressive thyroid cancer with a very poor prognosis.

Medullary carcinoma of the thyroid (MCT) arises from C cells (parafollicular cells). **Plasma calcitonin** is elevated and useful for diagnosis. Most cases of medullary carcinoma are sporadic. However, MCT is a component of **MEN 2A and 2B**, as well as **familial MCT syndrome**, which are all caused by mutations of different regions of the *RET* proto-oncogene.

Clinical Presentation and Diagnosis

Thyroid cancer usually presents as an asymptomatic single nodule. It is not painful or tender, and does not cause hyperthyroidism or hypothyroidism. Clinical findings that increase the probability of carcinoma in a nodule are listed in this chapter in the section, Single Thyroid Nodules. The diagnostic procedure of choice is **FNAC**.

Treatment of Papillary and Follicular Thyroid Carcinoma

The initial treatment of papillary and follicular carcinoma is **total thyroidectomy**. In all patients with follicular carcinoma, and in patients with papillary carcinoma who have characteristics that place them at increased risk of tumor recurrence (Table 7-3), **thyroid remnant ablation** is performed. Radioactive iodine (RAI) is taken up by tumor cells only if TSH levels are elevated, so levothyroxine therapy is withheld until plasma TSH is >30 μU/mL (usually about 2 weeks); then 30 to 100 mCi of RAI is given. A **whole body RAI (WBI) scan** is usually performed several days after the ablation dose. The purpose of remnant ablation is to destroy remaining normal and malignant thyroid tissue, to reduce the risk of tumor recurrence, and facilitate monitoring patients for recurrence.

To inhibit growth of residual tumor cells, patients are then treated with **levothyroxine at a dose that suppresses plasma TSH to below the normal range**. In patients with risk

TABLE 7-3	FACTORS THAT INCREASE RISK OF RECURRENCE OR MORTALITY IN PAPILLARY THYROID CANCER
Tumor diameter >2 cm	
Invasion through the thyroid capsule	
Cervical lymph node metastases	
Distant metastases	
Age >45 years	

factors for recurrence or with known metastatic disease, plasma TSH should be maintained at about 0.1 μU/mL. In low-risk patients, plasma TSH should be maintained between 0.1 and 0.5 μU/mL.

WBI scans are then done at 6 to 12 month intervals. Usually the required elevation of plasma TSH is achieved by stopping levothyroxine therapy for about 2 weeks, although recombinant human TSH can be injected instead. **If RAI uptake by functioning thyroid tissue is detected, patients are treated with RAI** (usually 100–200 mCi). One or more RAI treatments usually eradicate remaining tumor. **WBI scanning can be discontinued after two consecutive negative scans.**

Patients require lifelong monitoring, since papillary thyroid cancer may recur after a long interval. **Plasma thyroglobulin** is measured at the time of WBI scanning (when TSH levels are elevated and secretion by remaining tumor is stimulated), and then at 6 to 12 month intervals while the patient is taking suppressive levothyroxine therapy. A rising thyroglobulin level indicates tumor recurrence and the need for further RAI therapy.

Most differentiated thyroid carcinomas can be cured, even if metastatic at the time of diagnosis. Only about 5% of patients with papillary thyroid carcinoma die of the disease.

Treatment of Medullary Carcinoma

The primary therapy for medullary carcinoma is total thyroidectomy. Early detection by genetic testing for the *RET* mutation is critical in kindreds with familial MCT, MEN 2A, or MEN 2B. Plasma calcitonin is used to monitor patients for recurrence. Levothyroxine replacement should be adjusted to keep plasma TSH level within the normal range. RAI therapy is not useful.

INCIDENTALLY DETECTED THYROID NODULES

Given their high prevalence, thyroid nodules are often found incidentally by imaging tests done for unrelated reasons. There is general agreement that nodules <1 cm in diameter do not require FNAC; a reasonable policy is to monitor such patients by annual thyroid palpation and to perform FNAC if a nodule becomes palpable. The management of incidental, nonpalpable thyroid nodules >1 cm in diameter is controversial. Some advocate the use of FNAC in all such nodules, but there is no evidence that this policy improves clinical outcomes. Given the excellent prognosis of thyroid carcinoma diagnosed when it becomes palpable, there is little reason to believe that earlier diagnosis will improve survival.

KEY POINTS TO REMEMBER

- Euthyroid diffuse goiter is almost always caused by Hashimoto's thyroiditis.
- Multinodular goiters are usually asymptomatic, but require treatment when compressive symptoms or hyperthyroidism occur.
- Single thyroid nodules are usually benign, but about 5% are thyroid carcinomas.
- FNAC is the best test for evaluation of a solitary thyroid nodule.
- Incidental thyroid nodules can be detected by US in 20%–60% of the general population, and most nodules have no clinical importance.
- Initial treatment of differentiated thyroid carcinoma includes thyroidectomy, and remnant ablation with RAI in high risk patients.
- Long-term management of differentiated thyroid carcinoma includes suppression of plasma TSH to below the normal range, monitoring of plasma thyroglobulin, and WBI scans.

REFERENCES AND SUGGESTED READING

American Thyroid Association Guidelines Taskforce. Management guidelines for patients with thyroid nodules and differentiated thyroid cancer. *Thyroid* 2006;16:1–33.

Ball DW. Medullary thyroid cancer: monitoring and therapy. *Endocrinol Metab Clin North Am* 2007;36:823–837.

Frates; MC, Benson CB, Charboneau JW, et. Al. Management of thyroid nodules detected at ultrasound: Society of Radiologists in US consensus conference statement. *Radiology* 2005;237:794–800.

Ross DS. Nonpalpable thyroid nodules—managing an epidemic. *J Clin Endocrinol Metab* 2002;87:1938–1940.

Sherman SI. Thyroid carcinoma. *Lancet* 2003;361:501–511.

Topliss D. Thyroid incidentaloma: the ignorant in pursuit of the impalpable. *Clin Endocrinol* 2004;60:18–20.

Tuttle RM, Leboeuf R, Mortorella AJ. Papillary thyroid cancer: monitoring and therapy. *Endocrinol Metab Clin North Am* 2007;36:753–778.

Van Nostrand D, Wartofsky L. Radioiodine in the treatment of thyroid cancer. *Endocrinol Metab Clin North Am* 2007;36:807–822.

Weetman AP. Radioiodine treatment for benign thyroid diseases. *Clin Endocrinol* 2007;66:757–764.

Hyperthyroidism

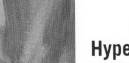

8

William E. Clutter

INTRODUCTION

Hyperthyroidism is the syndrome caused by thyroid hormone excess. Thyrotoxicosis is a synonym. It affects about 2% of women and 0.2% of men.

CAUSES

Graves' disease is the most common cause of hyperthyroidism, especially in young patients. This autoimmune disorder may also cause **proptosis** (exophthalmos) or **pretibial myxedema**, neither of which is found in other causes of hyperthyroidism (Table 8-1).

Toxic multinodular goiter (MNG) is a common cause of hyperthyroidism in older patients. Unusual causes of hyperthyroidism include **iodine-induced hyperthyroidism** (usually precipitated by drugs such as **amiodarone** or radiographic contrast media), **thyroid adenomas**, **subacute thyroiditis** (a painful tender goiter with transient hyperthyroidism), **painless thyroiditis** (a nontender goiter with transient hyperthyroidism, most often seen in the postpartum period), and **factitious hyperthyroidism** (surreptitious ingestion of thyroid hormone). The other causes of hyperthyroidism are extremely rare.

Pathophysiology

Graves' disease is an autoimmune disorder in which autoantibodies (**thyroid-stimulating immunoglobulins, TSIs**) bind to the thyroid-stimulating hormone (TSH) receptor and mimic the effects of TSH. Graves' disease is much more common in women. It occurs at any age, but is most common in young adults. A family history of Graves' disease or Hashimoto's disease is common. Patients have a **diffuse goiter,** which is soft and nontender. Increased blood flow sometimes causes a thyroid bruit or thrill. There is diffuse hyperplasia of follicular cells with a lymphocytic infiltrate. The natural history of Graves' disease may be marked by exacerbations and remissions of hyperthyroidism.

Graves' disease and Hashimoto's disease are clearly related. Both are autoimmune in origin and cluster in the same families, and antithyroid antibodies are present in both. Sometimes, one evolves into the other (e.g., patients with Graves' disease may later become hypothyroid even if treated only with antithyroid drugs).

Graves' disease includes two extrathyroidal signs caused by the underlying autoimmune disease, not by thyroid hormone excess. They are not seen with other causes of hyperthyroidism.

Graves' ophthalmopathy, characterized by inflammation and edema of retroorbital tissues (extraocular muscles and fat), causes forward protrusion of the globe (proptosis or exophthalmos). **Pretibial myxedema**, a rare plaque-like thickening of the skin over the shins, is due to accumulation of glycosaminoglycans in the dermis.

TABLE 8-1	CAUSES OF HYPERTHYROIDISM

Graves' disease

Toxic multinodular goiter

Toxic adenoma

Iodine and iodine-containing drugs (e.g., amiodarone, iodinated contrast agents)

Painless thyroiditis

Subacute thyroiditis

Factitious hyperthyroidism

Ectopic thyroid tissue (struma ovarii)

Chorionic gonadotropin-induced (choriocarcinoma, hydatidiform mole)

TSH-secreting pituitary adenoma

TSH, thyroid-stimulating hormone.

In **toxic multinodular goiter** (**MNG**), areas of autonomous function (i.e., not regulated by TSH) develop within a MNG and produce excess thyroid hormone. Patients are usually elderly and have a longstanding MNG. **Thyroid adenomas** occasionally cause hyperthyroidism. Thyroid carcinomas produce hormone very inefficiently and almost never cause hyperthyroidism, so a thyroid nodule in a hyperthyroid patient is almost certainly benign.

Certain forms of **thyroiditis** disrupt follicles, release stored hormone, and cause transient hyperthyroidism (lasting from a few weeks to a few months), often followed by a similar period of hypothyroidism. **Subacute thyroiditis** is a granulomatous inflammation that causes a painful, tender goiter. **Painless thyroiditis** is a form of lymphocytic thyroiditis that may cause hyperthyroidism, especially in the postpartum period (i.e., the first few months after delivery). Patients often have a small diffuse nontender goiter, and may be suspected of having Graves' disease. Although some authors refer to Hashimoto's thyroiditis as a rare cause of hyperthyroidism, these patients likely have coexisting Graves' disease.

Iodine-induced hyperthyroidism (jod-Basedow phenomenon; German for iodine plus German eponym for Graves' disease) usually occurs in patients with euthyroid goiters after large doses of iodine (e.g., **x-ray contrast medium** or **amiodarone**). Presumably, areas of autonomous function in these glands produce excess thyroid hormone only when high iodine levels permit. After iodine exposure ends, hyperthyroidism gradually resolves. Amiodarone also produces direct toxic effects on the thyroid.

Factitious use of thyroid hormone is usually for the purpose of weight loss. Recently, hyperthyroidism due to thyroid hormone-containing "nutritional supplements" has been reported.

Very high levels of chorionic gonadotropin (which weakly cross-reacts with the TSH receptor) secreted by trophoblastic tumors can cause hyperthyroidism.

PRESENTATION

Symptoms include heat intolerance and weight loss (due to increased metabolic rate), weakness, palpitations, oligomenorrhea, and anxiety (Table 8-2). Signs include brisk tendon reflexes, fine tremor, proximal weakness, stare, and eyelid lag. Cardiac abnormalities may be prominent,

TABLE 8-2	MANIFESTATIONS OF HYPERTHYROIDISM

Symptoms

Heat intolerance, increased sweating

Weight loss (often with increased appetite)

Anxiety, irritability

Palpitations

Oligomenorrhea

Increased stool frequency

Dyspnea

Fatigue, weakness

Signs

Brisk reflexes, fine tremor

Lid lag, stare

Sinus tachycardia

Atrial fibrillation

Warm, moist skin

Palmar erythema, onycholysis

Hair loss

Muscle weakness and wasting

Exacerbation of heart failure or coronary artery disease

Periodic paralysis (primarily in Asian men)

including sinus tachycardia, atrial fibrillation, and exacerbation of coronary artery disease or heart failure. **In the elderly**, hyperthyroidism may present with only atrial fibrillation, heart failure, weakness, or weight loss, and a high index of suspicion is needed to make the diagnosis.

Graves' disease may cause additional findings that are not due to hyperthyroidism (Table 8-3). Symptoms of ophthalmopathy include increased lacrimation, foreign body sensation, conjunctival redness, and periorbital edema. Fibrosis of extraocular muscles can

TABLE 8-3	MANIFESTATIONS OF GRAVES' DISEASE

Diffuse goiter

Ophthalmopathy

    Retrobulbar pressure or pain

    Periorbital edema, scleral injection

    Exophthalmos (proptosis)

    Extraocular muscle dysfunction

    Exposure keratitis

    Optic neuropathy (rare)

Pretibial myxedema (localized dermopathy)

cause diplopia. Rarely proptosis threatens vision by corneal exposure (due to incomplete lid closure) or compression of the optic nerve.

Diagnosis

Hyperthyroidism should be suspected in any patient with compatible symptoms, as it is a readily treatable disorder that may become very debilitating.

Plasma TSH is the best initial diagnostic test, as a TSH level >0.1 μU/mL excludes clinical hyperthyroidism. If plasma TSH is <0.1 μU/mL, plasma free thyroxine (T_4) should be measured to determine the severity of hyperthyroidism and as a baseline for therapy. If plasma free T_4 is elevated, the diagnosis of clinical hyperthyroidism is established.

If plasma TSH is <0.1 μU/mL but free T_4 is normal, the patient may have clinical hyperthyroidism due to elevation of plasma triiodothyronine (T_3) alone (T3 toxicosis); plasma T_3 should be measured in this case. TSH may also be suppressed by severe nonthyroidal illness (see Chapter 6). A third-generation TSH assay with a detection limit of 0.02 μU/mL may be helpful in patients with suppressed TSH and nonthyroidal illness. Most patients with clinical hyperthyroidism have plasma TSH levels that are <0.02 μU/mL in such assays, whereas nonthyroidal illness rarely suppresses TSH to this degree. Finally, mild (or subclinical) hyperthyroidism may lower TSH to <0.1 μU/mL and, therefore, suppression of TSH alone does not confirm that symptoms are caused by hyperthyroidism.

Thyroid imaging with ultrasound or radionuclide scan is not useful in diagnosing hyperthyroidism.

Differential Diagnosis

The cause of hyperthyroidism should be determined, since this affects the choice of therapy (Table 8-4). Differential diagnosis is based on:

- Palpation of the thyroid. Almost all hyperthyroid patients with a diffuse nontender goiter have Graves' disease, but this is also rarely due to postpartum or painless thyroiditis. Patients without palpable thyroid enlargement almost always have Graves' disease, but the possibility of factitious hyperthyroidism should be considered if there is no goiter. The diagnosis of toxic MNG or hyperthyroidism due to a thyroid adenoma is made by palpating multiple nodules or a single nodule. A painful, tender thyroid indicates subacute thyroiditis.
- The presence of proptosis or pretibial myxedema, which indicate Graves' disease (although many patients with Graves' disease lack these signs).
- Recent pregnancy, neck pain, or iodine administration, which suggest other causes.

TABLE 8-4	DIFFERENTIAL DIAGNOSIS OF HYPERTHYROIDISM
Type of Goiter	**Diagnosis**
Diffuse, nontender goiter	Graves' disease or painless thyroiditis
Multiple thyroid nodules	Toxic multinodular goiter
Single thyroid nodule	Thyroid adenoma
Tender painful goiter	Subacute thyroiditis
Normal thyroid gland	Graves' disease, painless thyroiditis, or factitious hyperthyroidism

TABLE 8-5	DIFFERENTIAL DIAGNOSIS OF HYPERTHYROIDISM BASED ON RAIU

Increased RAIU	Decreased RAIU
Graves disease	Subacute thyroiditis
Toxic multinodular goiter	Painless thyroiditis
Thyroid adenoma	Iodine-induced hyperthyroidism
	Factitious hyperthyroidism

RAIU, radioactive iodine uptake.

Most cases are due to Graves' disease or toxic MNG, and the diagnosis is usually obvious from the clinical findings and palpation of the thyroid. In a few patients with a diffuse goiter or with no thyroid enlargement, **24-hour radioactive iodine uptake (RAIU**, Table 8-5) is needed to distinguish Graves' disease (in which RAIU is elevated), from diseases in which RAIU is low.

MANAGEMENT

Some forms of hyperthyroidism (subacute or postpartum thyroiditis) are transient and require only symptomatic therapy. Three methods are available for definitive therapy (none of which controls hyperthyroidism rapidly): RAI, thionamides, and subtotal thyroidectomy. **During treatment, patients are followed by clinical evaluation and measurement of plasma free** T_4. Plasma TSH is useless in assessing the initial response to therapy, as it remains suppressed until after the patient becomes euthyroid. Regardless of the therapy used, all patients with Graves' disease require lifelong follow-up for recurrent hyperthyroidism or development of hypothyroidism.

Symptom Relief

A **β-adrenergic antagonist** (such as **atenolol** 25–100 mg daily) is used to relieve symptoms such as palpitations, tremor, and anxiety, until hyperthyroidism is controlled by definitive therapy, or until transient forms of hyperthyroidism subside. The dose is adjusted to alleviate symptoms and tachycardia, and then reduced gradually as hyperthyroidism is controlled. Verapamil at an initial dose of 40 to 80 mg PO tid can be used to control tachycardia in patients with contraindications to β-adrenergic antagonists.

Choice of Definitive Therapy

In Graves' disease, RAI therapy is the treatment of choice for almost all patients. It is simple and highly effective, but it **cannot be used during pregnancy or lactation. Propylthiouracil (PTU) should be used to treat hyperthyroidism in pregnancy.** Long-term control of Graves' disease with thionamides is achieved in less than one half of patients, and these drugs carry a small risk of life-threatening side effects. Thyroidectomy should be used in patients who refuse RAI therapy and who relapse or develop side effects with thionamide therapy.

Other Causes of Hyperthyroidism

Toxic MNG and toxic adenoma should be treated with RAI (except in pregnancy). Transient forms of hyperthyroidism caused by thyroiditis should be treated symptomatically with atenolol. Iodine-induced hyperthyroidism is treated with thionamides and atenolol until the patient is euthyroid. Although treatment of some patients with **amiodarone-induced hyperthyroidism** with glucocorticoids has been advocated, **nearly all patients with amiodarone-induced hyperthyroidism respond well to thionamide therapy.**

RAI Therapy

A single dose of iodine-131 permanently controls hyperthyroidism in about 90% of patients, and further doses can be given if necessary. A **pregnancy test** is done immediately before therapy in potentially fertile women. A 24-hour RAIU is usually measured and used to calculate the dose. Thionamides interfere with RAI therapy and should be discontinued 3 to 7 days before treatment. If iodine therapy has been given, it should be discontinued at least 2 weeks before RAI therapy. Most patients with Graves' disease are treated with 8 to 10 mCi; treatment of toxic MNG requires higher doses.

Follow-up

Usually several months are needed to restore euthyroidism. Patients are evaluated at 4- to 6-week intervals, with assessment of clinical findings and plasma free T_4. **If thyroid function stabilizes within the normal range**, the interval between follow-up visits is increased gradually to annual intervals. **If symptomatic hypothyroidism develops**, thyroxine therapy is started. Mild hypothyroidism after RAI therapy may be transient, and asymptomatic patients can be observed for an additional 4 to 6 weeks to determine whether hypothyroidism will resolve spontaneously. **If symptomatic hyperthyroidism persists after 6 months, RAI treatment is repeated.**

Side Effects

Hypothyroidism occurs in more than half of patients within the first year and continues to develop at a rate of approximately 3% per year thereafter. Because of the release of stored hormone, a slight rise in plasma T_4 may occur in the first 2 weeks after therapy. This development is important only in **patients with severe cardiac disease**, which may worsen as a result. Such patients should be treated with thionamides to restore euthyroidism and to deplete stored hormone before treatment with RAI. No convincing evidence has been found that RAI has a clinically important effect on the course of Graves' eye disease. It does not increase the risk of malignancy. No increase in congenital abnormalities has been found in the offspring of women who conceive after RAI therapy, and the radiation exposure to the ovaries is low, comparable to that from common diagnostic radiographs. Unwarranted concern for potential teratogenic effects should not influence physicians' advice to patients.

Thionamides

Methimazole and PTU inhibit thyroid hormone synthesis by thyroid peroxidase. PTU also inhibits extrathyroidal conversion of T_4 to T_3 by type 1 deiodinase. Once thyroid hormone stores are depleted (after several weeks to months), T_4 levels decrease. These drugs have no permanent effect on thyroid function. **In the majority of patients with Graves' disease, hyperthyroidism recurs within 6 months after therapy is discontinued.** Spontaneous remission of Graves' disease occurs in approximately one-third of patients during thionamide therapy, and in this minority, no other treatment may be needed. Remission is more likely in mild hyperthyroidism of recent onset, and if the goiter is small.

Initiation of Therapy

Before starting therapy, patients must be warned of side effects and precautions. Usual starting doses are PTU, 100 to 200 mg PO tid, or methimazole, 10 to 40 mg PO daily; higher initial doses can be used in severe hyperthyroidism.

Follow-up

Restoration of euthyroidism takes up to several months. Patients are evaluated at 4-week intervals with assessment of clinical findings and plasma free T_4. If plasma free T_4 levels do not fall after 4 to 8 weeks, the dose should be increased. Doses for PTU and methimazole, respectively, as high as 300 mg PO qid, or methimazole, 60 mg daily, may be required.

Once the plasma free T_4 level falls to normal, the dose is adjusted to maintain plasma free T_4 within the normal range. There is no consensus on the optimal duration of therapy, but periods of 6 months to 2 years are most common. Patients must be monitored carefully for recurrence of hyperthyroidism after the drug is stopped.

Side effects are most likely to occur within the first few months of therapy. Minor side effects include rash, urticaria, fever, arthralgias, and transient leukopenia. **Agranulocytosis** occurs in about 0.3% of patients treated with thionamides. Other life-threatening side effects include **hepatitis**, vasculitis, and drug-induced lupus erythematosus. These complications usually resolve if the drug is stopped promptly. **Patients must be warned to discontinue the drug immediately if jaundice or symptoms suggestive of agranulocytosis develop (e.g., fever, chills, sore throat)** and to contact their physician promptly for evaluation. Routine monitoring of the white blood cell (WBC) count is not useful for detecting agranulocytosis, which develops suddenly.

Subtotal Thyroidectomy

This procedure provides long-term control of hyperthyroidism in most patients. Surgery may trigger a perioperative exacerbation of hyperthyroidism, and patients should be prepared for surgery by one of two methods:

- **A thionamide** is given until the patient is nearly euthyroid. **Supersaturated potassium iodide (SSKI),** 40 to 80 mg (1–2 drops) PO bid, is then added 1 to 2 weeks before surgery. Both drugs are stopped postoperatively.
- **Atenolol** (50–100 mg daily) is started 1 to 2 weeks before surgery. The dose of atenolol is increased, if necessary, to reduce the resting heart rate below 90 beats/minute and is continued for 5 to 7 days postoperatively. SSKI is dosed as indicated previously.

Follow-up

Clinical findings and plasma free T_4 and TSH should be assessed 4 to 6 weeks after surgery. If thyroid function is normal, the patient is seen at 3 and 6 months, and then annually. If symptomatic hypothyroidism develops, thyroxine therapy is started. Mild hypothyroidism after subtotal thyroidectomy may be transient, and asymptomatic patients can be observed for an additional 4 to 6 weeks to determine whether hypothyroidism will resolve spontaneously. Hyperthyroidism persists or recurs in 3% to 7% of patients.

Complications of thyroidectomy include **hypothyroidism** in 30% to 50% of patients and **hypoparathyroidism** in 3%. Rare complications include permanent vocal cord paralysis, resulting from recurrent laryngeal nerve injury, and perioperative death. The complication rate appears to depend on the experience of the surgeon.

SPECIAL TOPICS

Mild (or subclinical) hyperthyroidism is diagnosed when the plasma TSH is suppressed to <0.1 μU/mL, but the patient has no symptoms that are definitely caused by hyperthyroidism, and plasma levels of free T_4 and T_3 are normal. Because subclinical hyperthyroidism increases the risk of **atrial fibrillation** in the **elderly** and those with **heart disease**; and predisposes to **osteoporosis** in **postmenopausal women**, it should be treated in these patients. Asymptomatic young patients with mild Graves' disease can be observed at semi-annual intervals for spontaneous resolution of hyperthyroidism, or the development of symptoms and increasing free T_4 levels that warrant treatment.

Urgent therapy is warranted when hyperthyroidism exacerbates heart failure or coronary artery disease and in rare patients with severe hyperthyroidism complicated by fever and delirium (thyroid storm). Concomitant diseases should be treated intensively, and confirmatory tests should be obtained before therapy is started, including serum TSH and free T_4.

- **PTU, 300 mg PO q6h,** should be started immediately.
- **Iodide (SSKI, 1–2 drops PO q12h)** should be started approximately 2 hours after the first dose of PTU, to inhibit thyroid hormone secretion rapidly.
- **Propranolol,** 40 mg PO q6h (or an equivalent dose of a parenteral β-antagonist), should be given to patients with angina or myocardial infarction, and the dose should be adjusted to control tachycardia. Propranolol may benefit some patients with heart failure and marked tachycardia but can further impair left ventricular systolic function. In patients with clinical heart failure, propranolol should be given only with careful monitoring of left ventricular function.
- Plasma free T_4 is measured every 3 to 7 days, and the doses of PTU and iodine are gradually decreased when free T_4 approaches the normal range. RAI therapy should be scheduled 2 weeks after iodine is discontinued.

Hyperthyroidism in Pregnancy

Hyperthyroidism increases the risk of miscarriage, preeclampsia, premature labor, and low birth weight, so it must be controlled. If hyperthyroidism is suspected, plasma TSH should be measured. Plasma TSH declines in early pregnancy owing to the thyroid-stimulating effects of human chorionic gonadotropin (hCG), but rarely to <0.1 μU/mL. If TSH is <0.1 μU/mL, the diagnosis should be confirmed by measurement of plasma free T_4. RAI therapy is contraindicated in pregnancy, and these patients should be treated with PTU. The dose should be adjusted at 4-week intervals to maintain the plasma free T_4 near the upper limit of the normal range. The dose required often decreases in the later stages of pregnancy. It is important to avoid overtreatment, since PTU crosses the placenta and can cause fetal hypothyroidism. Atenolol, 25 to 50 mg PO daily, can be used to relieve symptoms while awaiting the effects of PTU.

TSIs also cross the placenta and can cause fetal or neonatal hyperthyroidism. In pregnant women who have previously been treated with RAI or thyroidectomy and are no longer hyperthyroid, measurement of plasma TSI in the third trimester helps assess the risk of neonatal hyperthyroidism. Newborns should be monitored carefully for hyperthyroidism. Women treated with PTU may safely breast-feed.

Treatment of Graves' Ophthalmopathy

Mild or moderate ophthalmopathy often resolves spontaneously and may require no treatment. Symptoms of conjunctival irritation respond to lubricant eye drops (e.g., Refresh eye drops) and ointment at bedtime (e.g., Refresh PM), which also protect against exposure keratitis. More severe ophthalmopathy, with the risk of visual loss, should be treated with glucocorticoids in consultation with an experienced ophthalmologist.

KEY POINTS TO REMEMBER

- Graves' disease is the most common cause of hyperthyroidism.
- Proptosis and pretibial myxedema are seen only in Graves' disease.
- RAI is the preferred treatment for most forms of hyperthyroidism, except in pregnancy; close monitoring for hypothyroidism is required and some patients require retreatment.
- Thioamides may also be used for treatment of hyperthyroidism, but carry the risk of life-threatening side effects; they are the treatment of choice for amiodarone-induced hyperthyroidism.
- Propylthiouracil (PTU) is the drug of choice in pregnancy complicated by Graves' disease and is dosed to maintain free T_4 levels close to upper limit of normal.
- Mild or subclinical hyperthyroidism in the elderly increases the risk of atrial fibrillation and osteoporosis and should be treated.

REFERENCES AND SUGGESTED READINGS

Clutter WE. Endocrine disorders. In: Cooper DH, Krainik AJ, Lubner SJ, et al., eds. *Washington Manual of Medical Therapeutics*, 32nd ed. Philadelphia: Lippincott Williams & Wilkins; 2007.

Cooper DS. Antithyroid drugs. *N Engl J Med* 2005;352:905–917.

Cooper DS. Hyperthyroidism. *Lancet* 2003;362:459–468.

LeBeau SO, Mandel SJ. Thyroid disorders during pregnancy. *Endocrinol Metab Clin North Am* 2006;35:117–136.

Nayuk B, Burman K. Thyrotoxicosis and thyroid storm. *Endocrinol Metab Clin North Am* 2006;35:663–686.

Osman F, Franklyn JA, Sheppard MC, et al. Successful treatment of amiodarone-induced thyrotoxicosis. *Circulation* 2002;105:1275–1277.

Peearc EN, Farwell AP, Braverman LE. Thyroiditis. *N Engl J Med* 2003;348:2646–2655.

Toft AD. Subclinical hyperthyroidism. *N Engl J Med* 2001;345:512–516.

Weetman AP. Radioiodine treatment for benign thyroid diseases. *Clin Endocrinol* 2007; 66:757–764.

Hypothyroidism

William E. Clutter

9

INTRODUCTION

Hypothyroidism is the syndrome caused by thyroid hormone deficiency. It is common, especially in women, with a prevalence of about 2% (compared with 0.1% for men). The prevalence of subclinical hypothyroidism is about 7.5% in women and 3% in men, and increases with age. Congenital hypothyroidism is one of the most common congenital defects (about 1 in 5000 births).

CAUSES

Primary hypothyroidism (resulting from disease of the thyroid itself) accounts for more than 95% of cases (Table 9-1). **Chronic lymphocytic thyroiditis (Hashimoto's disease)** is by far the most common cause. It is an autoimmune disorder in which the thyroid is damaged by cell-mediated immunity. **Iatrogenic hypothyroidism** due to thyroidectomy or radioactive iodine (RAI, iodine-131) therapy is also common. **Transient hypothyroidism** occurs in painless (or postpartum) thyroiditis and subacute thyroiditis, usually after a period of hyperthyroidism. **Drugs that may cause hypothyroidism** (usually in patients with underlying autoimmune thyroiditis) include iodine-containing drugs such as **amiodarone**, lithium, interferon-α and interferon-β, interleukin-2, thalidomide, bexarotene, and sunitinib. Thionamide drugs used to treat hyperthyroidism can cause hypothyroidism if the dose is excessive.

Secondary hypothyroidism due to thyroid-stimulating hormone (TSH) deficiency is uncommon but may occur in any disorder of the pituitary or hypothalamus, including surgery, trauma, or radiation to the area. However, it rarely occurs without other evidence of pituitary disease.

Rare hemangiomas that express thyroid hormone deiodinase type 3 (which converts thyroxine [T_4] to inactive reverse triiodothyronine [rT_3]) have been reported to cause hypothyroidism, a syndrome called **consumptive hypothyroidism.**

Thyroid hormone resistance caused by mutations in the thyroid hormone receptor-beta gene usually does not cause symptoms of hypothyroidism, since increased levels of thyroid hormone compensate for defective responsiveness.

Pathophysiology

Hashimoto's thyroiditis (chronic lymphocytic thyroiditis) is much more common in women, and increases in prevalence with age. The disease gradually impairs the thyroid's ability to produce hormone, prompting a compensatory rise in TSH secretion. This additional stimulus maintains normal thyroid hormone levels for a time (a state called **subclinical hypothyroidism**). In many of these patients, hormone production eventually falls despite high TSH

TABLE 9-1	CAUSES OF HYPOTHYROIDISM

Primary hypothyroidism
    Chronic lymphocytic (Hashimoto's) thyroiditis
    Radioactive iodine treatment or external neck radiation
    Thyroidectomy
    Transient (during recovery from painless thyroiditis or subacute thyroiditis)
    Drugs
    Severe iodine deficiency (not seen in the United States)
    Congenital hypothyroidism (thyroid dysgenesis or genetic defects in thyroid
      hormone synthesis)
Secondary (central) hypothyroidism
    Any pituitary or hypothalamic disease
Other
    Consumptive hypothyroidism due to vascular tumors expressing deiodinase

levels, and frank clinical hypothyroidism develops. Patients usually have antithyroid antibodies (**antithyroid peroxidase** and **antithyroglobulin**), but cellular immunity is more important in thyroid destruction. They may have autoimmune disease of other endocrine glands (such as Addison's disease), and often have a family history of either Hashimoto's or Graves' disease. There is lymphocytic infiltration of the thyroid, fibrosis, and variable degrees of follicular destruction. Depending on the extent of follicular damage and lymphocytic infiltration, it causes an **atrophic, impalpable thyroid** or a **firm, nontender diffuse goiter**. (Hashimoto's disease is also the most common cause of euthyroid goiter in the United States.)

Iatrogenic hypothyroidism is a common complication of treatment for hyperthyroidism. After radioactive iodine therapy, it may occur quickly, or not until years later. Hypothyroidism always follows the complete or near-complete **thyroidectomy** done for thyroid cancer, and may occur after subtotal thyroidectomy for hyperthyroidism.

Most cases of **congenital hypothyroidism** are caused by dysplasia or aplasia of the thyroid, with little or no detectable thyroid tissue. Rarely, genetic defects of hormone synthetic enzymes, or maternal treatment with antithyroid drugs or iodine cause congenital hypothyroidism with a goiter.

Drug-induced hypothyroidism can occur during treatment of Graves' disease with **thionamides**. Occasionally **iodine excess** or **lithium** (which inhibit thyroid hormone secretion) cause hypothyroidism, usually in patients with underlying autoimmune thyroiditis. Most cases of hypothyroidism are permanent, but **self-limited forms of thyroiditis** (painless lymphocytic thyroiditis and subacute thyroiditis) cause transient hypothyroidism, usually after a period of hyperthyroidism. Painless thyroiditis is most common in the postpartum period. In **secondary hypothyroidism** there are usually other pituitary hormone deficiencies, and since TSH is not elevated, there is no goiter.

PRESENTATION

Hypothyroidism causes a variety of symptoms, many of which are nonspecific (Table 9-2). It usually develops gradually, and the onset of symptoms is insidious. The most specific findings are **cold intolerance** (feeling cold when others are comfortable) and **delayed relaxation of tendon reflexes**. Patients may or may not have a goiter. Other symptoms include

TABLE 9-2	SYMPTOMS AND SIGNS OF HYPOTHYROIDISM
Symptoms	**Signs**
Cold intolerance	Delayed tendon reflex relaxation
Lethargy, fatigue	Facial and periorbital puffiness
Weight gain (modest)	Bradycardia
Dry skin, hair loss	Poor memory, dementia
Constipation	Nonpitting edema (myxedema)
Myalgias, arthralgias	Pleural and pericardial effusions
Menorrhagia	Carpal tunnel syndrome
Hoarseness	Deafness
	Hypoventilation
	Hypothermia

mild weight gain (due to decreased metabolic rate), fatigue, somnolence, poor memory, constipation, menorrhagia and impaired fertility, myalgias, and hoarseness. Other signs include bradycardia, facial and periorbital edema, dry skin, and nonpitting edema (myxedema) that results from accumulation of glycosaminoglycans in interstitial spaces. **Hypothyroidism does not cause marked obesity.** Rare manifestations include hypoventilation, hypothermia, pericardial or pleural effusions, deafness, and carpal tunnel syndrome.

Laboratory findings may include **hyponatremia** and elevated plasma levels of cholesterol, triglycerides, and creatine kinase. Primary hypothyroidism may cause hyperprolactinemia. The electrocardiogram (ECG) may show low voltage and T-wave abnormalities.

MANAGEMENT

Diagnosis

Hypothyroidism is common, readily treatable, and should be suspected in any patient with compatible symptoms, especially in the presence of a diffuse goiter or a history of RAI therapy or thyroid surgery.

In suspected primary hypothyroidism, plasma TSH is the best initial diagnostic test. A normal value excludes primary hypothyroidism, and a markedly elevated value (>20 μU/mL) confirms the diagnosis. It is seldom necessary to measure thyroid autoantibodies, since Hashimoto's thyroiditis accounts for almost all spontaneous hypothyroidism.

Mild elevation of plasma TSH (<20 μU/mL) may be caused by **nonthyroidal illness,** but usually indicates **mild (or subclinical) primary hypothyroidism,** in which thyroid function is impaired but increased secretion of TSH maintains plasma free T_4 levels within the reference range. These patients may have nonspecific symptoms compatible with hypothyroidism and a mild increase in serum cholesterol and low-density-lipoprotein (LDL) cholesterol. They develop clinical hypothyroidism at a rate of about 2.5% per year. In patients with mildly elevated plasma TSH, the test should be repeated with measurement of plasma free T_4 to confirm the diagnosis.

If secondary hypothyroidism is suspected because of evidence of pituitary disease (e.g., a known sella turcica or hypothalamic mass, or a history of pituitary surgery, radiation, or trauma), **plasma free T_4 should be measured.** A low value is diagnostic of secondary hypothyroidism in this setting. **Plasma TSH levels are usually within the**

reference range in secondary hypothyroidism and cannot be used alone to make this diagnosis. Patients with secondary hypothyroidism should be evaluated for other pituitary hormone deficits and the pituitary should be imaged with magnetic resonance imaging (MRI).

Treatment

Levothyroxine is the drug of choice. The average replacement dose is 1.6 mcg/kg PO daily, and most patients require doses between 75 and 150 mcg daily. In elderly patients, the average replacement dose is lower. The need for lifelong treatment should be emphasized. Levothyroxine should be taken 30 minutes before a meal, since dietary fiber and soy products interfere with its absorption. It should not be taken together with **medications that inhibit its absorption** including **calcium carbonate, ferrous sulfate,** cholestyramine, sucralfate, and aluminum hydroxide. **Other drug interactions that increase thyroxine clearance and dose requirement** include estrogen, rifampin, some anticonvulsants (carbamazepine, phenytoin, and phenobarbital) and some anticancer drugs (imatinib and bexarotene). Newer anticonvulsants have not been reported to cause this interaction. **Amiodarone** blocks conversion of T_4 to T_3, and also increases levothyroxine dose requirements.

Initiation of Therapy

Young, otherwise healthy adults should be started on 75 to 100 mcg daily. This regimen gradually corrects hypothyroidism, since thyroxine has a half-life of 7 days, and several weeks are required to reach steady-state plasma levels of T_4. Symptoms begin to improve within a few weeks. In otherwise healthy **elderly patients,** the initial dose should be 50 mcg daily. Patients with **cardiac disease** should be started on 25 to 50 mcg daily and monitored carefully for exacerbation of cardiac symptoms.

Dose Adjustment and Follow-Up

In primary hypothyroidism, the goal of therapy is to maintain plasma TSH within the normal range. Plasma TSH should be measured 6 to 8 weeks after initiation of therapy. The dose of levothyroxine should be adjusted in 12 to 25-mcg increments at intervals of 6 to 8 weeks until plasma TSH level is normal. Thereafter, annual TSH measurement is adequate to monitor therapy. TSH should also be measured frequently in the **first trimester of pregnancy,** since the thyroxine dose requirement increases at this time (see below).

In secondary hypothyroidism, plasma TSH cannot be used to adjust therapy. The goal of therapy is to **maintain the plasma free T_4 near the middle of the reference range.** The dose of levothyroxine should be adjusted at 6- to 8-week intervals until this goal is achieved. Thereafter, annual measurement of plasma free T_4 is adequate to monitor therapy.

Side Effects of Levothyroxine Therapy

Overtreatment produces **iatrogenic hyperthyroidism,** indicated by a subnormal TSH level, and should be avoided since it increases the risk of **osteoporosis** and **atrial fibrillation. Coronary artery disease** may be exacerbated by treatment of hypothyroidism. The dose of levothyroxine should be increased slowly, with careful attention to worsening angina, heart failure, or arrhythmias. In patients with concomitant **adrenal failure,** correction of hypothyroidism may exacerbate the symptoms and signs of adrenal failure. In patients with **pituitary disease** and secondary hypothyroidism, the pituitary–adrenal axis should be assessed and treatment of secondary adrenal failure started before treatment of hypothyroidism.

SPECIAL TOPICS

Mild (or Subclinical) Hypothyroidism

Patients with mild hypothyroidism should be treated with levothyroxine if any of the following are present: (a) **symptoms compatible with hypothyroidism**, (b) a **goiter**, (c) **hypercholesterolemia** that warrants treatment, (d) **pregnancy**, or (e) the **plasma TSH is >10 μU/mL**. Untreated patients should be monitored annually, and levothyroxine should be started if symptoms develop or serum TSH increases to >10 μU/mL.

Pregnancy

Thyroxine dose increases by an average of 50% in the first half of pregnancy owing to accelerated conversion of T_4 to reverse T_3 by placental deiodinase type 3. In women with primary hypothyroidism, **plasma TSH level should be measured as soon as pregnancy is confirmed and monthly thereafter through the second trimester**. The levothyroxine dose should be increased as needed to maintain plasma TSH level within the normal range. After delivery, the prepregnancy dose should be resumed.

Problems with Treatment

Treatment of most cases of hypothyroidism is simple and straightforward. Occasionally, it is difficult to achieve a levothyroxine dose that normalizes TSH level, or a dose that was adequate no longer maintains a normal TSH level. Common explanations for this include:

- **Poor or erratic medication compliance.** Directly observed therapy at weekly intervals may be necessary in some cases.
- **Drug interactions** (see Treatment in this chapter).
- **Pregnancy**, in which the dose requirement increases in the first trimester.
- **Gradual failure of remaining endogenous thyroid function** after RAI treatment of hyperthyroidism.

Diagnosis of Hypothyroidism in Severely Ill Patients

In severe nonthyroidal illness, the diagnosis of hypothyroidism may be difficult (see Chapter 6). Plasma total T_4 and free T_4 measured by routine assays may be low. **Plasma TSH is the best initial diagnostic test. A normal TSH value is strong evidence that the patient is euthyroid**, except when there is evidence of pituitary or hypothalamic disease or in patients treated with **dopamine** or high doses of **glucocorticoids**. **Marked elevation of plasma TSH (>20 μU/mL) establishes the diagnosis of primary hypothyroidism.**

Moderate elevations of plasma TSH (<20 μU/mL) may occur in euthyroid patients with nonthyroidal illness and are not specific for hypothyroidism. Plasma free T_4 should be measured if TSH is moderately elevated, or if secondary hypothyroidism is suspected, and patients should be treated for hypothyroidism if plasma free T_4 is low. Thyroid function in these patients should be reevaluated after recovery from illness.

Emergent Therapy

Emergent therapy for hypothyroidism is rarely necessary. Most patients with hypothyroidism and concomitant illness can be treated in the usual manner. However, hypothyroidism may impair survival in critical illness by contributing to **hypoventilation, hypotension, hypothermia, bradycardia, or hyponatremia.** Little evidence supports the contention that severe hypothyroidism alone causes coma or shock; most reports of **myxedema coma** predate recognition that nonthyroidal illness itself lowers thyroid hormone levels (see Diagnosis of Hypothyroidism in Severely Ill Patients in this chapter).

Hypoventilation and hypotension should be treated intensively, along with any concomitant diseases. Confirmatory tests (plasma TSH and free T_4) should be obtained before thyroid hormone therapy is started in a severely ill patient.

Levothyroxine, 50 to 100 mcg IV, can be given q6 to 8h for 24 hours, followed by 75 to 100 mcg IV daily until oral intake is possible. Replacement therapy should be continued in the usual manner if the diagnosis of hypothyroidism is confirmed. No clinical trials have determined the optimum method of thyroid hormone replacement, but this method rapidly alleviates thyroxine deficiency while minimizing the risk of exacerbating underlying coronary disease or heart failure. Such rapid correction is warranted only in extremely ill patients. Vital signs and cardiac rhythm should be monitored carefully to detect early signs of exacerbation of heart disease. Hydrocortisone, 50 mg IV q8h, is usually recommended during rapid replacement of thyroid hormone, because such therapy may precipitate adrenal crisis in patients with adrenal failure.

Hypothyroidism and Surgery

Urgent surgery can be performed on untreated hypothyroid patients without an increased risk of major adverse events. Elective surgery should be deferred until euthyroidism is achieved. Hypothyroid patients undergoing surgery can have their levothyroxine dose held for several days until they are able to eat (owing to the 7-day half-life of the drug). However, IV replacement should be considered if oral intake is delayed by more than 1 week after surgery. The IV replacement dose is approximately 80% of the oral dose.

THYROIDITIS

Autoimmune or Hashimoto's Thyroiditis

(See the section Pathophysiology in this chapter)

Painless Thyroiditis

Painless thyroiditis (also known as postpartum or silent thyroiditis) is an autoimmune disorder that is most common in the first 6 months of the postpartum period. The incidence is believed to be approximately 10% in the United States. It is characterized by a small, nontender diffuse goiter, and transient hyperthyroidism followed by hypothyroidism, although only one phase may be recognized clinically. Hypothyroidism is usually transient, but may be permanent. Hyperthyroidism results from follicular damage and release of stored hormone by a lymphocytic infiltrate. Consequently, **radioactive iodine uptake (RAIU) is very low.** Antithyroid peroxidase antibodies may be present.

The diagnosis should be suspected in women with symptoms of hyperthyroidism or hypothyroidism within 6 months of delivery. Plasma TSH and free T_4 should be measured to confirm the functional state. The hyperthyroid phase can be distinguished from Graves' disease by (a) the absence of proptosis (which is seen only in Graves' disease), (b) measurement of RAIU (if the patient is not nursing), and (c) repeating thyroid function tests after several weeks to assess for spontaneous improvement. Symptoms of hyperthyroidism should be treated with a β-**adrenergic antagonist.** Thionamides are not useful, since thyroid hormone synthesis is already suppressed. Symptomatic hypothyroidism is treated with replacement therapy with levothyroxine for 2 to 3 months followed by discontinuation for 4 to 6 weeks and measurement of plasma TSH level. Women with a history of postpartum thyroiditis have a higher risk of developing hypothyroidism in later life.

Subacute Thyroiditis

Subacute thyroiditis (also known as de Quervain's or granulomatous thyroiditis) is characterized by a painful, tender goiter and transient hyperthyroidism resulting from release of stored thyroid hormone, followed by transient hypothyroidism. It is the most common cause of thyroid pain. It frequently occurs after an upper respiratory tract infection and is thought to have a viral etiology. Symptoms of hyperthyroidism occur in ~50% of patients and can be treated with a β-adrenergic antagonist. Pain should be treated with nonsteroidal anti-inflammatory drugs (NSAIDs); corticosteroid treatment may be needed in severe cases. Thionamides or RAI are not useful. Transient hypothyroidism may be treated with levothyroxine for 3 to 6 months.

Acute Infectious Thyroiditis

Infection of the thyroid by bacteria, fungi, mycobacteria, or parasites is rare. It may occur in immunosuppressed, elderly, or debilitated patients, or in patients with underlying thyroid disease. Patients are acutely ill, with fever, chills, dysphagia, anterior neck pain, and swelling. The thyroid is tender. Patients are usually biochemically euthyroid. Diagnosis is made by fine-needle aspiration, with Gram's staining and culture of the aspirate. Antibiotics and drainage of abscess are the mainstays of treatment.

Reidel's Thyroiditis

Reidel's thyroiditis is a very rare fibrosing thyroiditis that may be part of a systemic fibrosing process. Patients present with a painless, hard, fixed goiter. Patients are initially euthyroid, but hypothyroidism eventually develops. Treatment is primarily surgical, although therapy with glucocorticoids and methotrexate may be tried early in the course of the disease.

KEY POINTS TO REMEMBER

- Hashimoto's thyroiditis is the most common cause of hypothyroidism in the United States.
- A normal plasma TSH concentration rules out primary hypothyroidism.
- Secondary hypothyroidism is diagnosed by measurement of plasma free T_4, not TSH
- The levothyroxine dose should be adjusted at 6–8 week intervals, based on plasma TSH in primary hypothyroidism and plasma free T_4 in secondary hypothyroidism.
- Worsening of symptoms of coronary disease may occur during levothyroxine therapy for hypothyroidism.
- The levothyroxine dose requirement increases during the first trimester of pregnancy.
- Painless thyroiditis may cause hyperthyroidism or hypothyroidism in the postpartum period.
- Nonthyroidal illness can change thyroid function tests and make diagnosis of hypothyroidism difficult.

REFERENCES AND SUGGESTED READINGS

Abalovich M, Amino N, Barbour LA, et al. Management of thyroid dysfunction during pregnancy and postpartum: an Endocrine Society Clinical Practice Guideline. *J Clin Endocrinol Metab* 2007;92[Suppl]:S1–S47.

Adler SM, Wartofsky L. The nonthyroidal illness syndrome. *Endocrinol Metab Clin North Am* 2007;36:657–672.

Alexander EK, Marqusee E, Lawrence J, et al. Timing and magnitude of increases in levothyroxine requirements during pregnancy in women with hypothyroidism. *N Engl J Med* 2004;351:241–249.

Pearce EN, Farwell AP, Braverman LE. Thyroiditis. *N Engl J Med* 2003;348:2646–2655.

Roberts CG, Ladenson PW. Hypothyroidism. *Lancet* 2004;363:793–803.

Surks MI, Ortiz E, Daniels GH, et al. Subclinical thyroid disease. Scientific review and guidelines for diagnosis and management. *JAMA* 2004;291:228–238.

Adrenal Incidentaloma

Shaili K. Felton

INTRODUCTION

Adrenal incidentalomas are masses found incidentally during radiographic imaging of the abdomen. By definition, patients do not present for evaluation of signs or symptoms of adrenal disease. Ready access to and use of high-resolution radiographic imaging for evaluation of nonspecific symptoms has led to increasing discovery of adrenal incidentalomas. Using computed tomography (CT) scanning, the prevalence of adrenal incidentalomas in the general population is ~3%, and increases with age.

In evaluating such a mass, the major concerns to address are:

- Is the mass benign or malignant?
- Does the mass secrete hormones, or is the mass nonfunctioning?

CAUSES

In one of the largest databases to date with 786 adrenal incidentalomas, the National Italian Study Group has confirmed that the most common finding (89%) on evaluation with hormone testing is a nonfunctioning mass (cortical adenoma, myelolipoma, cyst, ganglioneuroma, or other). Evaluation of the remaining masses revealed subclinical Cushing's syndrome (6.2%), pheochromocytoma (3.4%), aldosterone-secreting adenoma (0.89%), and a single virilizing tumor. Of note, most of the adrenocortical carcinomas found in this series were non–hormone secreting. Table 10-1 lists several common diagnoses associated with adrenal incidentalomas.

PRESENTATION

Although, by definition, patients with incidentalomas do not present with clinical evidence of hormone excess, a thorough history and physical examination for any signs and symptoms of hormonal dysfunction should be completed. Special effort should be made to elicit any subtle signs or symptoms suggestive of specific hormonal hyperfunction or malignancy. This inquiry should include investigation for Cushing's syndrome (weight gain, moon facies, supraclavicular fat pads, thinned skin, easy bruising, or proximal muscle weakness), pheochromocytoma (hypertension, paroxysms of pain, palpitations, perspiration, and/or pallor), aldosterone-secreting adenoma (hypertension or hypokalemia), and malignancy (weight loss, primary nonadrenal cancers, lymphoma, and virilizing signs or symptoms suggestive of adrenocortical carcinoma). A known history of malignancy makes metastasis to the adrenal gland more likely.

TABLE 10-1	DIFFERENTIAL DIAGNOSIS OF ADRENAL INCIDENTALOMA

Benign
  Nonhormone secreting
    Nonfunctioning adenoma
    Lipoma/myelolipoma
    Cyst
    Ganglioneuroma
    Hematoma
    Infection (tuberculosis, fungal)
  Hormone secreting
    Pheochromocytoma
    Aldosterone-secreting adenoma
    Subclinical Cushing's syndrome
Malignant
  Adrenocortical carcinoma
  Metastatic neoplasm
  Lymphoma
  Malignant pheochromocytoma

MANAGEMENT

Biochemical Testing

Biochemical testing should assess possible hormone secretion by the adrenal mass. Appropriate studies include:

- Serum potassium and plasma aldosterone concentration/plasma renin activity ratio (PAC/PRA) to address aldosterone excess
- Plasma metanephrines or 24-hour urine metanephrines and/or catecholamines to rule out subclinical pheochromocytoma
- A 1-mg dexamethasone suppression test to rule out subclinical Cushing's syndrome
- A dehydroepiandrosterone sulfate (DHEA-S) level should be determined if virilizing signs or symptoms are present

Any positive results on these screening tests should prompt further evaluation. Please refer to chapters on Conn's syndrome (Chapter 13), Cushing's syndrome (Chapter 14), and Pheochromocytoma (Chapter 15) for more detailed discussions of these tests and their interpretation.

Radiologic Assessment

The probability of an adrenal mass being malignant **directly correlates with its size.** Tumor diameters ranging from 3 to 6 cm have been proposed as cutoffs that should lead to surgical resection. A Mayo Clinic retrospective analysis of 342 adrenal masses removed over a 5-year period revealed that all adrenocortical carcinomas were ≥4 cm in diameter. In a larger retrospective series from Italy, a 4-cm cutoff was 93% sensitive for adrenocortical carcinoma, but 76% of lesions >4 cm were benign.

CT scan may be useful in establishing whether an adrenal mass is benign or malignant. A homogeneous adrenal mass <4 cm with smooth borders and an attenuation value <10 Hounsfield units strongly suggests a benign lesion. Diagnostic criteria are not as clear for lesions measuring 4 to 6 cm, but if they are hormonally inactive and have a benign appearance on CT scan, such lesions can be monitored. Lesions >6 cm, regardless of appearance on CT scan, are more likely to be malignant, and surgical referral is warranted. Magnetic resonance imaging (**MRI**) appears to be as effective as CT scanning in distinguishing benign and malignant masses, with benign adenomas exhibiting signal drop on chemical shift imaging with intensity similar to that of T2-weighted images of the liver. Pheochromocytomas generally exhibit hyperintensity on T2-weighted imaging. Again, lesions >6 cm in diameter by MRI are more likely to be malignant, even if they have a benign appearance on MRI, and should prompt surgical referral.

Fine-Needle Aspiration and Tissue Biopsy

Generally, a thorough history and physical examination, biochemical testing, and radiologic assessment are sufficient for clinical decision making in cases of adrenal incidentaloma. Biopsy of the adrenal mass is generally not advised, as it is rarely helpful. The major exception is a patient with a known extraadrenal primary malignancy. In this case, biopsy may help distinguish recurrence and metastasis of cancer from a benign adenoma. However, biopsy should be done only if pheochromocytoma has been ruled out by biochemical testing, as biopsy of a pheochromocytoma can precipitate a hypertensive emergency.

Treatment

At the completion of the clinical, biochemical, and radiologic evaluation described previously, any mass that suggests primary adrenocortical malignancy by size or radiologic characteristics warrants **surgical removal,** as long as the patient is a good surgical candidate. If, however, the evaluation suggests that the mass is a metastasis or a primary nonadrenal cancer, such as lymphoma, generally no surgical removal is needed, but rather treatment of the primary cancer. Adrenal function is unlikely to be hindered by tumor invasion, because more than 70% to 80% of the gland function must be interrupted to pose any risk for adrenal crisis.

Hypersecreting adrenal incidentalomas found to be **pheochromocytomas** or **aldosterone-secreting adenomas** should be considered for surgical removal as well, on the basis of criteria for their respective diagnoses. Resection of a pheochromocytoma requires preoperative α-adrenergic blockade and volume expansion with oral salt or IV saline. However, surgical treatment for subclinical Cushing's syndrome remains controversial.

Prior to surgical excision of an adrenal mass, it is important to determine whether there is excessive cortisol secretion. The diagnoses of a hormonally hypersecreting adrenal mass and adrenocortical carcinoma are not mutually exclusive. It is common for adrenocortical carcinomas to release excessive cortisol. If there is any suspicion of excessive cortisol secretion, one should be aware of the possibility of **adrenal crisis** during or after the surgery. It has been reported several times in the literature that even mild cortisol hypersecretion of one adrenal gland may atrophy the contralateral adrenal gland. When the hyperfunctioning adrenal gland is removed, the atrophied gland may not be able to compensate in the setting of postsurgical recovery. These patients should be covered with stress-dose steroids during surgery and receive a corticotropin stimulation test after surgery to diagnose any resulting adrenal insufficiency. Patients who fail postoperative testing may require months of glucocorticoid replacement before recovery of the hypothalamic-pituitary–adrenal axis. Thus, even if the size of the mass warrants its removal, the patient should still undergo a complete biochemical workup to rule out subclinical Cushing's syndrome or pheochromocytoma.

FOLLOW-UP

If the history, physical examination, and hormonal and radiologic evaluations are not suggestive of either a primary adrenal carcinoma or a hypersecreting adenoma, then it is reasonable to conclude that the incidentaloma is benign, but follow-up is necessary. Schedules for follow-up by repeat radiologic imaging and biochemical analyses remain controversial. Most of these schedules recommend repeat imaging at 3 months and again during the following year. A significant increase in the size of the mass (e.g., >1 cm) should raise the possibility of malignancy and lead to surgical referral. Patients should also be evaluated annually with a thorough history and physical examination for development of overt signs of hypersecretion or malignancy. Many practitioners continue to follow adrenal incidentalomas with radiographic imaging every few years. As the data to support such a practice are limited, its utility remains controversial.

KEY POINTS TO REMEMBER

- Size is important. Adrenal masses >4 cm in diameter are more likely to be malignant, and surgical resection should be considered. Adrenal masses >6 cm should be resected owing to the unacceptably high risk of malignancy, even if the radiologic appearance is otherwise benign.
- The great majority (~89%) of adrenal incidentalomas are nonfunctioning masses.
- A full biochemical workup should be completed before any surgery is undertaken. Findings suggestive of pheochromocytoma warrant preoperative α-blockade as described in Chapter 15. Testing suggestive of Cushing's syndrome or subclinical Cushing's syndrome warrants perioperative stress-dose steroid coverage and postoperative corticotropin stimulation testing.

REFERENCES AND SUGGESTED READINGS

Boland GW, Lee MJ, Gazelle GS, et al. Characterization of adrenal masses using unenhanced CT: an analysis of the CT literature. *AJR Am J Roentgenol* 1998;171:201–204.

Bülow B, Ahrén B. Adrenal incidentaloma—experience of a standardized diagnostic programme in the Swedish prospective study. *J Intern Med* 2002;252:239–246.

Dunnick NR, Korobkin M. Imaging of adrenal incidentalomas: current status. *AJR Am J Roentgenol* 2002;179:559–568.

Grumbach MM, Biller BMK, Braunstein GD, et al. Management of the clinically inapparent adrenal mass ("incidentaloma"). *Ann Intern Med* 2003;138:424–429.

Herrera MF, Grant CS, van Heerden JA, et al. Incidentally discovered adrenal tumors: an institutional perspective. *Surgery* 1991;110:1014–1021.

Kloos RT, Gross MD, Francis IR, et al. Incidentally discovered adrenal masses. *Endocrine Rev* 1995;16(4): 460–484.

Mantero F, Masini AM, Opocher G, et al. Adrenal incidentaloma: an overview of hormonal data from the national Italian study group. *Horm Res* 1997;47:284–289.

Mantero F, Terzolo M, Arnoldi G, et al. A survey on adrenal incidentaloma in Italy. *J Clin Endocrinol Metab* 2000; 85:637–644.

McLeod MK, Thompson NW, Gross MD, et al. Sub-clinical Cushing's syndrome in patients with adrenal gland incidentalomas: pitfalls in diagnosis and management. *Am Surg* 1990;56:398–403.

Young WF. Management approaches to adrenal incidentalomas: a view from Rochester, Minnesota. *Endocrinol Metab Clin North Am* 2000;29:159–185.

Young WF. The incidentally discovered adrenal mass. *N Engl J Med* 2007;356:601–610.

Adrenal Insufficiency

Manu V. Chakravarthy

11

INTRODUCTION

The adrenal axis is a complex balance of hormones from the hypothalamus, pituitary, and adrenal glands. A defect in any one of these locations can lead to hypofunction of the adrenals. In 1855, Thomas Addison first described his eponymous syndrome, which was characterized by wasting and hyperpigmentation, and identified its cause as destruction of the adrenal gland. Primary adrenal insufficiency (Addison's disease) corresponds to dysfunction at the level of the adrenal gland from any cause. Secondary adrenal insufficiency refers to loss of adrenocorticotropic hormone (ACTH) from the pituitary. Tertiary adrenal insufficiency refers to loss of corticotropin-releasing hormone (CRH) from the hypothalamus.

Depending on the series, the estimated prevalence of chronic primary adrenal insufficiency is 60 to 120 per million in Caucasian populations, with a peak age of diagnosis in the fourth decade of life. Secondary adrenal insufficiency has an estimated prevalence of 150 to 280 per million with a peak age of diagnois in the sixth decade of life. Both conditions are more prevalent in women than in men.

CAUSES

The causes of adrenal insufficiency can be broadly grouped as primary (adrenal) and central (pituitary and hypothalamus)—see Table 11-1. When Thomas Addison described his initial case in 1855, the most common etiology was tuberculosis infiltration of the adrenal glands. Over the years, autoimmune destruction of the adrenal gland (**autoimmune adrenalitis**) has emerged as the leading cause of primary adrenal insufficiency in the United States, although tuberculosis remains a major factor in the developing world. Autoimmune adrenalitis can be isolated or can occur as part of an autoimmune polyglandular syndrome (APS, types I and II) (see Chapter 35).

Other etiologies to consider for primary adrenal insufficiency include disseminated fungal infections, human immunodeficiency virus (HIV)-related opportunistic infections [most commonly cytomegalovirus (CMV)], bilateral adrenal hemorrhage associated with coagulopathies or sepsis, metastatic cancer involving more than 80% to 90% of the total adrenal mass, and X-linked adrenoleukodystrophy (the most common cause in children). Some medications can also potentially precipitate symptomatic adrenal insufficiency in a person with limited adrenal reserve. For example, rifampin and phenytoin increase cortisol metabolism, whereas ketoconazole, aminoglutethimide, etomidate, and suramin decrease cortisol secretion by inhibiting cortisol biosynthesis.

Secondary adrenal insufficiency results when the pituitary is involved, affecting ACTH secretion (Table 11-1). Decreased ACTH stimulation of the adrenal glands results

TABLE 11-1   CAUSES OF ADRENAL INSUFFICIENCY

Primary (Adrenal)

Autoimmune (70%–90%)
  Isolated adrenal insufficiency
    (associated with HLA-DR3)
  Polyglandular autoimmune syndrome
    type I (mutation in the *AIRE* gene)
  Polyglandular autoimmune syndrome
    type II (associated with HLA-DR3)

Infectious and infiltrative
  Tuberculosis (7%–20%)
  Disseminated pseudomonas,
    histoplasmosis
  HIV and its opportunistic infections
    (CMV, *Mycobacterium avium* complex
    *Cryptococcus, Pneumocystis
    carinii* pneumonia, toxoplasmosis)
  Syphilis
  Amyloidosis
  Sarcoidosis

Metastatic carcinoma
  Lung, breast, colon cancer, melanoma

Medications
  Rifampin, phenytoin, barbiturates,
    ketoconazole, etomidate

Adrenal hemorrhage/infarction
  Meningococcal sepsis with Waterhouse-
    Friderichsen syndrome
  Primary antiphospholipid syndrome
  Disseminated intravascular coagulopathy

Genetic disorders
  Adrenoleukodystrophy (mutation in the
    ABCD1 gene)
  Congenital adrenal hyperplasia
    (deficiencies in steroidogenic acute
    regulatory protein, 21-hydroxylase,
    11-β-hydroxylase, 3-β-hydroxyl-Δ-
    5-steroid dehydrogenase)
  Mutations in *DAX-1* and *SF-1*
    transcription factors
  Smith-Lemli-Opitz syndrome (*DHCR7*
    gene mutation)
  Kearns-Sayre syndrome (mitochondrial
    DNA deletions)
  Familial glucocorticoid deficiency-
    Allgrove's syndrome (*AAAS* gene
    mutation)

Central (Pituitary or hypothalamus)

Prolonged use of exogenous
  glucocorticoids

Pituitary/hypothalamic tumors
  Pituitary adenoma
  Craniopharyngioma
  Rathke's cleft cyst
  Pituitary stalk lesions

Infectious and infiltrative
  Tuberculosis
  Histoplasmosis
  Neurosarcoidosis
  Metastasis

Infarction, hemorrhage/apoplexy
  Sheehan's syndrome
  Large intracranial artery aneurysms

Head trauma

Lymphocytic hypophysitis

Genetic pituitary abnormalities from
  mutations in *PROP-1* and other
  pituitary transcription factors

Isolated ACTH deficiency

Familial cortisol-binding globulin
  deficiency

Abrupt withdrawal of megesterol (a
  progestin with some glucocorticoid
  activity)

ACTH, adrenocorticotropic hormone; CMV, cytomegalovirus.
Adapted from Oelkers W. Adrenal insufficiency. *N Engl J Med* 1996;335:1206–1212; Arlt W, Allolio B.
Adrenal insufficiency. *Lancet* 2003;361:1881–1893, with permission.

in adrenal atrophy over several weeks. If loss of pituitary ACTH secretion is caused by a pituitary mass, then deficiencies of other pituitary hormones are usually present. Isolated ACTH deficiency is rare. Tertiary adrenal insufficiency is caused by processes that affect the hypothalamus and that interfere with CRH secretion, such as craniopharyngioma, sarcoidosis, or cranial radiation. The most common cause of tertiary adrenal insufficiency is suppression of the hypothalamic–pituitary-adrenal (HPA) axis by high-dose exogenous glucocorticoids. Those at highest risk of developing adrenal insufficiency from exogenous glucocorticoid use are patients who have received more than 10 mg of prednisone daily, especially if doses are taken at night. Megastrol acetate (Megace) can suppress the HPA axis to cause adrenal insufficiency; affected patients need to be supported with exogenous glucocorticoids until the axis recovers following discontinuation of megastrol acetate.

PRESENTATION

The clinical presentation of adrenal insufficiency can be variable and is dependent on the level of the hypothalamic–pituitary-adrenal axis that is affected, as well as the rate and extent of loss of adrenal function. Patients may remain undiagnosed for quite some time until a significant physical stressor precipitates an adrenal crisis—an endocrine emergency.

Acute Adrenal Insufficiency

Acute adrenal insufficiency (adrenal crisis) most often occurs in patients with primary adrenal insufficiency (rarer in patients with secondary adrenal insufficiency, unless there is pituitary apoplexy) and is precipitated by acute stress (surgery, infection, or bilateral adrenal hemorrhage). It is characterized by shock including severe volume depletion and hypotension that is out of proportion to the severity of the current illness. Other presenting features may include nausea and vomiting with a history of weight loss and anorexia, abdominal pain ("acute abdomen" if the etiology is acute adrenal infarction or hemorrhage), fatigue, fever, confusion or coma, electrolyte abnormalities (especially hyperkalemia), and eosinophilia. Although many of these symptoms are nonspecific, it is critical to recognize the clinical syndrome because acute adrenal crisis is an endocrine emergency that requires prompt treatment.

Chronic Primary Adrenal Insufficiency

Chronic primary adrenal insufficiency is more insidious in its onset. A significant illness can transform latent chronic primary adrenal insufficiency into a life-threatening adrenal crisis. Hence, early recognition and diagnosis is essential, even though in its early stage the diagnosis may be difficult given the nonspecific nature of the presenting symptoms (chronic malaise, fatigue, generalized weakness, myalgias, nausea, vomiting, anorexia, abdominal pain, and weight loss). Destruction of the adrenal gland generally leads to the loss of all adrenal hormones, including cortisol and aldosterone. The resulting lack of feedback inhibition on the pituitary by cortisol leads to increased ACTH secretion. This series of defects leads to the distinguishing findings in primary adrenal insufficiency—generalized hyperpigmentation of the skin and mucosa (increased ACTH levels stimulate the melanocortin receptor to upregulate melanin synthesis), renal salt wasting with resultant salt craving, hyponatremia and hyperkalemia, as well as volume depletion and hypotension (which are largely a manifestation of decreased aldosterone levels).

Furthermore, as autoimmune disease is the most common etiology of primary adrenal insufficiency in the United States, it is common for patients with autoimmune adrenalitis to have evidence of other autoimmune diseases such as hypo- or hyperthyroidism, type 1 diabetes, or vitiligo (see Chapter 35). Patients with longstanding adrenal insufficiency can also manifest psychiatric symptoms, ranging from impairment in memory to depression and psychosis.

Central Adrenal Insufficiency

In secondary and tertiary adrenal insufficiency, patients have inadequate pituitary ACTH and hypothalamic CRH secretion, respectively. This defect rarely occurs in isolation and is usually associated with other pituitary hormone losses especially that of growth hormone deficiency, which is typically present in more one third of the patients with isolated ACTH deficiency. Patients with pituitary ACTH deficiency may present with many of the same symptoms as primary adrenal insufficiency, including general malaise, fatigue, myalgias, arthralgias, and weight loss. In addition, because of the loss of other pituitary hormones, patients may experience amenorrhea, decreased libido, or cold intolerance. Mass effects (headaches or visual field defects) from a pituitary or hypothalamic tumor may also be present.

Patients with secondary or tertiary adrenal insufficiency, in contrast to those with primary adrenal insufficiency, do not manifest hyperpigmentation, because their ACTH is not elevated. Patients with a central defect also have less prominent volume depletion and hypotension, because the renin–angiotensin-aldosterone system is usually intact. Secretion of aldosterone is normal, and consequently they are not hyperkalemic. Hyponatremia or hypoglycemia may be present.

MANAGEMENT

Diagnosis

Given the subtle and sometimes vague symptoms of chronic adrenal insufficiency, its diagnosis is often difficult and depends on a high index of clinical suspicion for the disease that is further corroborated by biochemical evidence. **Treatment should be started immediately before the diagnosis is fully established in any patient suspected to be in adrenal crisis.**

A multistep approach is needed to document whether there is inadequate cortisol secretion by the adrenals and whether the cause of adrenal insufficiency is lack of ACTH. Once adrenal insufficiency is documented, a primary cause should be sought and treated as appropriate.

Documentation of Inadequate Cortisol Secretion

Inappropriately low cortisol production is the *sine qua non* finding in the diagnosis of adrenal insufficiency of any cause. Because peak cortisol values are present normally between 4 AM and 8 AM, basal early morning cortisol values <3 mcg/dL suggest a diagnosis of adrenal insufficiency. However, given the lower sensitivity (~36%) of early morning cortisol measurements, this test cannot be used exclusively to rule out adrenal insufficiency. Random serum cortisol levels at other times of the day are also not informative unless they are in the high-normal range, which would be consistent with an intact HPA axis. It is for these reasons that the **cosyntropin stimulation test** has become the most widely used dynamic test to assess adrenal function. Serum cortisol levels >18 mcg/dL (500 nmol/L) to 20 mcg/dL (550 nmol/L) obtained 30 or 60 minutes after IV or IM injection of 250 mcg cosyntropin, a synthetic ACTH, excludes primary adrenal insufficiency and most cases of secondary adrenal insufficiency. Although a subnormal response (<18 mcg/dL) confirms adrenal insufficiency, its type and cause require further studies. Most steroid replacements (e.g., cortisone, hydrocortisone, and prednisone) interfere with the radioimmunoassay for serum cortisol; therefore, patients already receiving such replacement should have their dose delayed on the day of testing until after the cosyntropin stimulation test. If the clinical situation permits, it may be useful to hold the glucocorticoid dosing on the day before the scheduled test or at least to reduce the dose to the lowest tolerated.

More recently, the low-dose cosyntropin stimulation test (using 1 mcg) has been suggested as a more sensitive and specific test. It is performed in the same manner with the same cutoff criteria as the standard-dose (250 mcg) test. Head-to-head comparison of the standard-dose and low-dose tests showed only minor improvements in sensitivity (at 95% specificity, the sensitivity of the low-dose test was 61% compared to 57% in the standard-dose test). Cosyntropin is available only in 250 mcg vials, making a dilution to 1 mcg less convenient and potentially fraught with errors. In short, the appropriate dose of cosyntropin for the accurate diagnosis of adrenal insufficiency remains controversial.

It is important to note that the cosyntropin stimulation test may be normal if administered in recent-onset secondary adrenal insufficiency, as it takes several weeks for the adrenals to atrophy after acute disruption of ACTH secretion (e.g., after pituitary injury). Furthermore, chronic partial secondary adrenal insufficiency may not be detected by the cosyntropin stimulation test. Therefore, in such settings, neither the standard-dose nor the low-dose cosyntropin stimulation test accurately diagnoses the condition given their similar receiver-operating characteristic curves. Instead, an insulin tolerance test (ITT) or metyrapone stimulation test may be needed and is reliable in these patients (see subsequent text).

If **adrenal crisis** is suspected, intravenous saline and dexamethasone, 4 mg IV q6h, should be started until the cosyntropin stimulation test can be performed. If the clinical situation permits, both cortisol and ACTH levels should be obtained before initiating therapy. In this acute setting, dexamethasone is the preferred glucocorticoid, because it does not cross-react with the cortisol in the assay and permits subsequent testing.

Inappropriately low cortisol levels can also be seen during **critical illness** (septic shock) with a structurally normal HPA axis ("relative" adrenal insufficiency). Because critical illness can raise basal cortisol levels, a further increase in response to cosyntropin may not occur. Recent studies have suggested that critically ill patients with a basal cortisol level of <25 mcg/dL or an incremental response <9 mcg/dL after cosyntropin stimulation have poorer outcomes and benefit from glucocorticoid treatment. Nevertheless, these data need to be interpreted in the context that severely ill patients also have decreased cortisol binding proteins. In light of these issues, there is currently no consensus regarding the precise diagnostic criteria in critical care settings.

Screening with the cosyntropin stimulation test for adrenal insufficiency **after pituitary surgery** should be done at least 4 to 6 weeks after the surgery, since adrenal atrophy develops only gradually after the onset of ACTH deficiency. Patients tested prior to the development of adrenal atrophy may have a false-negative test and be incorrectly presumed to have an intact HPA axis. Patients can be maintained on glucocorticoid replacement with the dose withheld for 24 hours before scheduled testing of adrenal function. Impairment of other hormonal axes after pituitary surgery increases the likelihood of ACTH deficiency, whereas isolated deficiency is uncommon.

Differentiating Primary versus Secondary Adrenal Insufficiency

The cosyntropin stimulation test is fast, accurate, and safe for diagnosing adrenal insufficiency, but it does not definitively differentiate between primary and secondary disease. An ACTH level obtained at the same time as a basal cortisol level can be helpful in this regard. A disproportionately elevated plasma ACTH level with a concurrently low serum cortisol suggests primary adrenal insufficiency. On the other hand, patients with secondary adrenal insufficiency have low serum cortisol with a low or low-normal plasma ACTH level. Accurate interpretation of the ACTH result depends on the reliability of the assay being performed, as well as on the assurance that no exogenous glucocorticoid treatment was given before ACTH determination (as this suppresses endogenous ACTH secretion).

As mentioned previously, other tests to differentiate primary from secondary adrenal insufficiency include the ITT and metyrapone stimulation test. Although the ITT has long been considered the gold standard, it is uncomfortable for the patient and requires close monitoring because the significant hypoglycemia resulting from the test is potentially dangerous. The ITT is contraindicated in patients with susceptibility to seizure, history of prior seizure, cerebrovascular disease, and cardiovascular disease.

Metyrapone is an inhibitor of the adrenal 11-β-hydroxylase and, therefore, blocks the final step in cortisol biosynthesis, resulting in hypocortisolemia, accumulation of serum 11-deoxycortisol, and consequent stimulation of ACTH secretion by feedback regulation. Because hypocortisolemia is not as strong a stimulus of ACTH secretion as is hypoglycemia, the metyrapone test is able to detect partial ACTH deficiency that may be missed by the standard-dose cosyntropin stimulation test or the ITT. However, its use is limited as metyrapone is not readily available and must be obtained by special arrangement from the pharmacist. In addition, the metyrapone stimulation test should not be performed in patients who have known severe cortisol deficiency, as metyrapone can precipitate an adrenal crisis.

Despite the various testing options available, no single test, including the ITT, classifies all patients accurately. Mild secondary adrenal insufficiency can yield normal tests results, and some healthy individuals might fail any single test by a small margin. Thus the diagnosis of adrenal insufficiency requires clinical judgment, and as more than one biochemical test is often needed, it is important to look for internal consistency among the various tests. The presence of persistent signs and symptoms, such as fatigue and orthostasis, should prompt repeat biochemical evaluation.

Determining the Cause of Adrenal Insufficiency

Identifying the cause of adrenal insufficiency is dependent on the level of the defect (primary vs. secondary vs. tertiary disease). Radiologic imaging should only be performed once laboratory diagnosis of adrenal insufficiency is made using one of the stimulation tests. The laboratory tests should identify whether the patient has primary or secondary adrenal insufficiency.

If the patient's clinical presentation is suggestive of autoimmune adrenalitis, radiologic evaluation is usually unnecessary. Autoimmune adrenalitis is diagnosed by measuring antibodies against 21-hydroxylase (CYP21A2), which are present in more than 80% of patients with recent onset of isolated autoimmune adrenalitis. However, autoantibodies against other steroidogenic enzymes and other endocrine cells are also present in some patients. Evaluation of other endocrine gland dysfunction associated with autoimmune adrenal insufficiency should be sought by measuring serum calcium, glucose, and TSH, and running tests of gonadal function.

In boys who have isolated primary adrenal insufficiency without neurologic symptoms, serum concentrations of very-long-chain fatty acids (>24 carbon chain length) should be measured to exclude adrenoleukodystrophy.

For patients with biochemical diagnosis of primary adrenal insufficiency, CT of the adrenal glands is helpful in identifying inflammation suggestive of infection, hemorrhage, or malignancy. In patients with laboratory evaluation suggestive of secondary adrenal insufficiency, a brain MRI with coned-down views of the pituitary is the method of choice to look for a space-occupying lesion in the pituitary or hypothalamus.

Treatment

Acute Treatment

Adrenal crisis is a life-threatening condition requiring immediate treatment. Therapy should not be delayed to perform diagnostic studies or await laboratory results. If there is no history suggestive of adrenal insufficiency, other causes of shock also need to be considered. Volume replacement using normal saline is essential to reverse hypotension and electrolyte abnormalities. While blood for serum cortisol, ACTH, and serum chemistry is drawn, "stress-dose" steroids should be started without delay. If the diagnosis is unclear, 4 mg IV dexamethasone (instead of hydrocortisone) should be given first, followed by cosyntropin stimulation testing. In patients with a clearly identified history of adrenal insufficiency, either dexamethasone or hydrocortisone (50–100 mg IV q6–8h) can be given until their condition has stabilized. In the acute setting, mineralocorticoid replacement is not useful, as it takes several days for its sodium-retaining effects to become apparent; intravenous saline alone will suffice. In adrenal crisis, any signs or symptoms should resolve quickly, generally over the following 1 to 2 hours. Once the stressor has been alleviated, steroid doses can be tapered over 1 to 3 days to an oral maintenance daily dose.

Maintenance Treatment
Maintenance therapy involves glucocorticoid replacement at physiologic levels. Many maintenance treatment regimens have been suggested. Chronic therapy for patients with either primary or secondary adrenal insufficiency requires glucocorticoid replacement with hydrocortisone 15 to 30 mg/day PO or its equivalent (prednisone 5.0–7.5 mg/day PO or dexamethasone 0.75–1.25 mg/day PO). The glucocorticoids can be administered in 1 to 3 divided doses. It is best to give a single dose in the morning to mimic the physiologic diurnal variation. If the patient thinks he or she could benefit from a split-dose regimen, usually the larger dose is given in the morning and the smaller dose later in the day. Treatment should be tailored (using the lowest dose possible) to the patient's symptoms so as to avoid fatigue, weight loss, hyponatremia, and, in primary adrenal insufficiency, hyperpigmentation. ACTH levels should not be used as a marker for glucocorticoid dose adjustment because the ACTH is not only invariably high in primary adrenal insufficiency, but also rapidly decreases after glucocorticoid ingestion. However, one should also avoid the complications of excess glucocorticoid replacement, such as weight gain, osteoporosis, and immune compromise. Patients with primary adrenal insufficiency should also receive mineralocorticoid replacement. Fludrocortisone is given at a dose of 0.05 to 0.2 mg PO daily, and is titrated to the patient's symptoms of orthostasis, normalization of potassium levels, and suppression of plasma renin activity to the middle to upper end of the normal range.

All patients with adrenal insufficiency should be given a medical-alert bracelet indicating the diagnosis of steroid dependence, and a physician's number to call. In addition, every patient should have with them pre-filled syringes of dexamethasone (4 mg/mL in saline solution); the patient and one or more responsible family or household members should be instructed on how to inject the dexamethasone in case of emergency (e.g., massive blood loss, inability to maintain oral intake, or presence of any of the symptoms of adrenal crisis). Instruction should also include the need to be brought to medical attention immediately after the injection.

Treatment for Specific Situations

- **Stress Dosing**. Patients and their families should be advised that development of febrile illness, upper respiratory infection, nausea, vomiting, or any other undue physical stress may warrant increases in their daily glucocorticoid requirements. In addition to aggressive hydration, the usual daily dose can initially be doubled and then doubled again if symptoms of adrenal insufficiency such as nausea, vomiting, or orthostasis persist. If at this point the patient's symptoms still do not resolve, an injectable dexamethasone kit can be prescribed for home use. If at any time there is uncertainty regarding the status or safety of the patient, the patient should be immediately brought to the nearest hospital for intravenous steroids. When the acute illness has resolved, patients may return to their usual daily replacement doses within 1 to 3 days.

- **Perioperative Dosing.** Determining the appropriate coverage for surgical procedures is dependent on the complexity and duration of the procedure. Patients on chronic glucocorticoid therapy or with a known diagnosis of adrenal insufficiency will likely require additional coverage during their procedure. For patients undergoing local anesthesia for <1 hour, the patient's usual daily dose should suffice. For surgery limited to the limbs involving general anesthesia, patients should continue their usual daily steroid dose preoperatively and then receive the dose again intravenously during the procedure. Patients undergoing surgery involving the thoracic or abdominal cavities should be given their baseline daily dose preoperatively and then receive the equivalent of hydrocortisone, 50 mg IV q6 to 8h during the procedure and for 2 to 3 days after surgery. The dose can be rapidly tapered to the patient's usual daily dose over the following 1 to 2 days. During the perioperative and postsurgical period, inadequate steroid coverage may be manifested by signs and symptoms of impending adrenal crisis such as hypotension, nausea, vomiting, or fever. If adrenal insufficiency is the cause of these signs and symptoms, they should resolve quickly once the patient is covered with adequate steroid doses.
- **Central adrenal insufficiency.** Because aldosterone secretion is not typically affected with secondary adrenal insufficiency, there is no need for mineralocorticoid replacement. However, other pituitary hormone deficiencies may need to be replaced.
- **Thyroid disease.** If a patient is concurrently diagnosed with both adrenal insufficiency and hypothyroidism, the patient must first receive adequate glucocorticoid replacement before initiating thyroid hormone therapy to avoid precipitating adrenal crisis. In patients with adrenal insufficiency and unresolved hyperthyroidism, glucocorticoid replacement should be doubled or tripled, since hyperthyroidism increases cortisol clearance.
- **Drug interactions.** Glucocorticoid dose may also need to be increased in patients taking drugs that accelerate hepatic steroid metabolism such as phenytoin, barbiturates, and rifampin.
- **Pregnancy.** Increased cortisol-binding globulin, antimineralocorticoid action of increased progesterone, and increased plasma renin activity are characteristic physiologic changes that occur in the later stages of pregnancy. Therefore, in the third trimester, glucocorticoid replacement doses may need to be doubled. Fludrocortisone is adjusted according to blood pressure and serum potassium level. During labor, adequate normal saline hydration and hydrocortisone 25 mg IV q6h should be administered. At the time of delivery, or if labor is prolonged, hydrocortisone should be administered intravenously in a dose of 100 mg q6h or as a continuous infusion. After delivery, the dose can be tapered rapidly to maintenance within 2 to 3 days.

Prognosis

Prior to the availability of glucocorticoids, nearly all patients with primary adrenal insufficiency died within a few years after diagnosis. Presently, the prognosis for patients with adrenal insufficiency depends mostly upon the underlying cause. For example, patients with autoimmune adrenalitis can expect a normal life-span and lifestyle, including participation in vigorous exercise programs, with adequate steroid replacement. On the other hand, prospective data indicate excess mortality in hypopituitarism, including secondary adrenal insufficiency, because of vascular and respiratory disease, as well as defects in other hormonal axes. The adverse effect of chronic secondary adrenal insufficiency on health-related quality of life is comparable to that of congestive heart failure.

KEY POINTS TO REMEMBER

- Symptoms and signs of adrenal insufficiency are nonspecific and variable, requiring a high degree of clinical suspicion for timely diagnosis.
- Autoimmune adrenalitis is the leading cause of primary adrenal insufficiency in the United States, although tuberculosis remains a major factor in the developing world.
- Prolonged use of exogenous glucocorticoids is the most common cause of secondary adrenal insufficiency, as chronic glucocorticoid use induces atrophy of pituitary corticotroph cells and decreases ACTH secretion.
- The cosyntropin stimulation test is the most widely used dynamic test to assess adrenal function. Obtain a baseline serum ACTH and cortisol. Obtain a second serum cortisol level precisely 30 minutes after administration of the 250 mcg of cosyntropin IV or IM. A level <18–20 mcg/dL is consistent with a diagnosis of adrenal insufficiency.
- If adrenal crisis is suspected, first treat the patient with 4 mg IV dexamethasone. The cosyntropin stimulation test can then be performed safely and properly without delay in treating the patient.
- Adrenally insufficient patients should be instructed in how to adjust glucocorticoid dosing during physically stressful illnesses or medical procedures.
- All patients with adrenal insufficiency should wear medical-alert bracelets or necklaces at all times.

REFERENCES AND SUGGESTED READINGS

Abdu TA, Elhadd TA, Neary R, et al. Comparison of the low dose short synacthen test (1 mcg), the conventional dose short synacthen test (250 mcg), and the insulin tolerance test for assessment of the hypothalamo-pituitary-adrenal axis in patients with pituitary disease. *J Clin Endocrinol Metab* 1999;84:838–843.

Arlt W, Allolio B. Adrenal insufficiency. *Lancet* 2003;361:1881–1893.

Axelrod L. Perioperative management of patients treated with glucocorticoids. *Endocrinol Metab Clin North Am* 2003;32:367–383.

Betterle C, Dalpra C, Mantero F, et al. Autoimmune adrenal insufficiency and autoimmune polyendocrine syndromes: autoantibodies, autoantigens and their applicability in diagnosis and disease prediction. *Endocr Rev* 2002;23:327–364.

Cooper MS, Stewart PM. Corticosteroid insufficiency in acutely ill patients. *N Engl J Med* 2003;348:727–734.

Coursin DB, Wood KE. Corticosteroid supplementation for adrenal insufficiency. *JAMA* 2002;287:236–240.

Dorin RI, Qualls CR, Crapo LM. Diagnosis of adrenal insufficiency. *Ann Intern Med* 2003;139:194–204.

Grinspoon SK, Biller BK. Laboratory assessment of adrenal insufficiency. *J Clin Endocrinol Metab* 1994;79:923–931.

Guttman PH. Addison's disease. *Arch Pathol* 1930;10:742–935.

Lamberts SW, Bruining HA, de Jong FH. Corticosteroid therapy in severe illness. *N Engl J Med* 1997;337: 1285–1292.

Laureti S, Vecchi L, Santeusanio F, et al. Is the prevalence of Addison's disease underestimated? *J Clin Endocrinol Metab* 1999;84:1762.

Mayo J, Collazos J, Martinez E, et al. Adrenal function in the human immunodeficiency virus-infected patient. *Arch Intern Med* 2002;162:1095–1098.

Minneci PC, Deans KJ, Banks SM, et al. Meta-analysis: the effect of steroids on survival and shock during sepsis depends on the dose. *Ann Intern Med.* 2004;141:47–56.

Nieman LK. Adrenal insufficiency. In: *UpToDate*, Rose, BD, ed. Waltham, MA: UpToDate; 2007.

Oelkers W. Adrenal insufficiency. *N Engl J Med* 1996;335:1206–1212.

Oelkers W. Hyponatremia and inappropriate secretion of vasopressin (antidiuretic hormone) in patients with hypopituitarism. *N Engl J Med* 1989;321:492–496.

Salem M, Tanish RE Jr, Bromberg J, et al. Perioperative glucocorticoid coverage. A reassessment 42 years after emergence of a problem. *Ann Surg* 1994;219:416–425.

Seidenwurm DJ, Elmer EB, Kaplan LM, et al. Metastases to the adrenal glands and the development of Addison's disease. *Cancer* 1984;43:552–557.

Thaler LM, Blevins LS. Adrenocorticotropin stimulation test in the evaluation of patients with suspected central adrenal insufficiency. *J Clin Endocrinol Metab* 1998;83: 2726–2729.

Zelissen PM, Bast EJ, Croughs RJ. Associated autoimmunity in Addison's disease. *J Autoimmun* 1995;8: 121–130.

Adult Congenital Adrenal Hyperplasia

12

Dominic N. Reeds

INTRODUCTION

Congenital adrenal hyperplasia (CAH) consists of a group of autosomal recessive genetic disorders characterized by functional abnormalities of adrenal steroid biosynthetic enzymes, leading to impaired cortisol biosynthesis. In response to low cortisol levels, there is a compensatory increase in serum adrenocorticotropic hormone (ACTH). These high ACTH levels induce hyperplastic changes of the dysfunctional adrenal tissue and increase production of virilizing steroids with little or no increase in cortisol production. Among the variety of genetic defects that result in CAH, only two result in virilization. Ninety-five percent of the cases result from **21-hydroxylase deficiency** and 5% are due to 11-hydroxylase deficiency. The incidence of classic 21-hydroxylase deficiency is thought to be 1 per 14,000 births. The majority of cases of classic CAH are discovered during childhood; however, better understanding of the genetics and pathophysiology of CAH has led to frequent discoveries of its milder, nonclassic forms during adulthood. The overall incidence of CAH is not known but appears to be 1% to 6% in adolescents and adults with hyperandrogenism. 11-Hydroxylase deficiency occurs in 1 per 100,000 births. Therapy for all forms of CAH consists of a balance between sufficient glucocorticoid replacement to suppress the overproduction of androgens and to prevent adrenal crises, while avoiding complications related to glucocorticoid excess. Discussion of CAH in this chapter is limited to 21-hydroxylase deficiency.

CAUSES

Deficient cortisol production is the key aberration in CAH, and mastery of the adrenal steroid biosynthesis pathway is essential to understanding the pathogenesis of the disease and the rationale behind treatment (Fig. 12-1).

Differing mutations occurring within the gene encoding 21-hydroxylase affect the severity and expression of the disease. Mutations associated with large reductions in enzyme activity result in severe deficiencies of aldosterone and cortisol; whereas, mutations associated with milder reductions result in less severe hormone abnormalities and a nonclassic course. Some patients with nonclassic CAH have one allele of the 21-hydroxylase gene with a "severe" mutation and one allele with a "mild" mutation. Thus, the severity of the phenotype in compound heterozygotes is determined by the less severe mutation. The reduction in cortisol levels stimulates ACTH release by the pituitary, in turn causing increased production of cortisol precursors, such as progesterone and 17-OH progesterone (17-OHP), which may be metabolized to androgen precursors (see Fig. 12-1).

Three-fourths of patients with classic CAH are "salt wasters," as they have no 21-hydroxylase activity and produce insufficient aldosterone to retain sodium. The remaining

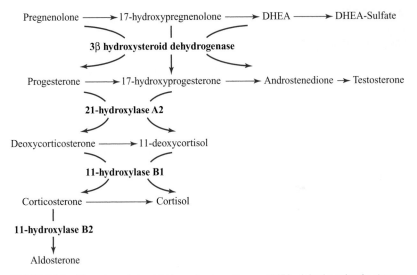

FIGURE 12-1. The adrenal steroid biosynthesis pathway. DHEA, dehydroepiandrosterone.

one-fourth of patients, who produce low but detectable enzyme activity, retain enough ability to produce aldosterone, and, although virilized, do not sodium waste, and so are known as "simple virilizers." Those who retain 20% to 60% of enzymatic activity typically present in adulthood with more subtle, nonclassic forms. All patients with classic 21-hydroxylase deficiency are at high risk for development of adrenal insufficiency without exogenous glucocorticoid administration, but acute adrenal crisis is uncommon in nonclassic forms.

PRESENTATION

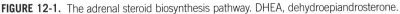

History

Classic 21-hydroxylase deficiency presents at or within several weeks of birth with hypotension as a result of adrenal insufficiency and virilization of female external genitalia (hypospadias, cryptorchidism, and clitoral enlargement) due to excess fetal adrenal androgens. The symptoms of nonclassic 21-hydroxylase deficiency may be subtle or even absent ("cryptic nonclassic CAH"). In women it may mimic polycystic ovary syndrome, with symptoms of cystic acne, hirsutism, infertility, and irregular menses. Male pattern hair loss is less frequently seen. Males with nonclassic CAH may experience infertility and acne. In children of both sexes, nonclassic CAH may be diagnosed during a work-up for premature pubarche or accelerated linear growth with advanced bone age.

The differential diagnosis for nonclassic CAH in adults is limited but includes polycystic ovarian syndrome, virilizing adrenal or ovarian tumors, and exogenous anabolic steroid use.

Physical Examination

Hyperandrogenic features dominate the physical examination, with temporal hair loss, hirsutism, and acne. Patients with classic CAH may have reduced height owing to androgen excess during puberty or from overreplacement of glucocorticoids, or both.

However, with more modern hormone replacement regimens, most patients attain their predicted adult height as adjusted for parental height. In nonclassic CAH, final adult height may be reduced owing to premature closure of epiphyses.

MANAGEMENT

Laboratory Diagnosis

Classic 21-hydroxylase deficiency is characterized by significantly elevated levels of 17-OHP in infancy, with varying degrees of virilization that may not become apparent until later in childhood. Nonclassic CAH may have borderline or normal 17-OHP. Ideally, 8 AM 17-OHP levels should be drawn in the follicular phase in women. A 17-OHP of <2 ng/mL makes CAH unlikely, and a value >4 ng/mL has been reported to have 100% specificity and 90% sensitivity. Values between 2 and 4 ng/mL require ACTH stimulation by administration of 250 mcg of synthetic ACTH IV and checking the plasma concentrations of 17-OHP before and 60 minutes after the drug is given; values may be compared with standard curves, which are easily obtainable. If the post-ACTH cortisol level is <20 mcg/dL, the patient should be made aware of the need to take additional glucocorticoids during times of physiologic stress. It should be noted that there are no reports of death from adrenal insufficiency as a result of nonclassic CAH in the medical literature. First-generation family members of affected patients should be screened for CAH because of the potential absence of clinical signs and potential harm that may result if a patient does not receive therapy.

Treatment

Treatment of adults with nonclassic 21-hydroxylase deficiency consists of administering the lowest dose of glucocorticoid replacement to suppress excess androgen production. **Dexamethasone** (Decadron) given in the evening is often considered to be the most effective treatment in adults, although there is an increased risk of overtreatment. Hydrocortisone is the preferred treatment in children because of improved clinical outcomes with respect to final adult height. Typical glucocorticoid replacement doses are 0.25–0.75 mg PO daily of dexamethasone or 10 to 25 mg/m^2 PO daily of hydrocortisone in two or three divided doses. Nocturnal dosing of hydrocortisone appears to be most effective in suppressing ACTH. Final adult height may be improved in children with advanced bone age, predicted to be at least one standard deviation below midparental target height, with the use of growth hormone and luteinizing hormone releasing hormone agonists (leuprolide). Adults with classic, salt-wasting CAH require glucocorticoid AND mineralocorticoid replacement. Generally, as little as 0.1 mg of fludrocortisone is sufficient.

 Monitoring the effects of steroid replacement is crucial. 17-OHP levels are relatively resistant to suppression by glucocorticoids, and, thus, a normal 17-OHP level often represents overtreatment. 17-OHP levels should be maintained at the upper end of normal to mildly supranormal levels. Androstenedione levels are more sensitive to suppression and may be a better indicator of replacement dosing, with a goal of keeping the androstenedione levels in the upper one-third of normal range. Mineralocorticoid replacement may be monitored by following potassium levels. Elevated renin levels or hypotension may signify insufficient mineralocorticoid replacement.

 Adrenal crisis in patients with CAH is managed with glucocorticoid replacement and volume repletion as described in Chapter 11.

 Pregnancy in classic CAH should be managed by an endocrinologist experienced in this area. Women with nonclassic CAH generally do not require glucocorticoid therapy during pregnancy unless prenatal evaluation suggests there is increased risk for a virilized female fetus (such as when the mother is a compound heterozygote for a severe mutation and the father is a heterozygous carrier). Discussion of prenatal counseling, diagnosis, and treatment of CAH is beyond the scope of this chapter, and the reader is referred to a recent review by Nimkarn and New (see full reference in References).

KEY POINTS TO REMEMBER

- Classic CAH typically presents at birth, however symptoms of nonclassic CAH may occur much later in life.
- It may be necessary to determine ACTH-stimulated 17-OH progesterone levels in patients with equivocal 17-OH progesterone levels and symptoms suggestive of nonclassic CAH.
- The lowest possible effective dose of steroids should be used to minimize the adverse effects of glucocorticoids on bone density.
- Pregnant patients with CAH should be followed by an experienced endocrinologist.

REFERENCES AND SUGGESTED READINGS

Augarten A, Weissenberg R, Parienta C, et al. Reversible male infertility in late onset congenital adrenal hyperplasia. *J Endocrinol Invest* 1991;14:237–240.

Bode HH, Rivkees SA, Cowley DM, et al. Home monitoring of 17 hydroxyprogesterone levels in congenital adrenal hyperplasia with filter paper blood samples. *J Pediatr* 1999;134:185–189.

Carroll MC, Campbell RD, Porter RR. Mapping of steroid 21-hydroxylase genes adjacent to complement component C4 genes in HLA, the major histocompatibility complex in man. *Proc Natl Acad Sci USA* 1985;82:521–525.

Culter GB, Laue L. Congenital adrenal hyperplasia due to 21-hydroxylase deficiency. *N Engl J Med* 1990;323:1806–1813.

Dewailly D. Nonclassic 21-hydroxylase deficiency. *Semin Reprod Med* 2002;20:243–248.

Horrocks PM, London DR. A comparison of three glucocorticoid suppressive regimes in adults with congenital adrenal hyperplasia. *Clin Endocrinol* 1982;17:547–556.

Horrocks PM, London DR. Effects of long term dexamethasone treatment in adult patients with congenital adrenal hyperplasia. *Clin Endocrinol* 1987;27:635–642.

Hughes IA. Management of congenital adrenal hyperplasia. *Arch Dis Child* 1988;63: 1399–1404.

Kohn B, Levine LS, Pollack MS, et al. Late-onset steroid 21-hydroxylase deficiency: a variant of classical congenital adrenal hyperplasia. *J Clin Endocrinol Metab* 1982; 55:817–827.

Levine LS, Dupont B, Lorenzen F, et al. Genetic and hormonal characterization of cryptic 21-hydroxylase deficiency. *J Clin Endocrinol Metab* 1981;53:1193–1198.

Lin-Su K, et al. Treatment with growth hormone and luteinizing hormone releasing hormone analog improves final adult height in children with congenital adrenal hyperplasia. *J Clin Endocrinol Metab* 2005;90:3318–3325.

Lopes LA, Dubuis JM, Vallotton MB, et al. Should we monitor more closely the dosage of 9 alpha-fluorohydrocortisone in salt-losing congenital adrenal hyperplasia? *J Pediatr Endocrinol Metab* 1998;11: 733–737.

Merke DP, Cutler GB. New approaches to the treatment of congenital adrenal hyperplasia. *JAMA* 1997;277:1073–1076.

Miller WL. Congenital adrenal hyperplasia in the adult patient. *Adv Intern Med* 1999;44: 155–173.

New MI. Nonclassic 21-hydroxylase deficiency. *J Clin Endocrinol Metab* 2006;91: 4205–4214.

Nimkarn S, New MI. Prenatal diagnosis and treatment of congenital adrenal hyperplasia. *Horm Res* 2007;67:53–60.

Pang SY, et al. Worldwide experience in newborn screening for classical congenital adrenal hyperplasia due to 21-hydroxylase deficiency. *Pediatrics* 1988;81:866–874.

Speiser PW, et al. Disease expression and molecular genotype in congenital adrenal hyperplasia due to 21-hydroxylase deficiency. *J Clin Invest* 1992;90:584–595.

Speiser PW. Congenital adrenal hyperplasia owing to 21-hydroxylase deficiency. *Endocrinol Metab Clin North Am* 2001;30:31–59.

White PC, Curnow KM, Pascoe L. Disorders of steroid 11-beta-hydroxylase isozymes. *Endocrinol Rev* 1994;15:421.

White PC, New MI, Dupont B. Congenital adrenal hyperplasia: part 1. *N Engl J Med* 1987;316:1519.

White PC, New MI, Dupont B. Congenital adrenal hyperplasia: part 2. *N Engl J Med* 1987;316:1580.

Conn's Syndrome

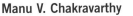

13

Manu V. Chakravarthy

INTRODUCTION

Jerome W. Conn in 1955 reported a 34-year-old woman with hypertension, intermittent paralysis, and biochemical analyses showing hypokalemia, metabolic alkalosis, and increased activity of urinary mineralocorticoid. This classical presentation represents **primary aldosteronism**, defined as renin-independent hypertension with nonsuppressible hypersecretion of aldosterone.

Prior to the measurement of the ratio of plasma aldosterone concentration (PAC) to plasma renin activity (PRA) as a screening test for primary aldosteronism, its prevalence among hypertensive patients was <3.5%. However, with the routine use of the PAC/PRA ratio, the prevalence of primary aldosteronism among all hypertensive persons is reported to be ~10% (range 5%–13%), which incidentally is the same estimate that was initially proposed by Conn. The prevalence appears to increase with the severity of hypertension and in populations with resistant hypertension, but is unaffected by ethnicity, although African Americans tend to have lower renin levels (which affects the PAC/PRA ratio) than Caucasian subjects. Compared to essential hypertension, primary aldosteronism is more common among younger patients.

CAUSES

Aldosterone is produced in the zona glomerulosa and is synthesized and released in response to renin-dependent production of angiotensin II. However, serum potassium, adrenocorticotropic hormone (ACTH), dopamine, and atrial natriuretic peptide (ANP) also affect its production and secretion. Aldosterone exerts its effect by binding to the nuclear mineralocorticoid receptor, which in turn binds to regulatory regions on DNA to affect gene expression. The end result is increased blood volume due to enhanced renal sodium reabsorption and potassium excretion.

Aldosterone-induced sodium retention and potassium wasting are of limited duration and do not lead to generalized edema or profound hypokalemia in the steady state because of "*aldosterone escape*," in which an increase in urinary sodium and decrease in urinary potassium excretion counteracts the acute effects of excess aldosterone. This phenomenon is thought to be mediated by increased secretion of ANP induced by the hypervolemia, decreased abundance of the thiazide sensitive NaCl co-transporter, and pressure natriuresis. In general, aldosterone production and secretion is tightly regulated by feedback from serum potassium levels and renin activity.

The two main causes of primary aldosterone excess are **idiopathic hyperaldosteronism** (IHA), which is usually due to bilateral adrenal hyperplasia and accounts for approximately two-thirds of cases, and **aldosterone-producing adenomas** (APA), which constitute about one-third of cases. IHA compared with APA is generally associated with milder aldosterone excess, milder hypertension and hypokalemia, and older age, The other causes of primary aldosteronism are generally much rarer (1%–3%) and include unilateral primary adrenal hyperplasia (PAH), aldosterone-producing adrenocortical carcinomas, aldosterone-producing ovarian tumor, and familial hyperaldosteronism (FH), types 1 and 2.

FH type 1 is also called **glucocorticoid-remediable aldosteronism** (GRA), which is inherited in an autosomal-dominant fashion and is usually associated with bilateral adrenal hyperplasia. It is caused by recombination between the promoter regions of 11-β-hydroxylase (*CYP11B1)* and the coding regions of 18-hydroxylase (*CYP11B2),* such that in the chimeric gene, ACTH (rather than renin or serum potassium) drives the expression of aldosterone synthase and aldosterone production. Type 2 is ACTH-independent and has an autosomal-dominant familial occurrence of APA, IHA, or both. Although the exact genetic defect is unknown, a locus on chromosome 7p22 has been implicated.

PRESENTATION

Patients may have few, if any, symptoms. Symptoms related to hypokalemia, such as muscle weakness and cramping, can occur. Other symptoms are nonspecific and may include headache, fatigue, palpitations, and polyuria. There are no specific physical findings in primary aldosteronism. Although excess sodium retention and volume expansion are thought to mediate the hypertension, edema is rare due to the phenomenon of aldosterone escape.

The majority of patients have hypertension, which may be mild to severe. But rarely, hypertension can be absent and, in such cases, resolution of hyperaldosteronism can lead to very low blood pressures. Hypervolemia is not only responsible for the hypertension but also for the marked suppression of renin release, leading to the very low plasma renin activity, the *sine qua non* of primary aldosteronism. This finding is of diagnostic importance in distinguishing primary from secondary hyperreninemic forms of hyperaldosteronism as seen with renovascular hypertension or diuretic therapy.

Patients with primary aldosteronism are found to have more severe end-organ damage than comparable patients with essential hypertension. Moreover, primary aldosteronism adversely affects kidney and cardiovascular function, independent of blood pressure. Glomerular filtration rate, renal perfusion pressure, and urinary albumin excretion are increased. When matched for age, blood pressure, and the duration of hypertension, patients with primary aldosteronism not only have greater left ventricular mass measurements compared to patients with other types of hypertension (essential hypertension, pheochromocytoma, and Cushing's syndrome), but also manifest increased cardiovascular risk (higher rates of stroke, nonfatal myocardial infarction, and atrial fibrillation), highlighting the deleterious effects of excess aldosterone.

Laboratory findings include hypokalemia, metabolic alkalosis, mild hypernatremia, and hypomagnesemia. Hypokalemia in primary aldosteronism may be spontaneous, become pronounced when patients are placed on diuretics, or be completely absent (in one series more than 60% of patients with primary aldosteronism with adequate sodium intake had no hypokalemia). The decrease in the serum potassium levels is accompanied by metabolic alkalosis, largely due to increased urinary H^+ excretion mediated by both hypokalemia and the direct stimulatory effect of aldosterone on distal acidification. Because of the mild persistent volume expansion, the osmostat regulating antidiuretic hormone release is reset upward with resulting stable plasma sodium concentrations between 143 and 147 mEq/L.

As opposed to patients with primary aldosteronism who develop hypertension between the third and fifth decades, GRA patients develop hypertension at birth or in early childhood. Patients with GRA are usually normokalemic because their aldosterone release has the same circadian pattern as that of ACTH, and, therefore, aldosterone secretion is above normal for only part of the day. However, these patients show marked hypokalemia when treated with thiazide diuretics. Patients with GRA also tend to have an increased prevalence of early cerebrovascular complications, especially hemorrhagic strokes from ruptured intracerebral aneurysms. The family history in patients with GRA may not consistently reveal hypertension, as environmental factors such as sodium intake may be modifying factors.

MANAGEMENT

Diagnosis

The evaluation for hyperaldosteronism consists of three main components: (a) screening, (b) confirmation, and (c) localization to establish the diagnosis.

Screening Tests

Screening of all hypertensive patients for primary aldosteronism is not currently recommended. Screening is recommended for hypertensive patients with at least one of the following:

- Spontaneous hypokalemia, easily provoked hypokalemia on modest diuretic doses, or refractory hypokalemia on standard potassium replacement doses;
- Hypertension that suggests a secondary cause, for example, on the basis of its severity, resistance to standard medical therapy, or accelerated clinical course;
- Adrenal incidentaloma; or
- Family history of primary aldosteronism.

In addition, William Young of the Mayo Clinic recommends screening younger (<30 years old) patients with stage 1 hypertension who are not obese and do not have a family history of hypertension. The absence of hypertension or hypokalemia *per se* does not preclude screening. Screening is generally not recommended in the elderly with mild hypertension and a normal serum potassium. The differential diagnosis for patients with hypertension and hypokalemia includes the general categories of primary or secondary aldosteronism, as well as states of real or apparent mineralocorticoid excess. A summary of these conditions is provided in Table 13-1. These categories can be distinguished by measuring morning **PAC** and **plasma PRA** on simultaneously obtained blood samples. Low PRA separates primary from secondary hyperaldosteronism. Low PRA and low PAC characterize states of real or apparent mineralocorticoid excess.

The **PAC/PRA ratio** (reported as ng/dL per ng/mL/hour) is the screening test of choice for primary aldosteronism. Ratios of >20 to >50 have been reported as supportive of primary aldosteronism. A PAC/PRA ratio >30 *and* PAC >20 ng/dL yield ~90% sensitivity and specificity. Use of the ratio alone without consideration of the absolute value for PAC may be misleading. For example, a subset of patients with essential hypertension may have elevated ratios by virtue of very low PRA without concomitant elevation in PAC.

Biochemical testing of the renin–angiotensin-aldosterone axis should occur in a sodium and volume replete state. Serum potassium levels should be normalized prior to testing. Potassium loading at the time of testing may increase aldosterone secretion.

Antihypertensive medications may affect the PAC or PRA. Patients must be off aldosterone receptor blockers (spironolactone or eplerenone) for at least 6 weeks prior to testing. Angiotensin-converting enzyme (ACE) inhibitors and angiotensin receptor blockers (ARBs) may raise the PRA and lead to a false-negative result for the PAC/PRA ratio in patients with primary aldosteronism. An undetectable PRA, however, in the context of ACE-inhibitor or ARB treatment, is suggestive of primary aldosteronism. β-blockers,

TABLE 13-1	DIFFERENTIAL DIAGNOSIS FOR HYPERTENSION AND HYPOKALEMIA		
↑ PAC and ↓ PRA **Primary aldosteronism**	**↑ PRA and ↑ PAC** **Secondary aldosteronism**	**↓ PRA and ↓ PAC** **Real or apparent mineralocorticoid excess states**	
Aldosterone producing adrenal adenomas	Renal artery stenosis	17-α-Hydroxylase deficiency	
Idiopathic hyperaldosteronism	Renin-secreting tumor Malignant hypertension	17-, 20-Hydroxlyase deficiency	
Glucocorticoid-remediable aldosteronism	Chronic renal disease Aortic coarctation	11-β-Hydroxylase deficiency	
Primary adrenal hyperplasia	Aortic stenosis Congestive heart failure	Deoxycorticosterone-secreting tumors	
Adrenocortical carcinoma	Cirrhosis[a] Diuretic abuse[a]	Deficient 11-β-hydroxysteroid dehydrogenase type 2	
Extraadrenal tumors with ectopic aldosterone secretion	Volume depletion[a] Bartter's syndrome[a] Gitelman's syndrome[a]	Chronic licorice ingestion (glycyrrhizic and glycyrrhetinic acid)	
		Exogenous mineralocorticoid use	
		Severe Cushing's syndrome (ectopic ACTH)	
		Cortisol resistance	
		Liddle's syndrome	

PAC, plasma aldosterone concentration; PRA, plasma renin activity.
[a]May not present with hypertension.

α-blockers, potassium-sparing diuretics other than spironolactone, and calcium channel blockers can generally be continued without compromising the results of screening. Some of these drugs may affect the PAC or PRA but do not appreciably alter the PAC/PRA ratio.

Confirmatory Tests

Confirmation of primary aldosteronism is made by documenting **nonsuppression of aldosterone during sodium loading**. The principle underlying aldosterone suppression testing is that an increase in intravascular volume should decrease renin release and subsequent aldosterone production in patients without primary aldosteronism. Both oral and intravenous sodium loading tests are available. In the **oral sodium loading** test, the patient is instructed to consume 5 to 6 g/day of sodium, either from dietary sources or sodium chloride tablets. A 24-hour urine collection is undertaken starting no sooner than the third day and assayed for urine aldosterone, sodium, and creatinine. Urine aldosterone excretion >14 mcg per 24 hours confirms nonsuppressibility of aldosterone. Adequacy of the sodium loading is documented by urinary excretion of sodium >200 mEq/day. During the oral sodium load, electrolytes must be measured daily and potassium replaced as needed, because sodium loading in patients with primary aldosteronism leads to potassium wasting. Potassium should be adequately replaced prior to initiation of the test. **Intravenous sodium loading** is an alternative test. Two liters of normal saline is infused intravenously over 4 hours to the recumbent patient. A PAC >10 ng/dL at 4 hours confirms the diagnosis of primary aldosteronism. These sodium loading tests may lead to volume overload, especially in patients with compromised left ventricular function, and must be closely monitored.

Localization Tests to Determine the Subtype

Once the diagnosis of primary aldosteronism is established, studies are then undertaken to differentiate unilateral disease (primarily APA), which is addressed surgically, from bilateral disease (primarily IHA), which is treated with aldosterone receptor blockade. The differential diagnosis of primary aldosteronism subtypes is summarized in Table 13-2. After biochemical confirmation of the diagnosis, the first imaging test is either **computed tomography (CT) or magnetic resonance imaging (MRI) of the adrenal glands.**

The presence of a unilateral adrenal mass on CT or MRI in a patient with primary aldosteronism does not establish a cause-and-effect relationship, because benign, nonfunctioning adrenal masses detected by CT or MRI are common (see Chapter 10). Moreover, failure to detect an adrenal mass by imaging does not rule out APA, and detection of bilateral lesions is not diagnostic of hyperplasia. Despite the limitations of adrenal imaging, it is not unreasonable to proceed to unilateral adrenalectomy if a solitary adenoma of >1 cm is detected in a young patient with confirmed primary aldosteronism and a completely normal contralateral adrenal gland. The likelihood of a solitary adrenal mass being a nonfunctioning adenoma increases with age. In many cases it is necessary to proceed to **adrenal venous sampling** (AVS). For example, it has been recommended that patients older than 40 years undergo AVS prior to a decision about surgery. AVS is technically difficult and requires a radiologist experienced in the technique. Adrenal vein blood samples are

TABLE 13-2	DIFFERENTIAL DIAGNOSIS OF PRIMARY ALDOSTERONISM SUBTYPES		
	APA	**IHA**	**GRA**
Adrenal venous sampling	Lateralization	No lateralization	No lateralization
Postural stimulation test	Decrease in PAC	Increase or no change in PAC	Decrease in PAC
Adrenal scintigraphy	Lateralization	No lateralization	No lateralization
Plasma 18-hydroxycorticosterone	>100 ng/dL	<50 ng/dL	<50 ng/dL
Urinary 18-hydroxycortisol, 18-oxocortisol	Mildly elevated	No change	Greatly elevated
Dexamethasone suppressibility	No	No	Yes

APA, aldosterone producing adrenal adenoma; IHA, idiopathic hyperaldosteronism; GRA, glucocorticoid-remediable aldosteronism; PAC, plasma aldosterone concentration.

obtained for the measurement of plasma aldosterone and cortisol to distinguish between an adenoma (greater than fourfold difference between the left and right samples) and hyperplasia (little difference between the two sides). Cortisol serves as a control because it should vary little between the two samples. Other tests include postural stimulation (APA shows a paradoxical fall in PAC from a supine 8 AM sample and a sample obtained after 4 hours of upright posture), adrenal scintigraphy with the ^{131}I-labeled cholesterol analog (6 β-[^{131}I]iodomethyl-19-norcholesterol), and dexamethasone suppression testing (PAC suppresses to <4 ng/dL in GRA). Measurement of plasma 18-hydroxycorticosterone (elevated in APA) or of urinary 18-hydroxycortisol and 18-oxocortisol (elevated in GRA) can also be used to differentiate between the subtypes. GRA can also be confirmed by PCR-based genetic testing.

When large adrenal masses (>4 cm) that have atypical features (dense, irregular, or mixed attenuation) are found in patients with biochemical evidence of primary aldosteronism, adrenocortical carcinoma is more likely.

Treatment

The main therapeutic goals in primary aldosteronism are not only the adequate control of blood pressure and correction of hypokalemia, but also the normalization of PAC and/or blockade of aldosterone activity given the known end-organ complications of hyperaldosteronism itself.

Unilateral laparoscopic adrenalectomy is the treatment of choice in APA and PAH. Laparoscopic adrenalectomy is associated with shorter hospital stays and lower morbidity than an open approach. Adequate blood pressure control and correction of hypokalemia with an aldosterone receptor antagonist before surgery is recommended. PAC should be measured the day after surgery to confirm surgical cure. Serum potassium levels should be analyzed the day after the operation, as hypokalemia is corrected rapidly after adrenalectomy for APA. Because aldosterone production in the contralateral adrenal might be suppressed during the first few postoperative weeks, a sodium-rich diet should be recommended and serum potassium levels should be monitored weekly for 4 weeks. Although blood pressure improves and serum potassium levels normalize in most patients with surgically treated APA, the presence of preexisting essential hypertension, end-organ damage, changes in vascular tone, or nephrosclerosis may contribute to postoperative hypertension, which persists in up to 40% of patients despite complete correction of the hyperaldosteronism.

Medical management is reserved for patients with bilateral disease (IHA, GRA) or patients with APA or PAH who refuse surgery or are poor surgical candidates. Surgical approaches have generally been ineffective for IHA, as only a minority of patients have significant improvements in hypertension, which has led to the notion that perhaps IHA is a variant of essential hypertension. Patients generally require lifelong therapy. There is little risk for malignant transformation of aldosterone-secreting adenomas. Effective pharmacologic agents include:

- **Spironolactone** at doses of 200 to 400 mg PO daily, taken with food in divided doses is rapidly effective in correcting hypokalemia, but its antihypertensive effects may not be apparent for several weeks. Antiandrogenic side effects, including gynecomastia, erectile dysfunction, impotence, and decreased libido in men and menstrual irregularities in women, limit its tolerability.
- **Eplerenone**, a highly selective mineralocorticoid receptor antagonist with fewer side effects (because of its extremely low binding affinity to both the androgen and progesterone receptors), represents a newer alternative. Eplerenone is approved for the treatment of uncomplicated essential hypertension (maximum approved dose, 100 mg daily). Eplerenone is 25% to 50% less potent than spironolactone, milligram per milligram, and is also much more expensive.

- **Amiloride and triamterene**, potassium-sparing diuretics that block the aldosterone-sensitive sodium channel in the collecting tubules, are alternatives to spironolactone. Amiloride doses of 10 to 30 mg PO daily and triamterene doses of 200 to 300 mg PO daily, in divided doses, block the renal effects of aldosterone, thereby lowering blood pressure and raising the serum potassium concentration. However, they do not decrease aldosterone levels per se and are ineffective antihypertensive agents. Adjunctive therapy with low doses of thiazide diuretics is usually needed to adequately control blood pressure because hypervolemia is a major reason for the resistance to amiloride. Side effects include dizziness, fatigue, and nausea.

Potassium supplements should not be given routinely with the agents previously noted, as hyperkalemia may result. Other second-line agents include dihydropyridine calcium channel blockers, diuretics, ACE inhibitors, and angiotensin II receptor antagonists. Patients with GRA may be treated with glucocorticoids at the lowest effective dose to avoid iatrogenic Cushing's syndrome. Alternatively, such patients may be treated with a mineralocorticoid antagonist as monotherapy with similar results.

KEY POINTS TO REMEMBER

- Primary aldosteronism (Conn's syndrome) is a condition of autonomous aldosterone excess that leads to suppressed renin levels.
- Symptoms, if at all present, may be related to hypokalemia (muscle weakness and cramping) or may be nonspecific (headache and fatigue).
- The majority of patients with Conn's syndrome have hypertension. Laboratory findings may include hypokalemia, metabolic alkalosis, and mild hypernatremia.
- Paired measurements of the PAC and PRA should be obtained; both the PAC/PRA ratio and the absolute PAC should be used as part of the screening test for Conn's syndrome. If abnormal, they should be followed by a confirmatory test to demonstrate nonsuppression of aldosterone by sodium loading.
- Unilateral total adrenalectomy is the treatment of choice in APA and PAH.
- Medical management is reserved for patients with bilateral disease (IHA, GRA) or for patients with APA or PAH who refuse surgery or are poor surgical candidates.

REFERENCES AND SUGGESTED READINGS

Blumenfeld JD, Sealey JE, Schlussel Y, et al. Diagnosis and treatment of primary hyperaldosteronism. *Ann Intern Med* 1994;121:877–885.

Dluhy RG, Lifton RP. Glucocorticoid-remediable aldosteronism. *J Clin Endocrinol Metab* 1999;84:4341–4344.

Gordon RD, Stowasser M, Klemm SA, et al. Primary aldosteronism and other forms of mineralocorticoid hypertension. In Swales J, ed. *Textbook of Hypertension*. Oxford: Blackwell Scientific; 1994:865–892.

Jonsson JR, Klemm SA, Tunny TJ, et al. A new genetic test for familial hyperaldosteronism type I aids in the detection of curable hypertension. *Biochem Biophys Res Commun* 1995;207:565–571.

Lim PO, Young WF, MacDonald TM. A review of the medical treatment of primary aldosteronism. *J Hypertens* 2001;19:353–361.

Lim PO, Dow E, Brennan G, et al. High prevalence of primary aldosteronism in the Tayside Hypertension Clinic population. *J Hum Hypertens* 2000;14:311–315.

Litchfield WR, Dluhy RG. Primary aldosteronism. *Endocrinol Metab Clin North Am* 1995; 24:593–612.

Litchfield WR, New MI, Coolidge C, et al. Evaluation of the dexamethasone suppression test for the diagnosis of glucocorticoid-remediable aldosteronism. *J Clin Endocrinol Metab* 1997;82:3570– 3573.

Litchfield WR, Anderson BF, Weiss RJ, et al. Intracranial aneurysm and hemorrhagic stroke in glucocorticoid-remediable aldosteronism. *Hypertension* 1998;31:445–450.

Mattsson C, Young WF. Primary aldosteronism: diagnostic and treatment strategies. *Nat Clin Pract Nephrol* 2006;2:198–208.

Schirpenbach C, Reincke M. Primary aldosteronism: current knowledge and controversies in Conn's syndrome. *Nat Clin Pract Endocrinol Metab* 2007;3:220–227.

Snow MH, Nicol P, Wilkinson R, et al. Normotensive primary aldosteronism. *BMJ* 1976;1:1125–1126.

Torpy DJ, Gordon RD, Lin JP, et al. Familial hyperaldosteronism type II: description of a large kindred and exclusion of the aldosterone synthase (*CYP11B2*) gene. *J Clin Endocrinol Metab* 1998;83:3214–3218.

Ulick S, Blumenfeld JD, Atlas SA, et al. The unique steroidogenesis of the aldosteronoma in the differential diagnosis of primary aldosteronism. *J Clin Endocrinol Metab* 1993;76:873–878.

Weinberger MH, Fineberg NS. The diagnosis of primary aldosteronism and separation of two major subtypes. *Arch Intern Med* 1993;153:2125–2129.

Young WF. Minireview: primary aldosteronism—changing concepts in diagnosis and treatment. *Endocrinology* 2003;144:2208–2213.

Young WF. The incidentally discovered adrenal mass. *N Engl J Med* 2007;356:601–610.

Cushing's Syndrome

Manu V. Chakravarthy

INTRODUCTION

Cushing's syndrome is a clinical condition resulting from prolonged exposure to excessive glucocorticoids from either endogenous or exogenous sources. The most common cause of Cushing's syndrome is from therapeutic administration of exogenous glucocorticoids. The most common endogenous cause of the syndrome is Cushing's disease, originally described by Harvey Cushing in 1932. Cushing's disease is usually caused by an adrenocorticotropic hormone (ACTH)–secreting pituitary adenoma. Other endogenous causes of the syndrome include ectopic secretion of ACTH or corticotropin-releasing hormone (CRH) by nonpituitary tumors and primary adrenal tumors. Frequent clinical findings include weight gain, truncal obesity, striae, hypertension, glucose intolerance, and infections. The nonspecific nature of these signs and symptoms coupled with the inherent limitations of the commonly used laboratory tests makes the diagnosis of Cushing's syndrome one of the most challenging in endocrinology.

CAUSES

Determining the cause of Cushing's syndrome requires an understanding of the pathophysiology of hypercortisolemia which, in turn, is critical to accurately diagnose and treat the condition. Broadly, Cushing's syndrome can be thought of as being either ACTH-dependent or ACTH-independent (see Table 14-1). A third category of pseudo-Cushing's syndrome is also considered in the appropriate clinical setting.

The **ACTH-dependent** form represents ~80% of all cases of Cushing's syndrome, of which the majority are due to ACTH-secreting pituitary microadenomas (Cushing's disease). Cushing's disease has an annual incidence of 5 to 25 per million, and women of reproductive age are 3 to 8 times more likely to have the disease. Ectopic ACTH syndrome accounts for ~10% of cases, and the ectopic secretion of ACTH causes bilateral adrenocortical hyperplasia and hyperfunction. Small cell carcinoma of the lung is the most common cause of ectopic ACTH secretion and accounts for >50% of cases. Tumors of the pancreas and thymus may also cause the ectopic ACTH syndrome. Ectopic CRH syndrome is a rare cause in which CRH secretion by the primary tumor causes hyperplasia of pituitary corticotrophs and consequent hypersecretion of ACTH, cortisol hypersecretion, and bilateral adrenal hyperplasia. Ectopic production of ACTH or CRH by neuroendocrine tumors, such as pheochromocytomas and carcinoid tumors, can also cause Cushing's syndrome.

The most common causes of the **ACTH-independent** form of Cushing's syndrome are adrenal adenoma and carcinoma, which represent 10% and 5% of cases, respectively. Most adrenocortical tumors are monoclonal, suggesting that they result from accumulated genetic abnormalities such as activation of proto-oncogenes and inactivation of tumor

TABLE 14-1   CAUSES OF CUSHING'S SYNDROME

Diagnosis	% of Patients
ACTH-dependent	
Cushing's disease (pituitary hypersecretion of ACTH)	70
Ectopic ACTH syndrome (nonpituitary tumors)	10
Ectopic CRH syndrome (nonhypothalamic tumors causing pituitary hypersecretion of ACTH)	<1
ACTH-independent	
Adrenal adenoma	10
Adrenal carcinoma	5
Micronodular hyperplasia	1
Macronodular hyperplasia	<2
Pseudo-Cushing's syndrome[a]	
Major-depressive disorder	1
Alcoholism	<1

[a]The prevalence of pseudo-Cushing's syndrome depends upon the individual physician's threshold of clinical suspicion.
Adapted from Newell-Price J, et al. Cushing's syndrome. *Lancet* 2006;367:1605–1617; Nieman LK. Cushing's syndrome. In: Rose BD, ed. *UpToDate*. Waltham, MA: UpToDate; 2007.

suppressor genes. Adrenal carcinomas produce excessive amounts of cortisol and other adrenal steroids, mostly because of their size.

Other causes of ACTH-independent Cushing's syndrome are rare and include bilateral micronodular and macronodular adrenal hyperplasia. One-half of the cases of bilateral micronodular adrenal hyperplasia occur in **Carney's complex**, an autosomal-dominant syndrome associated with endocrine tumors such as pituitary adenomas, testicular and thyroid tumors, cardiac atrial myxomas, pigmented lentigines, blue nevi, and schwannomas. Macronodular hyperplasia is associated with very large adrenal glands (≥100–500 g) that contain multiple nonpigmented nodules. In some cases, the macronodules express increased numbers of receptors normally found in the adrenal or ectopic receptors (e.g., GIP receptors), such that normal levels of the ligand result in pathologic cortisol hypersecretion. Hypercortisolism from hyperplastic adrenal nodules can also occur in **McCune-Albright syndrome**, which is associated with multiple autonomous hyperfunctioning endocrinopathies, as well as café-au-lait spots and polyostotic fibrous dysplasia. Cushing's syndrome can be associated with indolent tumors and other states of hormone excess. One series reported Cushing's disease in 16% of patients with multiple endocrine neoplasia 1 (MEN1) and Zollinger-Ellison syndrome.

In the differential diagnosis, Cushing's syndrome must be distinguished from other conditions associated with elevated cortisol but without Cushing's syndrome. Depression, alcoholism, medications, obesity, anorexia nervosa, psychiatric illness, stress/trauma/acute illness, states of elevated cortisol-binding protein (pregnancy, estrogen therapy), familial generalized glucocorticoid resistance, and the metabolic syndrome can cause mild clinical and laboratory findings similar to those in Cushing's syndrome, termed **pseudo-Cushing's syndrome**. The laboratory and clinical findings of hypercortisolism disappear if the primary process is successfully treated. Metabolic syndrome may mimic Cushing's syndrome with central obesity, hypertension, and glucose intolerance. Women with the metabolic syndrome may also have features of polycystic ovarian syndrome and present with menstrual irregularities and hyperandrogenism (hirsutism, acne).

PRESENTATION

Patients present with a wide spectrum of manifestations ranging from subclinical to overt syndrome, depending on the duration and intensity of excess glucocorticoid production, the presence or absence of mineralocorticoid and androgen excess, and the cause of the hypercortisolism. Symptoms of Cushing's syndrome that occur in the setting of malignancy may be overshadowed by manifestations of the malignancy such as weight loss instead of weight gain. Patients with cyclical Cushing's syndrome may have intermittent symptoms. Cushing's syndrome during pregnancy can be difficult to diagnose as both conditions may be complicated by excessive weight gain, striae, hypertension, edema, and glucose intolerance. The degree of hypercortisolemia and many of the clinical manifestations tend to be less severe in older patients (>50 years of age). Some patients with incidentally discovered adrenal adenomas have subclinical Cushing's syndrome associated with glucose intolerance and hypertension.

Some of the major findings suggestive of Cushing's syndrome are presented in subsequent text of this chapter (also see Table 14-2). However, it is important to note that none of them are truly pathognomonic of the syndrome, and, therefore, a high degree of clinical suspicion is required to diagnose the condition.

- **Progressive central obesity** involving the abdomen, face, and neck (buffalo hump, moon facies, supraclavicular fat pads, and exophthalmos from retroorbital fat deposition).
- **Metabolic complications** include glucose intolerance (owing to stimulation of gluconeogenesis by cortisol and peripheral insulin resistance caused by obesity), and hypertension (through poorly understood multifactorial etiologies), both of which confer increased cardiovascular risk, a major cause of morbidity and death in patients with Cushing's syndrome. Severe hypertension and hypokalemia are more commonly

TABLE 14-2	SYMPTOMS AND SIGNS IN PATIENTS WITH CUSHING'S SYNDROME	
Sign/symptom		**% of Patients**
Truncal obesity		95
Facial fullness		90
Gonadal dysfunction (decreased libido)		90
Skin atrophy and bruising		80
Menstrual irregularity		80
Hypertension		75
Hirsutism, acne		75
Mood disorders		70
Muscle weakness		65
Diabetes or glucose intolerance		60
Osteopenia, osteoporosis, fractures		50

Adapted from Newell-Price J, et al. Cushing's syndrome. *Lancet* 2006;367:1605–1617.

seen in patients with ectopic ACTH syndrome because the very high serum cortisol levels overwhelm the capacity of the 11-β-hydroxysteroid dehydrogenase type 2 enzyme, which oxidizes cortisol to inactive cortisone, thereby resulting in activation of mineralocorticoid receptors.

- **Dermatologic manifestations** of skin atrophy (thinning of the stratum corneum), fragile skin with easy bruisability, wide purple striae (due to the stretching of fragile skin), cutaneous fungal infections, and hyperpigmentation (in ectopic ACTH syndrome).
- **Reproductive changes** include menstrual irregularities, hirsutism, oily facial skin with acne, and other signs of virilization (temporal balding, deepening voice), especially in women with adrenal carcinoma.
- **Musculoskeletal manifestations** are proximal myopathy, muscle wasting (resulting from the catabolic effects of excess glucocorticoid on skeletal muscle), and osteoporosis (caused by decreased bone formation, increased bone resorption, and decreased intestinal and renal calcium reabsorption). Vertebral compression fractures, pathologic fractures of the rib or long bones, and aseptic necrosis of the femoral heads may also be present.
- **Neuropsychiatric changes** can include labile mood, agitated depression, anxiety, panic attacks, mild paranoia, impaired short-term memory and cognition, and insomnia.

MANAGEMENT

Diagnosis

Because of the possibility of both pituitary and adrenal incidentalomas, it is essential for biochemical diagnosis to precede imaging studies. The biochemical diagnosis of Cushing's syndrome involves three critical steps: (a) documenting the presence of hypercortisolism (does the patient have Cushing's syndrome?), (b) determining if the cortisol excess is ACTH-independent or ACTH-dependent (does the patient have primary adrenal disease or an ACTH-secreting tumor?), and (c) determining the source of the ACTH in the ACTH-dependent form (does the patient have Cushing's disease or ectopic ACTH syndrome?).

Does the Patient Have Cushing's Syndrome?

The **24-hour urine free cortisol** measurement is the best screening test for Cushing's syndrome, as it provides the most direct and reliable practical index of cortisol secretion, given that it is an integrated measure of the serum free cortisol concentration. A complete 24-hour specimen and a reliable reference laboratory are critical for obtaining a valid result. The patient can be assumed to have Cushing's syndrome if basal urinary cortisol excretion is two to threefold higher than the normal range obtained on at least two separate occasions; the evaluation can then proceed to the next step of establishing the cause for the hypercortisolism. If it is equivocally increased, that is, above the upper limit of normal, but not quite 3 times as much, the patient needs to be reevaluated after several weeks or undergo further testing (see subsequent text and Table 14-3) to help differentiate among mild Cushing's, cyclic Cushing's, and pseudo-Cushing's syndrome. These tests are designed not only to detect excess cortisol secretion, but also to assess the loss of the normal feedback suppression of the hypothalamic–pituitary–adrenal (HPA) axis, and the loss of the normal diurnal rhythm of cortisol secretion.

Another commonly used screening test is the **1-mg overnight dexamethasone suppression test.** This low-dose test was designed to differentiate patients with Cushing's syndrome of any cause from patients who do not have Cushing's syndrome. However, because it has a high false-positive rate (Table 14-3), it should not be used as the sole criterion for making the diagnosis of Cushing's syndrome. In the case of a positive test, it may be informative to retain a serum sample collected at the time of cortisol measurement for

TABLE 14-3 BIOCHEMICAL TESTS FOR ESTABLISHING HYPERCORTISOLISM

Test	Protocol	Measurements	Interpretation	Sensitivity (%)	Specificity (%)
1 mg overnight DST	Dex, 1 mg PO at 11 PM	8 AM plasma cortisol	Normal, <5 mcg/dL	98	70–80
24-Hour UFC	24-hour urine collection	Cortisol, creatinine	Values 2- to 3-fold higher than the upper limit of normal suggest Cushing's syndrome	95–100	98
2-Day LDDST (urine)	Dex, 0.5 mg PO q6h for 48 hrs (last dose 6 AM)	24 hour urine for cortisol, 17-OHCS, creatinine during last 24 hour of dex administration.	UFC >36 mcg/day or urine 17-OHCS >4 mg/day suggests Cushing's syndrome	56–69	74–100
2-Day LDDST (serum)	Dex, 0.5 mg PO q6h for 48 hours (last dose 6 AM)	Plasma cortisol 2 hours after last dose of dex	Normal <1.4 mcg/dL	90	100
CRH/dex	Same as LDDST with first dose dex given at noon; CRH, 1 mcg/kg IV at 8 AM after last dose of dex	Plasma cortisol 15 min after CRH injection	Cortisol >1.4 mcg/dL suggests Cushing's syndrome	100	100
Late-evening salivary cortisol	11 PM sample	Salivary cortisol	Value <1.3 ng/mL excludes Cushing's syndrome	92	100
Midnight plasma cortisol	Indwelling catheter and hospitalization recommended	Midnight plasma cortisol	Cortisol >7.5 mcg/dL suggests Cushing's syndrome	96	100

CRH, corticotrophin-releasing hormone; UFC, urine free cortisol; dex, dexamethasone; DST, dexamethasone suppression test; LDDST, low-dose dexamethasone suppression test; 17-OHCS, 17-hydroxycorticosteroid.

measurement of the dexamethasone level. A low dexamethasone level suggests noncompliance, individual variation in dexamethasone metabolism, or drug effects on dexamethasone metabolism.

In some patients, an unequivocal conclusion cannot be reached, even after measurement of urinary free cortisol and use of the low-dose dexamethasone suppression tests. In such circumstances, either a late-evening salivary cortisol, midnight plasma cortisol, or the CRH after dexamethasone testing can be used. The **salivary cortisol** measurement has distinct advantages: it is noninvasive, saliva is easily collected, cortisol is stable in saliva even at room temperature for several days, and it can be performed by the patient at home. It is especially useful for patients suspected of having cyclical or intermittent Cushing's syndrome. However, it is important to choose a laboratory that provides a validated response range, because cortisol measurements of the same saliva sample using different assay techniques may yield different results. The **CRH after-dexamethasone test** is particularly useful to differentiate patients with Cushing's from those with pseudo-Cushing's syndrome. Compared to patients with Cushing's syndrome, depressed patients continue to show a suppressed plasma cortisol ($<$1.4 mcg/dL) even after CRH infusion, which reflects preserved sensitivity of ACTH secretion to dexamethasone suppression.

Regardless of which test is used, it is important to understand the inherent limitations of the tests and the causes of false-positive and false-negative test results (see Table 14-4).

TABLE 14-4	CAUSES OF FALSE-POSITIVE AND FALSE-NEGATIVE BIOCHEMICAL TESTS FOR CUSHING'S SYNDROME	
Test	**False-positive**	**False-negative**
1 mg overnight DST; 2-day LDDST	Error with timing of dex administration Meds increasing metabolism of dex Decreased absorption of dex Hypercortisolemia without Cushing's syndrome Pseudo-Cushing's syndrome	Chronic renal failure (GFR <30 mL/min) Increased sensitivity of the HPA axis to dex
24-hour UFC	High fluid intake Interference with carbamazepine in the HPLC assay Hypercortisolemia without Cushing's syndrome Pseudo-Cushing's syndrome	Cyclic Cushing's Early Cushing's Chronic renal failure Interference with fibrate-class of drugs
Midnight plasma cortisol; Late-evening salivary cortisol	Stress from hospitalization or blood draw Critically ill patients Patients with depression	Cyclic Cushing's

dex, dexamethasone; UFC, urine free cortisol; DST, dexamethasone suppression test; LDDST, low-dose dexamethasone suppression test; HPLC, high-performance liquid chromatography.

Does the Patient Have Primary Adrenal Disease or an ACTH-Secreting Tumor?

Once endogenous Cushing's syndrome has been confirmed, the second stage of the workup involves the differentiation of ACTH-dependent from ACTH-independent forms. This can be best accomplished by measuring **plasma ACTH levels using a two-site immunoradiometric assay.**

Undetectable or low levels of ACTH (<5 mcg/dL) in a patient with a serum cortisol concentration >15 mcg/dL characterizes a primary adrenal source (ACTH-independent Cushing's syndrome). Thin-section computed tomography (CT) or magnetic resonance imaging (MRI) of the adrenal glands looking for an adrenal mass is usually the next procedure. ACTH levels >15 mcg/dL typically indicate an ACTH-dependent cause, and the next step involves a search for the source of the high ACTH (pituitary vs. nonpituitary).

An ACTH level in the 5 to 15 mcg/dL range is considered indeterminate and should be repeated (as in most cases the cortisol secretion turns out to be ACTH-dependent). If the ACTH level remains consistently in the indeterminate range, a CRH-stimulation test can be performed. After CRH infusion, if the peak ACTH response is blunted (<10 mcg/dL), an ACTH-independent (adrenal) cause is likely. However, if there is >50% increase in mean plasma cortisol from baseline after CRH infusion, an ACTH-dependent cause is likely.

Does the Patient Have Cushing's Disease or Ectopic ACTH Syndrome?

There can be considerable overlap in ACTH levels between patients with Cushing's disease and ectopic ACTH syndrome, especially in those with occult malignancy or bronchial carcinoid tumors. The distinction between the two is critical as it significantly influences treatment. Several tests can be utilized to aid in the differentiation between pituitary Cushing's disease and nonpituitary (ectopic) ACTH syndrome (see Table 14-5).

One fundamental difference between the two conditions is the fact that Cushing's disease is usually suppressible (by dexamethasone) and stimulatable (by CRH), in contrast to ectopic ACTH syndrome. Therefore, a commonly used initial test is the **high-dose dexamethasone suppression test (HDDST)**, which takes advantage of the fact that ACTH secretion by pituitary adenomas that cause Cushing's disease is only relatively resistant to negative-feedback regulation by glucocorticoids. By contrast, nonpituitary tumors producing ectopic ACTH are completely resistant to such feedback (with the exception of bronchial carcinoids). The high-dose test can be administered as a standard 2-day test (2 mg, every 6 hours × 8 doses) or as a single overnight 8-mg dose (see Table 14-5). If the urine free cortisol suppresses >90%, or the plasma cortisol suppresses >50% from baseline, Cushing's disease is most likely. An MRI of the pituitary gland should be obtained next.

If Cushing's disease cannot be definitively differentiated from ectopic ACTH syndrome as described previously, additional studies may be useful. For example, in situations of either cortisol suppression on HDDST with a negative pituitary MRI or nonsuppression on HDDST with a positive pituitary MRI, **inferior petrosal sinus sampling (IPSS)** may demonstrate pituitary ACTH hypersecretion by documenting a central-to-peripheral ACTH gradient in the blood draining the tumor (see Table 14-5). If there is no conclusive central-to-peripheral gradient after IPSS, the search for an ectopic ACTH source must continue. ^{111}In-Octreotide or pentetreotide scintigraphy can detect some ectopic ACTH-secreting tumors, although neither is specific for ACTH-secreting tumors. Chest and upper abdominal CT or MRI should be performed to confirm any positive pentetreotide scans and to identify masses not detected by scintigraphy before IPSS is undertaken.

Treatment

As treatment is almost entirely based on the source of the hypercortisolism, the need for an accurate diagnosis cannot be overemphasized. Ideal treatment goals are to reverse the clinical manifestation of hypercortisolemia by decreasing cortisol secretion to normal

TABLE 14-5	TESTS TO DIFFERENTIATE CUSHING'S DISEASE FROM ECTOPIC ACTH SYNDROME			
Test	Protocol	Interpretation	Sensitivity (%)	Specificity (%)
2-day HDDST	Collect 24-hour urine for 17-OHCS or UFC, creatinine; give dex, 2 mg PO q6h for 48 hours; re-collect urine during last 24 hours of dex administration	Suppression of urine 17-OHCS >64% or UFC >90% compared to baseline suggests Cushing's disease	83	100
8 mg overnight dex	Measure plasma cortisol at 8 AM; give dex, 8 mg p.o. at 11 PM; re-draw blood for plasma cortisol next morning at 8 AM	Suppression of plasma cortisol by >50% compared to baseline suggests Cushing's disease	92	100
CRH	Place an indwelling venous catheter 2 hours prior to testing. Give CRH 1 mcg/kg i.v. bolus at 8 AM; draw plasma ACTH at −5, −1 minute before CRH and +15, +30 minutes after CRH	Increase of ACTH (mean of +15 and +30 minute values) by 35% greater than baseline (mean of −5 and −1 minute) suggests Cushing's disease	93	100
IPSS	Simultaneous bilateral inferior petrosal sinus sampling and peripheral sampling for ACTH before and after CRH, 100 mcg i.v.	Basal petrosal: peripheral ACTH ratio ≥2 or post-CRH petrosal: peripheral ACTH ratio ≥3 suggests Cushing's disease	97–100	100

17-OHCS, 17-hydroxycorticosteroid; ACTH, adrenocorticotropic hormone; CRH, corticotrophin-releasing hormone; dex, dexamethasone; HDDST, high-dose dexamethasone suppression test; IPSS, inferior petrosal sinus sampling; UFC, urine free cortisol.

levels, and to remove the tumor while avoiding permanent hormone deficiency and dependence on medications.

Exogenous Cushing's Syndrome
Gradual withdrawal of the glucocorticoid is important, because most patients on long-term therapy will have some degree of HPA-axis suppression with resultant adrenal insufficiency if therapy is abruptly discontinued.

ACTH-Independent Cushing's Syndrome

Adrenal imaging by either CT or MRI will demonstrate unilateral or bilateral disease. Patients with adrenal adenoma or carcinoma are treated with unilateral adrenalectomy. Bilateral adrenalectomy is recommended for patients with bilateral micronodular or macronodular disease. During and after unilateral adrenalectomy, patients should receive glucocorticoid replacement until the HPA axis recovers from the prolonged suppressive effects of glucocorticoid excess. Patients with bilateral adrenalectomy require lifelong glucocorticoid and mineralocorticoid replacement. In addition to adrenalectomy, patients with adrenal carcinomas typically require medications to control hypercortisolemia, which frequently recurs.

Cushing's Disease

Transsphenoidal microadenectomy is the treatment of choice for patients with Cushing's disease with a clearly circumscribed microadenoma. In other cases (especially if no adenoma is found during surgery), subtotal (85%–90%) resection of the anterior pituitary may be performed if future fertility is not a concern for the patient. Patients with incomplete resection of the tumor may undergo repeat surgery or pituitary irradiation with either conventional radiation or stereotactic radiation with the ^{60}Co gamma knife. Pituitary irradiation may not control the hypercortisolemia for months to years, and patients require medical therapy until the full effects of the radiation are seen. Bilateral adrenalectomy may need to be performed in patients with refractory disease. **Nelson's syndrome** occurs in up to 25% of patients with Cushing's disease who are treated with bilateral adrenalectomy. In this syndrome, the pituitary enlarges and the patient develops hyperpigmentation associated with high ACTH levels. Pituitary irradiation before bilateral adrenalectomy may prevent Nelson's syndrome.

Surgical cure with transsphenoidal adenomectomy can be assessed with postoperative morning cortisol and ACTH levels, which are undetectable with successful complete resection of the tumor. During and after transsphenoidal resection of the adenoma, patients require glucocorticoid replacement until recovery of the HPA axis.

Ectopic ACTH and CRH Syndrome

Tumors that can be localized by imaging studies should be removed surgically. Imaging studies include CT, MRI, and somatostatin receptor scintigraphy. Areas that may be imaged for the presence of tumor include the chest, abdomen, pelvis, and neck. If the source is an occult tumor or if there is metastatic disease, medical treatment is required. Tumors expressing somatostatin receptors may be responsive to somatostatin analogs. Bilateral adrenalectomy may be performed in refractory cases.

Medical Therapy with Adrenal Enzyme Inhibitors

Patients treated with these medications should have plasma cortisol and 24-hour urine free cortisol levels monitored and doses titrated to keep cortisol levels in the normal range. Glucocorticoid replacement is added as cortisol levels approach the low-normal range.

- **Ketoconazole** is an antifungal agent that inhibits 17-20 lyase, 11-β-hydroxylase, and cholesterol side-chain cleavage enzyme. It is usually the first-line medication. Its cortisol-reducing effects are dose-dependent and can be seen rapidly. The major side effect is liver toxicity. Other side effects include gynecomastia, impotence, and gastrointestinal symptoms. Doses range from 200 to 1200 mg orally daily in two to three divided doses.
- **Mitotane** inhibits cholesterol side-chain cleavage enzyme and 11-β-hydroxylase. Mitotane induces permanent destruction of adrenocortical cells and, therefore, can be used to achieve medical adrenalectomy as an alternative to surgical adrenalectomy.

Glucocorticoid replacement is started at initiation of mitotane treatment. Mineralo-corticoid treatment may eventually be required. Side effects are generally dose dependent and include gastrointestinal symptoms, weakness, lethargy, leukopenia, gynecomastia, and hypercholesterolemia. Doses start at 0.5 grams orally at bedtime and are increased slowly to 2 to 3 g/day in 3 to 4 divided doses for a total of 6 to 9 months.

- **Metyrapone** inhibits 11-β-hydroxylase. Major side effects include increased androgens, hypertension, and hypokalemia through increased 11-deoxycorticosterone. Doses range from 250 to 1000 mg orally, given every 6 hours. Lower doses of 500 to 750 mg orally daily can be used when given in combination with ketoconazole and/or aminoglutethimide.
- **Aminoglutethimide** is an anticonvulsant that inhibits the cholesterol side-chain cleavage enzyme. The usual dose is 250 mg 2 to 3 times a day. Side effects include gastrointestinal upset, lethargy, ataxia, hypothyroidism, headache, bone marrow suppression, and skin rash. It is not as effective a monotherapy as ketoconazole or metyrapone, and thus is frequently used in combination with other agents.

Medical Therapy with Other Agents

- *Mifepristone (RU486)*: This antiprogestin is a cortisol receptor antagonist at high doses.
- *Octreotide*: May be useful for ectopic ACTH syndrome.
- *Etomidate*: The only intravenous drug that can reduce cortisol levels. May be useful in hospitalized patients for acute management when used in nonsedation doses as a continuous infusion.
- *Bromocriptine*: Has only a modest effect in Cushing's disease.

Cushing's Syndrome During Pregnancy

Rare cases of Cushing's syndrome during pregnancy have been reported. Pregnant patients may be treated effectively with transsphenoidal surgery for Cushing's disease. Bilateral adrenalectomy may also be performed. Metyrapone and aminoglutethimide may be used during pregnancy, but mitotane and ketoconazole, which are teratogenic, are contraindicated.

Prognosis

Untreated Cushing's syndrome is often fatal, with most deaths resulting from cardiovascular/thromboembolic complications or bacterial/fungal infections. Effective therapy, either by surgical cure or by pharmacologic control of hypercortisolism, leads to gradual improvement in the symptoms and signs of Cushing's syndrome over a period of 2 to 12 months. Hypertension, glucose intolerance, osteoporosis, and psychiatric symptoms generally improve but may not resolve completely.

Cure rates after transsphenoidal surgery for Cushing's disease range from 80% to 90%, depending on the various criteria used to define a cure. Cure is likely if the patient develops hypocortisolism in the first few days to weeks after surgery. Postoperative random plasma cortisol levels of 1.8 to 5 mcg/dL have been used to designate a cure in several studies. Remission is also achieved in an additional 45% to 80% of the patients undergoing pituitary irradiation after unsuccessful pituitary surgery. Patients requiring a second pituitary surgery have a remission rate of 43% to 71%. Most patients are rendered hypoadrenal for months to years after the procedure. During this period, they require glucocorticoid replacement therapy.

It is difficult to predict residual pituitary function after partial hypophysectomy, as some patients have normal pituitary function even after subtotal hypophysectomy; nevertheless, the more extensive the resection, the greater the risk of loss of pituitary function. Thus long-term follow-up and monitoring for signs and symptoms of tumor recurrence is mandatory. The HPA axis must be evaluated 6 to 12 months after surgery to determine the potential need for lifetime exogenous steroid replacement therapy. Patients with pan-hypopituitarism subsequent to surgery require lifetime monitoring and titration of hormone replacement therapy.

Patients with adrenal adenomas and benign ACTH-secreting tumors that can be completely resected can be cured. However, patients with ectopic ACTH secretion or adrenocortical carcinoma may have a poor prognosis associated with the underlying malignancy. These patients are rarely cured, but the hypercortisolemia can be controlled with medications or bilateral adrenalectomy. These patients usually succumb to the underlying malignancy rather than to the effects of hypercortisolemia.

KEY POINTS TO REMEMBER

- The most common cause of Cushing's syndrome is iatrogenic, exogenous glucocorticoid use.
- Findings suggestive of Cushing's syndrome include central obesity, violaceous striae, skin atrophy, easy bruising, virilization, proximal muscle weakness, and unexplained osteoporosis.
- The evaluation of Cushing's syndrome consists of biochemical confirmation of hypercortisolism (before imaging) and differentiation between ACTH-dependent and ACTH-independent causes.
- The 24-hour urine free cortisol measurement is the best initial test for diagnosing Cushing's syndrome.
- Plasma ACTH levels differentiate ACTH-dependent from ACTH-independent causes.
- Patients with adrenal adenoma or carcinoma are treated with unilateral adrenalectomy.
- Transsphenoidal adenectomy is the treatment of choice for Cushing's disease.
- ACTH-secreting tumors that can be localized by imaging studies should be removed surgically. Occult tumors and metastatic disease require medical treatment.

REFERENCES AND SUGGESTED READINGS

Aron DC, Schnall AM, Sheeler LR. Cushing's syndrome and pregnancy. *Am J Obstet Gynecol* 1990;162: 244–252.

Boscaro M, Barzon L, Fallo F, et al. Cushing's syndrome. *Lancet* 2001;357:783–791.

Clark AJ, Metherell LA. Mechanisms of disease: the adrenocorticotropin receptor and disease. *Nat Clin Pract Endocrinol Metab* 2006;2:282–290.

Findling JW, Raff H. Cushing's syndrome: important issues in diagnosis and management. *J Clin Endocrinol Metab* 2006;91:3746–3753.

Flack MR, Oldfield EH, Cutler GB Jr, et al. Urine free cortisol in the high-dose dexamethasone suppression test for the differential diagnosis of the Cushing syndrome. *Ann Intern Med* 1992;116: 211–217.

Invitti C, Pecori Giraldi F, de Martin M, et al. Diagnosis and management of Cushing's syndrome: results of an Italian multicentre study. *J Clin Endocrinol Metab* 1999;84: 440–448.

Isidori AM, Kaltsas GA, Grossman AB. Ectopic ACTH syndrome. *Front Horm Res* 2006; 35:143–156.

Jenkins PJ, Trainer PJ, Plowman PN, et al. The long-term outcome after adrenalectomy and prophylactic pituitary radiotherapy in adrenocorticotropin-dependent Cushing's syndrome. *J Clin Endocrinol Metab* 1995;80:165–171.

Kirk LF, Hash RB, Katner HP, et al. Cushing's disease: clinical manifestations and diagnostic evaluation. *Am Fam Physician* 2000;62:1119–1127.

Koerten JM, Morales WJ, Washington SR 3rd, et al. Cushing's syndrome in pregnancy: a case report and literature review. *Am J Obstet Gynecol* 1986;154:626–628.

Makras P, Toloumis G, Papadogias D, et al. The diagnosis and differential diagnosis of endogenous Cushing's syndrome. *Hormones (Athens)* 2006;5:231–250.

Meier CA, Biller BM. Clinical and biochemical evaluation of Cushing's syndrome. *Endocrinol Metab Clin North Am* 1997;26:741–762.

Newell-Price J, Bertagna X, Grossman AB, et al. Cushing's syndrome. *Lancet* 2006;367: 1605–1617.

Nieman LK, Oldfield EH, Wesley R, et al. A simplified morning ovine ACTH-releasing hormone stimulation test for the differential diagnosis of adrenoACTH-dependent Cushing's syndrome. *J Clin Endocrinol Metab* 1993;77:1308–1312.

Nieman LK. Cushing's syndrome. In: Rose BD, ed. *UpToDate*. Waltham, MA: UpToDate; 2007.

Orth DN. Cushing's syndrome. *N Engl J Med* 1995;332:791–803.

Papanicolaou DA, Yanovski JA, Cutler GB Jr, et al. A single midnight serum cortisol measurement distinguishes Cushing's syndrome from pseudo-Cushing states. *J Clin Endocrinol Metab* 1998;83: 1163–1167.

Petersenn S, Unger N, Walz MK, et al. Diagnostic value of biochemical parameters in the differential diagnosis of an adrenal mass. *Ann N Y Acad Sci.* 2006;1073:348–357.

Raff H, Raff JL, Findling JW. Late-night salivary cortisol as a screening test for Cushing's syndrome. *J Clin Endocrinol Metab* 1998;83:2681–2686.

Sonino N, Zielezny M, Fava GA, et al. Risk factors and long-term outcome in pituitary-dependent Cushing's disease. *J Clin Endocrinol Metab* 1996;81:2647–2652.

Stewart PM. The adrenal cortex. In: Larsen PR, Kronenberg HM, Melmed S, et al., eds. *Williams Textbook of Endocrinology*, 10th ed. Philadelphia: WB Saunders; 2003:491–551.

Tyrrell JB, Findling JW, Aron DC, et al. An overnight high-dose dexamethasone suppression test for rapid differential diagnosis of Cushing's syndrome. *Ann Intern Med* 1986; 104:180–186.

Yanovski JA, Cutler GB Jr, Chrousos GP, et al. ACTH-releasing hormone stimulation following low-dose dexamethasone administration: a new test to distinguish Cushing's syndrome from pseudo-Cushing's states. *JAMA* 1993;269:2232–2238.

Pheochromocytoma

Manu V. Chakravarthy

INTRODUCTION

Pheochromocytoma is a tumor arising from catecholamine producing chromaffin cells in the adrenal medulla. Similar tumors within the sympathetic and parasympathetic ganglia are classified as extraadrenal paragangliomas. Although these tumors may have similar clinical presentations and are treated with similar approaches, the distinction between pheochromocytoma and paraganglioma is an important one because of implications for associated neoplasms, risk for malignancy, and genetic testing. Pheochromocytomas can occur from infancy to old age, with peak incidence in the third and fourth decades of life. It is a rare tumor and accounts for <0.2% of cases of hypertension. Pheochromocytoma may be fatal if undiagnosed and untreated.

Although most pheochromocytomas are benign, 10% to 15% of them are malignant, as defined by local invasion or distant metastases. Biochemical behavior and histologic appearance do not predict malignant potential. Malignant pheochromocytomas tend to be indolent and metastasize to bone, liver, lymph nodes, and lung.

CAUSES

Pathophysiology

Pheochromocytomas can be either sporadic (solitary, unilateral, and intraadrenal tumors) or familial (also typically intraadrenal, but often multicentric and bilateral). The frequency of familial pheochromocytoma in two large series was approximately 20%, and they can occur in the context of autosomal dominant hereditary syndromes. Hereditary disorders associated with pheochromocytoma can be caused by mutations in either oncogenes such as *RET* (multiple endocrine neoplasia (MEN) 2) or tumor suppressor genes such as *VHL* (von Hippel-Lindau syndrome) or *NF1* (neurofibromatosis type 1). Genetic screening is recommended for patients diagnosed with pheochromocytoma before age 20 years, bilateral adrenal tumors, multiple paragangliomas, or for those who have a family history of pheochromocytoma or paraganglioma.

As pheochromocytomas arise from the adrenal medulla, these tumors intermittently release biologically active quantities of catecholamines that result in the symptoms of net vasoconstriction with increase in both systolic and diastolic blood pressure and tachycardia. Norepinephrine and epinephrine within chromaffin cells are metabolized by catechol-*O*-methyl transferase to their respective *O*-methyl derivatives, normetanephrine and metanephrine, respectively. Because the intratumoral metabolism of catecholamines is independent of its release (which can be intermittent or occur at low rates), the measurement of catecholamine metabolites in the plasma or urine provides superior diagnostic sensitivity, and forms the basis for the diagnosis of pheochromocytoma.

Differential Diagnosis

Increased sympathetic activity is seen in several conditions other than pheochromocytoma, and includes the following:

- Essential hypertension
- Anxiety disorder (during therapy with tricyclic antidepressant drugs)
- Abrupt clonidine or propranolol withdrawal
- Monoamine oxidase (MAO)–inhibitor pressor crisis
- Cocaine and amphetamine abuse
- Over-the-counter decongestants and other sympathomimetic drugs
- Myocardial infarction
- Aortic dissection
- Incidental adrenal adenoma
- Autonomic dysfunction (Guillain-Barré syndrome)
- Neuroblastoma/ganglioneuroblastoma (malignant tumors of the adrenals and sympathetic chain; hypertension is uncommon and usually occurs in childhood)
- Ganglioneuroma (benign tumors of the sympathetic chain, usually found in the posterior mediastinum with clinical features similar to paragangliomas)
- Diencephalic epilepsy

Other causes of "spells" confused with pheochromocytoma include:

- Thyrotoxicosis
- Menopausal symptoms
- Idiopathic flushing disorder
- Hyperadrenergic spells
- Renovascular disease
- Hypoglycemia
- Mast cell disease
- Carcinoid syndrome

PRESENTATION

Patients with pheochromocytoma often experience a characteristic paroxysm or crisis caused by release of catecholamines. The **classic symptomatic triad** includes episodic **headache**, **sweating**, and **palpitations**. In the presence of **hypertension**, this triad is found to be 91% sensitive and 94% specific for pheochromocytoma (Table 15-1).

Paroxysms associated with pheochromocytoma may be precipitated by displacement of abdominal contents (e.g., lifting or palpation). Typically, paroxysms last 30 to 40 minutes and occur with sufficient frequency for an event to be observed within 1 to 2 days. Paroxysms tend to increase in frequency and severity over time. Blood pressure can be elevated, often to alarming levels, when measured during a paroxysm. Several medications may precipitate a **hypertensive crisis** in the setting of pheochromocytoma (Table 15-2). These drugs should be avoided until pheochromocytoma has been excluded, resected, or the patient has been pre-medicated with an α-adrenergic antagonist.

Hypertension, present in more than 90% of patients, is the most common physical examination finding in pheochromocytoma. It is usually severe, refractory to conventional therapy, and is associated with signs of end-organ damage such as proteinuria or retinopathy; however, it may also resemble essential hypertension in the absence of paroxysms. Despite the association of pheochromocytoma with paroxysms, only 25% to 40% of patients experience truly paroxysmal hypertension, and 5% to 10% of patients present with normal blood pressure.

TABLE 15-1	SYMPTOMS AND SIGNS IN PATIENTS WITH PHEOCHROMOCYTOMA

Symptoms	Signs
Headache (80%)	Hypertension (often severe)
Sweating (71%)	Postural hypotension
Palpitations (64%)	Resting tachycardia
Pallor (42%)	Fever
Nausea (42%)	Perspiration
Tremor (31%)	Pallor (especially of the face and chest)
Weakness/fatigue (28%)	Tremor
Anxiety (22%)	Abdominal mass
Epigastric pain (22%)	Hypertension and paroxysmal symptoms after abdominal palpation
	Hypertensive retinopathy
	Retinal angiomas (von Hippel-Lindau syndrome)
	Hyperplastic corneal nerves (slit lamp exam, MEN2B)
	Marfanoid body habitus; mucosal neuromas (MEN2B)
	Thyroid nodule (MEN2A or 2B)
	Café-au-lait spots (neurofibromatosis)

MEN, multiple endocrine neoplasia.
Data from Thomas JE, et al. The neurologist's experience with pheochromocytoma. A review of 100 cases. *JAMA* 1966;197:754–758; Young WF, Kaplan NM. Diagnosis and treatment of pheochromocytoma in adults. In: Rose BD, ed. *UpToDate*. Waltham, MA: UpToDate; 2007.

TABLE 15-2	DRUGS THAT MAY PRECIPITATE HYPERTENSIVE CRISIS IN THE SETTING OF PHEOCHROMOCYTOMA

Decongestants
Tricyclic antidepressants
MAO inhibitors
Phenothiazines
β-Blockers
Metoclopramide
Atropine
Glucagon
Cosyntropin (ACTH)
Radiographic contrast
Droperidol

ACTH, adrenocorticotropic hormone; MAO, monoamine oxidase.

Headache may vary in duration and intensity and can occur in up to 80% to 90% of symptomatic patients. Generalized sweating occurs in up to 60% to 70% of patients. Other less frequent symptoms include pallor, dyspnea, generalized weakness, blurry vision, and unexplained cardiopulmonary dysfunction. Rare presentations include episodic hypotension (when the tumor secretes only epinephrine) or rapid cyclic fluctuations of blood pressure. (See Table 15-1 for more symptoms and signs of pheochromocytoma.)

Patients with pheochromocytoma may also be completely asymptomatic. In a Mayo Clinic series of 150 patients, ~10% of patients with a pheochromocytoma were discovered serendipitously by abdominal computerized technology (CT) scanning. Another series from the Cleveland Clinic of 33 patients showed that nearly 58% of patients diagnosed with adrenal pheochromocytoma were asymptomatic and their adrenal tumors were discovered incidentally on imaging done for other reasons. Therefore, the diagnosis of pheochromocytoma requires a high index of suspicion, especially in patients with one or more of the following:

- Refractory hypertension and/or onset of hypertension before 20 years of age;
- Nonexertional palpitations, spells, diaphoresis, headache, or tremor;
- Familial syndrome (e.g., MEN2, NF1, VHL) or a family history of pheochromocytoma;
- Incidental adrenal mass with imaging characteristics consistent with pheochromocytoma [marked enhancement on contrast CT or high-signal intensity on T2-weighted magnetic resonance imaging (MRI)];
- Pressor response during anesthesia and surgery;
- Idiopathic dilated cardiomyopathy.

MANAGEMENT

Diagnosis

There are two essential components to the diagnosis of pheochromocytoma: (a) biochemical confirmation and (b) anatomic localization of the tumor.

Biochemical Testing

Confirming the clinical diagnosis requires biochemical evidence of inappropriate catecholamine production. On the basis of the current consensus statements from the First International Symposium on Pheochromocytoma, initial testing should include measurements of **fractionated metanephrines in urine or plasma**, or both, as available. Based on their much superior sensitivity and specificity, catecholamine metabolites, normetanephrine and metanephrine (NMN and MN) rather than the parent catecholamines norepinephrine and epinephrine (NE and E) are the preferred measurements. VMA has no significant role in the biochemical workup given its poor sensitivity. A summary of the performance characteristics of the plasma and urine tests are presented in Table 15-3.

Biochemical parameters are typically elevated more than twofold when a pheochromocytoma is present. Although there is no current consensus on whether plasma or urine measurements are preferred, it is generally agreed that the reference intervals for either of the measurements of fractionated metanephrines should ensure the highest diagnostic sensitivity, with specificity being a secondary consideration to avoid the deadly consequences of a missed diagnosis. From this standpoint, given a 97% to 99% sensitivity (Table 15-3), plasma free metanephrines are the best initial test in patients with a high pretest probability of disease (MEN2, von Hippel-Lindau syndrome, and previously surgically cured pheochromocytomas). Because of its high negative predictive value, normal plasma NMN and MN levels essentially rule out a diagnosis of pheochromocytoma. However, given a 85% to 89% specificity, elevated plasma NMN and MN levels, unless

TABLE 15-3	PERFORMANCE CHARACTERISTICS OF BIOCHEMICAL ASSAYS FOR PHEOCHROMOCYTOMA	
Test	Sensitivity (%)	Specificity (%)
NIH series		
Plasma		
Free metanephrines	99	89
Catecholamines	84	81
24 hour urine		
Fractionated metanephrines	97	69
Total metanephrines	77	93
Catecholamines	86	88
Vanillylmandelic acid	64	95
Mayo series		
Plasma free metanephrines	97	85
24 hour urine total metanephrines and catecholamine	90	98

NIH, National Institutes of Health.

Adapted from Lenders JW, et al. Biochemical diagnosis of pheochromocytoma: which test is best? *JAMA* 2002;287:1427–1434; Sawka AM, et al. A comparison of biochemical tests for pheochromocytoma: measurement of fractionated plasma metanephrines compared with the combination of 24-hour urinary metanephrines and catecholamines. *J Clin Endocrinol Metab* 2003;88: 553–558.

markedly increased, need to be further confirmed with more specific tests such as 24-hour urine metanephrines and catecholamines (98% specific), or plasma chromogranin A (96% specific).

If there is ambiguity in differentiating false-positive from true-positive results, further biochemical testing is necessary before proceeding to imaging. Prior to repeating the tests, careful consideration of the various causes of false-positive results from medications and other factors is warranted (Table 15-4). Although existing data regarding the effect of posture on plasma NMN and MN measurements are ambiguous, to further minimize the likelihood of false-positive results, ideally, blood samples should be collected from patients in the supine position with a venous catheter in place for at least 30 minutes.

The much improved biochemical assays for catecholamines and their metabolites have made pharmacologic tests for pheochromocytoma largely unnecessary. However, the **clonidine suppression test** and **glucagon stimulation test** are occasionally helpful. The clonidine suppression test may be useful when plasma catecholamines are elevated but nondiagnostic; a decrease in plasma norepinephrine by >50% is the normal expected response, whereas consistently elevated levels suggest pheochromocytoma. False-positive results can occur in patients taking tricyclic antidepressants or beta-blockers. A more than threefold rise in plasma norepinephrine after administration of glucagon diagnoses pheochromocytoma with high specificity, but the test has low sensitivity. Premedication

TABLE 15-4 FACTORS INTERFERING WITH BIOCHEMICAL TESTING

Stimulation of endogenous catecholamines	Exogenous catecholamines	Drugs that alter catecholamine metabolism	Drugs that interfere with biochemical assays
• Emotional and physical stress (surgery, trauma) • Drug withdrawal (alcohol, clonidine) • Drugs (vasodilators, caffeine, nicotine, theophylline, ephedrine, amphetamines) • Hypoglycemia • Obstructive sleep apnea • Myocardial ischemia • Stroke	• Bronchodilators • Appetite suppressants • Decongestants	• β-Blockers (falsely increases urine catecholamines and metanephrines) • Phenoxybenzamine (falsely increases plasma and urine norepinephrine and normetanephrine) • Tricyclic antidepressants (falsely increases plasma and urine norepinephrine and normetanephrine) • Levodopa • Methyldopa • Theophylline • MAO-inhibitors	• Labetalol, sotalol[a] • Acetaminophen[b] • Clofibrate • Quinidine

ACE, angiotensin-converting enzyme; HPLC, high performance liquid chromography; MAO, monoamine oxidase.; SSRI, selective serotonin uptake inhibitors.

[a]Interference only with the spectrophotometric assay for metanephrines; catecholamines measured by HPLC and metanephrines by mass spectrometry are not affected.

[b]Plasma free metanephrines measured by HPLC are not affected.

Diuretics, ACE inhibitors, and SSRIs generally do not interfere with the biochemical tests.

---

with an α-adrenergic blocker is necessary to limit the potential pressor response to norepinephrine.

Anatomic Localization

Radiologic evaluation should be initiated only after biochemical confirmation of catecholamine excess. In situations of a high-pretest probability, less compelling biochemical evidence might justify imaging studies. Based on the First International Symposium on Pheochromocytoma, there was no consensus on whether CT or MRI is preferred for initial localization of a tumor. Because ~95% of pheochromocytomas are intraabdominal, an abdominal CT or MRI scan is usually obtained first. Both modalities have high sensitivity (95%–100%), but relatively low specificity (~70%) owing to the higher prevalence of adrenal "incidentalomas." Hyperintensity on T2-weighted MRI images may distinguish pheochromocytoma from other adrenal tumors, which are isointense to liver.

If the CT or MRI scan does not detect an intraadrenal tumor despite strong clinical and biochemical evidence, then evaluation for extraadrenal pheochromocytoma should be undertaken with ^{123}I-MIBG. MIBG is a marker for norepinephrine storage that is concentrated in pheochromocytomas. MIBG scans have lower sensitivity (80%–90%), but higher specificity (~100%) than either CT or MRI. ^{123}I-MIBG is more sensitive than ^{131}I-MIBG. An octreoscan (^{111}In-octreotide) is insensitive (<30%) but may detect tumors in unusual locations when MIBG scans are negative, especially in metastatic pheochromocytoma. [18]Fluoro-dopamine PET scanning may be useful in identifying metastases, but its role is yet to be fully determined in identifying sporadic benign pheochromocytomas.

Treatment

Surgical resection is the definitive therapy for pheochromocytoma. Removing a pheochromocytoma is a high-risk surgical procedure, and an experienced surgeon–anesthesiologist team is required. In addition, patients must undergo appropriate medical preparation to control the effects of excessive adrenergic stimulation and prevent intraoperative hypertensive crisis. An endocrinologist or other physician experienced in the management of pheochromocytoma should supervise preoperative therapy.

Phenoxybenzamine is the preferred drug for preoperative preparation to control blood pressure. It is an irreversible, long-acting, nonspecific α-adrenergic antagonist. A starting dose of 10 mg orally once or twice a day is titrated (in divided doses to between 20 and 100 mg total daily dose) until the patient's blood pressure and symptoms are controlled and orthostasis occurs. Volume expansion (e.g., with oral salt supplements or intravenous fluids) helps minimize hypotension. Tachycardia may develop during α-blockade and require treatment with a β-blocker. However, **β-blockers should not be started until after adequate α-adrenergic blockade is achieved** (usually 2–3 days later) to prevent a paradoxical rise in blood pressure due to unopposed α-adrenergic receptor stimulation. Underlying cardiomyopathy (due to chronic catecholamine exposure) may also become evident with the initiation of β-adrenergic blockade, resulting in acute pulmonary edema. Therefore, when the β-blocker is administered, it should be used cautiously and at a low dose (e.g., 10 mg of propranolol every 6 hours to start), with the dose increased as necessary to control the tachycardia (goal heart rate is 60–80 beats per minute). Typically, the patient is ready for surgery in about 10 to 14 days following the preoperative medical treatment regimen described previously. α-Blockade may be started at a low dose as an outpatient, but patients may need to be admitted to the hospital for dose titration because of the expected development of orthostatic hypotension.

Preoperative treatment with a calcium channel blocker has also been demonstrated as an effective medical preparation before surgery. Calcium channel blockers can be used as supplements to α- and β-adrenergic blockade to achieve blood pressure control or as an alternative therapy if adrenergic blockade causes severe side effects. Metyrosine (1–2 g orally daily), an agent that inhibits catecholamine biosynthesis, may be added to phenoxybenzamine therapy, or used for patients who cannot be treated with the typical α- and β-adrenergic blockade protocol because of intolerance or cardiopulmonary reasons. Metyrosine is also useful for long-term management of inoperable patients.

Pheochromocytomas have traditionally been resected through a transabdominal approach. However, refinements in radiologic localization have permitted an increase in laparoscopic resections through a flank incision, which is currently the procedure of choice for patients with solitary intraadrenal pheochromocytomas. Laparoscopic approach usually results in less intraoperative blood loss, shorter operative time and length of hospital stay, and lower costs compared to open adrenalectomy. For intraadrenal sporadic pheochromocytoma, the entire gland should be removed. Patients with familial pheochromocytomas (MEN2 or von Hippel-Lindau disease) have a high incidence of bilateral disease and usually require bilateral adrenalectomies. When bilateral adrenalectomy is planned, the patient should receive perioperative "stress-dose" glucocorticoid coverage and appropriate postoperative glucocorticoid management.

Intraoperative hypertension and cardiac arrhythmias usually occur during anesthesia induction, intubation, or tumor manipulation. Acute hypertensive crises should be treated intravenously with sodium nitroprusside, phentolamine, or nicardipine. Lidocaine or esmolol can be used for cardiac arrhythmias. After tumor resection, patients may experience mild hypotension, but severe hypotension can be avoided with aggressive fluid replacement. Approximately 10% to 15% of patients may experience postoperative hypoglycemia that can be managed by short-term infusion of glucose.

Prognosis

In a large surgical series, overall perioperative mortality and morbidity rates were 2.4% and 24%, respectively. Risk factors for operative complications include large tumor, high urine catecholamine and metanephrine levels, prolonged surgery and anesthesia, and severe preoperative hypertension. Surgical removal of a pheochromocytoma does not always lead to long-term cure of pheochromocytoma or hypertension, even in patients with a benign tumor. In one series, pheochromocytoma recurred as a benign or malignant tumor in 14% of patients with an apparently benign tumor at the time of surgical resection. Hypertension-free survival in patients without recurrence was 74% at 5 years and 45% at 10 years. Survival does not appear to be affected by the site of the tumor. Patients with malignant pheochromocytoma have a 5-year survival of ~40%. Recurrence is more likely in patients with familial pheochromocytoma/paraganglioma, right-sided adrenal tumors, and extraadrenal tumors.

Long-term follow-up is indicated in all patients, even in those apparently cured. Catecholamines and metanephrines should be rechecked one week after surgery to assess the adequacy of tumor resection by monitoring for a return to the laboratory reference range. If levels are normal, patients should be screened annually for 5 years and biannually thereafter, or if symptoms suspicious for pheochromocytoma recur. Patients with familial tumor syndromes, bilateral tumors, or paragangliomas should be monitored annually.

Special Topics

Malignant Pheochromocytoma

Approximately 10% of all catecholamine-secreting tumors are malignant. Other than local invasion or distant metastases, there are no distinctive histologic or biochemical characteristics that differentiate benign from malignant pheochromocytomas. However, recent studies have shown that patients harboring a succinate dehydrogenase B mutation are more likely to develop malignant disease. Although a reduction in tumor size is palliative, a distinct survival advantage of debulking is unproven. Reduced tumor burden can help with subsequent radiation therapy, which may be useful for treatment of symptomatic bone metastases. Combination chemotherapy with cyclophosphamide, vincristine, and dacarbazine may result in tumor regression and symptom relief in up to 50% of patients, but the responses are short-lived. ^{131}I-MIBG therapy is the single most effective adjunct to surgical therapy for malignant pheochromocytomas.

Pregnancy

Pheochromocytoma is a rare but potentially lethal cause of hypertension during pregnancy, with features similar to those in the general population. However, if hypertension and proteinuria occur, pheochromocytoma may be difficult to distinguish from preeclampsia. Diagnosis is still made on the basis of elevated plasma and/or urinary fractionated metanephrines and anatomic localization by MRI. Nuclear scintigraphy and stimulation tests are considered unsafe during pregnancy. Women should be prepared for surgery with phenoxybenzamine followed by β-blockade as necessary for tachycardia. Although phenoxybenzamine is considered to be safe for the fetus, it does cross the placenta and can cause perinatal depression and transient hypotension. If the diagnosis of pheochromocytoma is made before 24 weeks of gestation, surgical resection is usually performed. After 24 weeks of gestation, medical management is continued until fetal maturation (as close to term as possible), at which time combined cesarean delivery and tumor resection are performed.

KEY POINTS TO REMEMBER

- Pheochromocytomas are catecholamine-hypersecreting tumors of chromaffin cells in the adrenal medulla. Neurochromaffin tumors arising in sympathetic and parasympathetic ganglia are called paragangliomas.
- Pheochromocytomas often cause severe hypertension. Patients may experience a classic triad of paroxysmal symptoms that includes severe headache, diaphoresis, and palpitations.
- Measurements of plasma or urinary fractionated metanephrines (normetanephrine and metanephrine) are the most accurate screening tests for pheochromocytoma.
- Tumors are typically located by CT or MRI, which should only be performed after obtaining reasonable clinical and/or biochemical evidence of a tumor. Pheochromocytomas have a characteristic bright appearance on T2-weighted MRI images. Nuclear scintigraphy is sometimes required when CT or MRI does not identify a tumor.
- Laproscopic surgery is the treatment of choice, and is the only cure for benign pheochromocytomas and paragangliomas. Patients must be pretreated with α-adrenergic blockade or combined α- and β-adrenergic blockade to avoid intraoperative complications (hypertensive crises or cardiac arrhythmias).
- Malignant pheochromocytoma cannot be diagnosed histologically and is defined by the presence of metastases. Accordingly, long-term follow-up is necessary after surgical resection to screen for recurrence.

REFERENCES AND SUGGESTED READINGS

Bravo EL, Tagle R. Pheochromocytoma: state-of-the-art and future prospects. *Endocr Rev* 2003;24:539–553.

Dluhy RG, Lawrence JE, Williams GH. Endocrine hypertension. In: Larsen PR, Kronenberg HM, Melmed S, et al., eds. *Williams Textbook of Endocrinology*, 10th ed. Philadelphia: WB Saunders; 2003:552–585.

Eisenhofer G, Lenders JW, Pacak K. Biochemical diagnosis of pheochromocytoma. *Front Horm Res* 2004;31:76–106.

Eisenhofer G, Goldstein DS, Walther MM, et al. Biochemical diagnosis of pheochromocytoma: how to distinguish true- from false-positive test results. *J Clin Endocrinol Metab* 2003;88:2656–2666.

Eisenhofer G, Kopin IJ, Goldstein DS. Catecholamine metabolism: a contemporary view with implications for physiology and medicine. *Pharmacol Rev* 2004;56:331–349.

Gimm O, Koch CA, Januszewicz A, et al. The genetic basis of pheochromocytoma. *Front Horm Res* 2004;31:45–60.

Goldstein RE, O'Neill JA Jr, Holcomb GW 3rd, et al. Clinical experience over 48 years with pheochromocytoma. *Ann Surg* 1999;229:755–764.

Ilias I, Pacak K. Current approaches and recommended algorithm for the diagnostic localization of pheochromocytoma. *J Clin Endocrinol Metab* 2004;89:479–491.

Kinney MA, Warner ME, vanHeerden JA, et al. Perianesthetic risks and outcomes of pheochromocytoma and paraganglioma resections. *Anesth Analg* 2000;91:1118–1123.

Lenders JW, Pacak K, Walther MM, et al. Biochemical diagnosis of pheochromocytoma: which test is best? *JAMA* 2002;287:1427–1434.

Neumann HP, Bausch B, McWhinney SR, et al. Germ-line mutations in nonsyndromic pheochromocytoma. *N Engl J Med* 2002;346:1459–1466.

Pacak K, Eisenhofer G, Ilias I. Diagnostic imaging of pheochromocytoma. *Front Horm Res* 2004;31: 107–120.

Pacak K, Eisenhofer G, Ahlman H, et al. Pheochromocytoma: recommendations for clinical practice from the First International Symposium. *Nat Clin Pract Endocrinol Metab* 2007;3:92–102.

Plouin PF, Chatellier G, Fofol I, et al. Tumor recurrence and hypertension persistence after successful pheochromocytoma operation. *Hypertension* 1997;29:1133–1139.

Roden M, Raffesberg W, Raber W, et al. Quantification of unconjugated metanephrines in human plasma without interference by acetaminophen. *Clin Chem* 2001;47: 1061–1067.

Sawka AM, Jaeschke R, Singh RJ, et al. A comparison of biochemical tests for pheochromocytoma: measurement of fractionated plasma metanephrines compared with the combination of 24-hour urinary metanephrines and catecholamines. *J Clin Endocrinol Metab* 2003;88:553–558.

Thomas JE, Rooke ED, Kvale WF. The neurologist's experience with pheochromocytoma. A review of 100 cases. *JAMA* 1966;197:754–758.

Ulchaker JC, Goldfarb DA, Bravo EL, et al. Successful outcomes in pheochromocytoma surgery in the modern era. *J Urol* 1999;161:764–767.

Yeo H, Roman S. Pheochromocytoma and functional paraganglioma. *Curr Opin Oncol* 2005;17:13–18.

Young WF, Kaplan NM. Diagnosis and treatment of pheochromocytoma in adults. In: Rose BD, ed. *UpToDate*, Waltham, MA: UpToDate; 2007.

Young WF. The incidentally discovered adrenal mass. *N Engl J Med* 2007;356:601–610.

Amenorrhea

16

Paraskevi Mentzelopoulos

INTRODUCTION

Beginning in puberty, pulsatile gonadotropin-releasing hormone (GnRH) production stimulates secretion and release of luteinizing hormone (LH) and follicle-stimulating hormone (FSH) from the pituitary gland. During the late luteal phase, GnRH is secreted episodically every 90 to 120 minutes, in response to a central nervous system "pulse generator." This rate of pulsatile release favors FSH secretion. FSH, in turn, stimulates ovarian follicles to develop. The follicle with the most FSH receptors becomes the dominant follicle, whereas the remaining follicles eventually undergo atresia. The theca cells surrounding the follicles produce androgens, which are aromatized to **estradiol** by neighboring granulosa cells. As the follicles develop, estradiol levels increase. The increasing level of estradiol provides negative feedback to the pituitary to suppress FSH. Estradiol is also involved in a positive feedback loop that increases the frequency of GnRH pulses (every 60 minutes) during the follicular phase and acts directly on the pituitary to stimulate LH secretion. LH further increases estradiol production, and this increases pituitary sensitivity to GnRH and results in a rapid elevation in LH production—the LH surge—which stimulates ovulation.

Progesterone levels start increasing just before ovulation. Approximately 36 hours after the LH surge, the oocyte is released from the dominant follicle at the surface of the ovary. After ovulation, the ruptured follicle (corpus luteum) continues to secrete progesterone. This hormone is involved in a negative feed-back loop to decrease GnRH pulsatility to every 3 to 5 hours, favoring FSH synthesis during the luteal-follicular transition. The granulosa cells continue to produce progesterone for approximately 14 days after ovulation, but then involute (luteolysis) unless pregnancy is established.

During the menstrual cycle the endometrium responds to hormones secreted from the ovaries. During the follicular phase, estrogens stimulate the proliferative phase of the endometrium. After ovulation, progesterone inhibits further endometrial proliferation and during the luteal phase causes several changes in the endometrium to prepare for implantation (secretory phase). If there is no implantation of an embryo, the endometrium enters the degenerative phase as a result of progesterone and estrogen withdrawal. The decline in estradiol and progesterone results in sloughing of the endometrium and the onset of menses.

Disturbance of this cycle at any level—the hypothalamus, pituitary, uterus, or ovary—can lead to disruption of the normal menstrual cycle, including cessation of menses.

Puberty is characterized by the onset of regular menstrual cycles and development of secondary sexual features. The average time between the onset of thelarche (breast development) and menarche (onset of menses) is 2 years. The age of menarche is variable depending on genetic and socioeconomic factors. The mean age of menarche in the United States is approximately 12 years. There are significant differences in the ages at menarche among racial groups.

An average adult **menstrual cycle** lasts approximately 28 days and usually has little cycle variability between the ages of 20 and 40 years. There is considerably more variation in a woman's menstrual cycle for the first 5 to 7 years after menarche and for the last 10 years before menopause. Most of the variations in the menstrual cycle are caused by changes in duration of the follicular phase. The luteal phase is not as variable and usually lasts 12 to 14 days after ovulation.

The mean age of **menopause** in the United States is 51 years but may occur earlier in women who smoke, have never had children, or have a family history of early menopause. Cessation of menses before age 40 is generally considered premature menopause. The 2 to 8 years before menopause are often characterized by irregular menses and breakthrough bleeding, as the normal ovulatory cycle is interspersed with anovulatory cycles of varying length.

Definition

Amenorrhea is the absence of menses or abnormal cessation of menses. Amenorrhea is further subdivided into primary or secondary amenorrhea.

Primary amenorrhea is defined as failure to menstruate by age 15 in the presence of normal secondary sexual development, or within 5 years after breast development that occurs before age 10.

Secondary amenorrhea is defined as the absence of menses for more than three cycles in women with previously regular menstrual cycles (after the exclusion of pregnancy) or for >6 months in women with previous oligomenorrhea.

Oligomenorrhea is defined as less than nine menstrual cycles a year.

Women who do not menstruate within 3 months after the discontinuation of oral contraceptives should be evaluated for amenorrhea.

Prevalence

The prevalence of amenorrhea not resulting from pregnancy, lactation, or menopause is 3% to 4%. Primary amenorrhea is seen in 10% to 15% of these cases.

CAUSES

The most common causes of amenorrhea are polycystic ovary syndrome (PCOS), hypothalamic amenorrhea, hyperprolactinemia, and ovarian failure.

Primary Amenorrhea

Primary amenorrhea usually results from an anatomic or genetic abnormality (Table 16-1), although most causes of secondary amenorrhea may also present as primary amenorrhea.

The most common cause of primary amenorrhea is chromosomal abnormalities causing **gonadal dysgenesis** (45%), such as Turner's syndrome. Turner's syndrome is caused by the absence of one of the X chromosomes (45,XO). Patients have normal development of external female genitalia, uterus, and fallopian tubes until puberty, at which time there is failure of sexual maturation owing to lack of estrogen. Gonadal failure in genetically XX females is known as premature ovarian failure (POF) and can occur at any age (see subsequent text). Individuals with XY gonadal dysgenesis (Swyer's syndrome) have female genitalia; the most frequent gene defect in these individuals is a mutation in the *SRY* gene (sex-determining region of the Y chromosome). In this case, gonads should be removed at the time of diagnosis because of the high risk for malignancy.

Congenital anatomic lesions of reproductive organs account for approximately 20% of primary amenorrhea. Menses cannot occur without an intact reproductive tract, including

TABLE 16-1   CAUSES OF PRIMARY AMENORRHEA

Congenital anatomic lesions

Müllerian agenesis, androgen insensitivity syndrome, vanishing testes syndrome, isolated vaginal or cervical agenesis

Outflow tract obstruction secondary to transverse vaginal septum or imperforate hymen

Enzyme deficiencies causing abnormalities in steroidogenesis

   5-α-reductase deficiency, 17-α-hydroxylase deficiency

   17,20-lyase deficiency, aromatase deficiency, galactosemia

Chromosomal abnormalities

Turner's syndrome (45,XO)

Swyer's syndrome (46,XY)

Fragile X

Trisomy X

Mixed gonadal dysgenesis 45,X/46,XY

Constitutional delay of puberty

Pregnancy

Ovarian etiologies

Premature ovarian failure

Mumps oophoritis

Tumors

Gonadotropin deficiency or defects in action

Idiopathic hypogonadotrophic hypogonadism or Kallmann's syndrome

FSH and LH receptor mutations

Damage to hypothalamus or pituitary from trauma, mass effect (adenoma, craniopharyngioma), infarction (Sheehan's syndrome), infiltrative or inflammatory diseases (sarcoidosis, lymphocytic hypophysitis)

Functional hypothalamic amenorrhea (exercise, eating disorders, stress, chronic illness)

Other endocrine diseases (hyperprolactinemia, hypothyroidism, Cushing's syndrome, polycystic ovary syndrome, nonclassic congenital adrenal hyperplasia)

the uterus, cervix, and vagina. An imperforate hymen can lead to obstruction of menstrual blood flow and lack of menses, and patients present with complaints of amenorrhea and cyclical abdominal pain.

Abnormal müllerian development secondary to various syndromes, such as müllerian agenesis, androgen insensitivity syndrome, and vanishing testes syndrome, can lead to primary amenorrhea. Müllerian agenesis is the most common of these disorders (~10% of primary amenorrhea cases). Patients are phenotypically and genetically female; they have normal secondary sexual characteristics, including pubic hair, but have congenital absence of a vagina and abnormal uterine development. Complete androgen insensitivity syndrome (also referred to as testicular feminization) is rare and is characterized by a 46,XY karyotype. Patients appear as phenotypically normal women, including breast development, but have minimal or no pubic hair and absence of uterus, fallopian tubes, and the upper two-thirds of the vagina. The syndrome is caused by a defect in the androgen receptor that results in resistance to the actions of testosterone. The external genitalia appear to be female, although the testes can often be palpated in the labia or inguinal region. It must be differentiated from müllerian agenesis, because in androgen insensitivity syndrome there is a high incidence of gonadal malignancy and gonads should be removed after the desired height has been achieved.

Less common causes of primary amenorrhea are **enzyme deficiencies** causing abnormalities in steroidogenesis, such as 5-α-reductase deficiency, 17-α-hydroxylase deficiency, 17,20-lyase deficiency, aromatase deficiency, or FSH and LH **receptor mutations**. There are multiple **hypothalamic causes** of primary amenorrhea, including functional hypothalamic amenorrhea, tumors, infiltrative lesions, and infections. Constitutional delay of puberty is the most common physiologic cause. Congenital GnRH deficiency resulting from idiopathic hypogonadotropic hypogonadism (IHH) or Kallmann's syndrome causes amenorrhea owing to deficiency or absence of GnRH secretion. Kallmann's syndrome is associated with anosmia, which distinguishes it from IHH.

Functional amenorrhea is caused by abnormal GnRH secretion, resulting in subsequent low GnRH pulsations, decreased serum LH, absent LH surge, anovulation, and low serum estradiol. Weight loss, anorexia nervosa, stress, and intense exercise are some of the common causes of functional hypothalamic amenorrhea. Three percent of adolescents presenting with primary amenorrhea will have hypothalamic dysfunction because of these reasons. Infiltrative diseases and tumors, such as craniopharyngioma, germinoma, and histiocytosis, can cause either primary or secondary amenorrhea, depending on the patient's age at presentation.

Hyperprolactinemia, whether from a pituitary adenoma or secondary source, can cause primary or secondary amenorrhea and may be associated with galactorrhea.

Physiologic causes, such as **pregnancy** or physiologic delay of puberty, should always be considered in the evaluation of primary amenorrhea.

Secondary Amenorrhea

Pregnancy is the most common cause of secondary amenorrhea. After pregnancy, ovarian disease (40%) and hypothalamic dysfunction (35%) are also common causes. Certainly, if the woman is of a typical age (>40 years) and/or manifests the usual associated symptoms (e.g., hot flashes, vaginal dryness), physiologic menopause should be considered.

Hyperandrogenism from any source can lead to amenorrhea due to chronic anovulation. Hyperandrogenic anovulation can be caused by late-onset congenital adrenal hyperplasia, Cushing's syndrome, PCOS, exogenous androgen use, or adrenal tumors. The most common cause is PCOS and is discussed in Chapter 20, Polycystic Ovary Syndrome (PCOS).

Other, less common, ovarian etiologies include ovarian tumors, premature ovarian failure (idiopathic, autoimmune, radiation, chemotherapy), and mosaic Turner's syndrome.

Premature ovarian failure (POF) is characterized by amenorrhea, estrogen deficiency and elevated FSH level in patients younger than 40 years of age. Ovarian function may fluctuate. Up to 40% of women with POF may have other autoimmune endocrinopathies such as autoimmune thyroiditis, type 1 diabetes mellitus, hypoparathyroidism, myasthenia gravis and, very rarely, Addison's disease (see Chapter 35, Autoimmune Polyendocrine Syndromes).

Women who are carriers of the permutation of fragile X syndrome can experience premature menopause.

All of the **hypothalamic lesions** that cause primary amenorrhea, except congenital GnRH deficiency, can also cause secondary amenorrhea. Of all of the hypothalamic etiologies, the most common cause of secondary amenorrhea is functional hypothalamic amenorrhea. Other less common hypothalamic causes are listed in Table 16-2.

Prolactin-secreting pituitary tumors are also a fairly common cause of secondary amenorrhea, comprising almost 20% of cases. Other, less common, pituitary causes of secondary amenorrhea are listed in Table 16-2.

Primary **hypothyroidism** can cause amenorrhea.

TABLE 16-2 CAUSES OF SECONDARY AMENORRHEA

Physiologic

Pregnancy

Menopause

Ovarian etiologies

Tumors

Prior chemotherapy, pelvic radiation, surgical trauma

Premature ovarian failure (autoimmune polyendocrinopathy, gene mutations, idiopathic)

Mosaic Turner's syndrome

Uterine etiologies

Asherman's syndrome (acquired scarring of the endometrial lining)

Pituitary etiologies

Prolactin-secreting pituitary tumor

Other nonlactotrophic pituitary adenomas

Space-occupying lesions

Empty sella syndrome

Pituitary infarction (Sheehan's syndrome)

Infiltrative lesions (lymphocytic hypophysitis)

Radiation, surgery

Hypothalamic etiologies

Functional hypothalamic amenorrhea (exercise, anorexia nervosa, weight loss, stress, chronic disease, depression)

Infiltrative diseases of the hypothalamus (sarcoidosis, lymphoma, Langerhans' cell histiocytosis, hemochromatosis)

Endocrine disorders

Primary hypothyroidism

Hyperprolactinemia from cause other than prolactin-secreting pituitary tumor (e.g., medication induced)

Cushing's syndrome

Polycystic ovary syndrome (PCOS)

Adrenal tumors with androgen overproduction

HAIRAN (hyperandrogenic, insulin resistance acanthosis nigricans) syndrome

Nonclassic congenital adrenal hyperplasia

Evaluation of Amenorrhea

The initial evaluation of the patient should include a detailed history; physical examination with thorough assessment of external and internal genitalia; FSH, prolactin, and TSH levels; and assessment of endogenous estrogen production (presence of secondary sexual characteristics, progesterone challenge test).

PRESENTATION

History

A careful history includes:

- Age of menarche
- Frequency and length of previous menstrual cycles
- Sexual activity
- Number of pregnancies and any complications
- Family history of pubertal development, menarche, and menstrual history (e.g., physiologic delay of puberty)
- Family history of genetic defects
- Weight changes, dietary habits
- Exercise regimen
- Psychosocial stressors
- Prescription medication or illicit drug use
- Gynecologic surgery/instrumentation or infection
- History of chemotherapy, central nervous system (CNS), or pelvic radiation

Review of Symptoms

- Symptoms of estrogen deficiency (e.g., hot flashes, vaginal dryness, decreased libido)
- Symptoms of endocrine diseases (e.g., hypothyroidism, galactorrhea)
- Symptoms of mass effect (e.g., headache, visual disturbance)
- History of anosmia (Kallmann's syndrome)
- Cyclic abdominal pain and breast changes (outflow obstruction or müllerian agenesis)

Physical Examination

Physical examination should include weight, height, breast examination, and pelvic examination. *In cases of primary amenorrhea it is very important to assess Tanner stage and the presence of secondary sexual characteristics that suggest exposure to estrogen action.*

Review of the growth chart may indicate constitutional delay of growth and puberty. Short stature, webbed neck, and widely spaced nipples should raise suspicion of Turner's syndrome.

A blind or absent vagina with breast development suggests müllerian agenesis, transverse vaginal septum (pubic hair present), or androgen insensitivity syndrome (minimal or no pubic hair). Patients with **hirsutism** or male pattern hair loss should have a free serum testosterone level checked. Signs of **virilization** (deepening of the voice, clitoromegaly, increased muscle mass) on physical examination should always prompt further evaluation for an androgen-secreting tumor.

Central obesity, supraclavicular fat pads, easy bruising, skin thinning, proximal muscle weakness, glucose intolerance, and hypertension should raise the suspicion of Cushing's syndrome.

Acanthosis nigricans is associated with insulin resistance, a feature of PCOS and hyperandrogenic insulin resistant acanthosis nigricans (HAIRAN) syndrome.

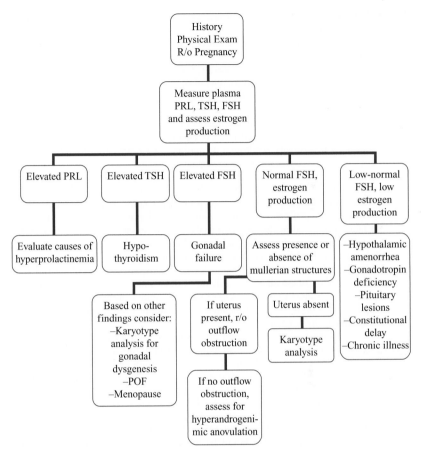

FIGURE 16-1. Diagnostic algorithm for amenorrhea.

Laboratory Evaluation and Imaging Studies

In primary amenorrhea a pelvic ultrasound should be done to confirm the presence of uterus and müllerian structures.

Absence of müllerian structures should prompt further evaluation with a karyotype analysis and serum testosterone level.

Rule out pregnancy by checking β-human chorionic gonadotropin (hCG). If the β-hCG is negative, other basic laboratory tests should include thyroid-stimulating hormone (TSH), prolactin (PRL) level, and FSH. Figure 16-1 provides an algorithm for the diagnostic workup of amenorrhea, listing the most common causes.

- **Elevated FSH levels** (hypergonadotropic amenorrhea ~40 % of cases)
    - If the FSH level is elevated, this suggests a **primary ovarian etiology and gonadal failure**. In the setting of primary amenorrhea and absence of secondary sexual characteristics, a karyotype analysis should be performed to rule out a chromosomal abnormality such as Turner's syndrome (45,XO) or premature ovarian failure (46,XX), or to rule out the presence of an occult Y chromosome, which is associated with an increased risk for gonadal tumors.

- In the setting of secondary amenorrhea, a karyotype analysis should also be performed to rule out mosaic Turner's syndrome. Other causes for premature ovarian failure such as ovarian lesions, prior trauma, radiation, and chemotherapy should be evaluated (see Table 16-1). Premature ovarian failure can be seen in the setting of polyglandular autoimmune syndromes but can also be idiopathic. If the patient is of an appropriate age and has associated symptoms, physiologic menopause can be diagnosed.
- **Normal FSH levels with evidence of estrogen production** (normogonadotropic amenorrhea ~30% of cases)
  - Normal gonadotropins with evidence of estrogen production (breast development) in primary amenorrhea could point to anatomic defects (like müllerian agenesis, androgen insensitivity syndrome) or outflow tract obstruction (like imperforate hymen, vaginal septum, cervical or vaginal agenesis).
  - In secondary amenorrhea if there is a history of uterine infection or instrumentation, the possibility of outflow obstruction (Asherman's syndrome) should be addressed.
  - Withdrawal bleeding in response to **progestin challenge test** (medroxyprogesterone, 10 mg orally daily for 10 days) rules out a uterine outflow tract obstruction.
  - Failure to respond to the progestin challenge with bleeding suggests either inadequate estrogen production to support endometrial proliferation or outflow tract obstruction. To differentiate these possibilities, the challenge is repeated with a combination of estrogen and progesterone (conjugated equine estrogen [Premarin] 1.25 mg orally daily or estradiol 2 mg daily for 21 days followed by progesterone as noted previously). Failure to bleed in response to this combination regimen strongly suggests outflow obstruction and should lead to anatomic investigation by hysterosalpingogram or hysteroscopy.
  - In the presence of hirsutism and other signs of androgen excess such as acne, seborrhea, and alopecia, causes of hyperandrogenic anovulation should be ruled out. Polycystic ovary syndrome is the most common cause of hyperandrogenic anovulation, but it is a diagnosis of exclusion (see Chapter 20, Polycystic Ovary Syndrome [PCOS]). A 17-hydroxyprogesterone level should be measured to rule out nonclassic congenital adrenal hyperplasia (CAH); 21-hydroxylase deficiency is the most common cause of nonclassic CAH (see also Chapter 20, Polycystic Ovary Syndrome [PCOS]). Testosterone and dehydroepiandrosterone sulfate (DHEA-S) should be measured, and, if elevated (total testosterone, >200 ng/dL; DHEA-S, >600 mcg/dL), appropriate imaging should be ordered to rule out the presence of an adrenal tumor. Cushing's syndrome can be ruled out with a 1-mg overnight dexamethasone suppression test or 24-hour urine free cortisol.
- **Low FSH levels and no evidence of estrogen production** (hypogonadotropic amenorrhea ~30% of cases)
  - Low gonadotropin levels point to a central etiology (hypothalamic or pituitary pathology), and a cranial MRI is indicated in most cases to rule out a hypothalamic or pituitary lesion before other etiologies are considered. In primary amenorrhea, the most common cause in this class of disorders is constitutional delay of puberty, and this accounts for almost 10% of cases. Other causes are hypothalamic or pituitary lesions, infiltrative diseases, idiopathic GnRH deficiency, Kallman's syndrome, or functional hypothalamic amenorrhea.
  - In secondary amenorrhea, the most common cause is functional hypothalamic amenorrhea. Panhypopituitarism secondary to space-occupying lesions, infiltrative diseases, pituitary apoplexy, previous surgery, or radiation would be other causes of hypogonadotropic amenorrhea with low estrogen production. A progesterone challenge test, as described previously, can help characterize endogenous estrogen production. No withdrawal bleeding after a 10-day administration of progestin would

suggest inadequate estrogen production to support endometrial proliferation. Unfortunately up to 20% of women with estrogen production will have a false-positive test and up to 40% of women with hypothalamic amenorrhea will have a false-negative test.

- Further evaluation and management for women with hyperprolactinemia is discussed in Chapter 2, Prolactinoma.
- Evaluation and treatment for patients with primary hypothyroidism is covered in Chapter 9, Hypothyroidism.

TREATMENT

Treatment for amenorrhea is directed at correcting the underlying etiology and, if possible and desired, achieving fertility.

Patients with a congenital or genetic cause for primary amenorrhea should be counseled about the underlying cause and their potential for achieving sexual maturation, induction of menses, and reproduction. Induction of puberty should be pursued under the direction of a specialist because the timing of menarche can greatly affect epiphyseal closure and final adult height. Patients with congenital anatomic abnormalities may require surgical correction. Patients with Y chromosomal material and residual testes should have their testes excised after puberty owing to the increased risk of testicular cancer after age 25.

Women with gonadal dysgenesis or failure can now carry a pregnancy on their own with the use of donor oocytes and new assisted reproductive technologies. For women with ovaries but no uterus, their own oocytes can be used and the embryos can be transferred to a gestational carrier.

Ovulation and fertility can often be restored in patients with hypothalamic amenorrhea through administration of pulsatile GnRH therapy. GnRH is injected every 1 to 2 hours by a programmable pump to simulate endogenous pulsatile GnRH secretion. Treatment with pulsatile GnRH achieves fertility in ~90% of women after six cycles and carries a low risk of multiple pregnancies.

Patients with anovulation due to pituitary disease do not respond to GnRH therapy and require therapy with exogenous gonadotropins if fertility is desired. Pure recombinant FSH and LH can be used in an effort to achieve fertility, but this should be done only under the direction of an experienced specialist, and patients should be warned that the chances of having a multiple pregnancy with this method are high.

Correcting the precipitating factors for functional hypothalamic disorders usually restores the normal menstrual cycle. In patients with amenorrhea caused by eating disorders or excessive exercise, a modest increase in caloric intake or decrease in athletic training can restore regular menses. Oral contraceptives may decrease bone turnover and preserve bone density. Adequate calcium and vitamin D should also be recommended.

Patients with either hypothalamic or pituitary disease who do not desire fertility and patients with secondary ovarian failure can simply be treated with hormone replacement therapy until the age of menopause, at which time continuing hormone replacement becomes controversial and will need to be addressed on an individual basis. Every woman should be counseled about the potential risks of hormone replacement therapy such as increased incidence of stroke, thromboembolic events, and breast cancer. Smoking cessation should be advised before the initiation of oral contraceptive agents because of the increased risk of deep venous thrombosis.

Specific therapy for PCOS is discussed in Chapter 20, Polycystic Ovary Syndrome (PCOS), and is aimed at controlling hirsutism, resuming menstruation, achieving fertility, and avoiding long-term sequelae of PCOS (glucose intolerance, endometrial hyperplasia, and possibly cardiovascular complications).

Management for patients with hyperprolactinemia or prolactinoma is discussed in Chapter 2, Prolactinoma.

KEY POINTS TO REMEMBER

- Amenorrhea is a symptom, not a diagnosis, and requires investigation into the underlying cause.
- The first step in the evaluation of either primary or secondary amenorrhea should be to rule out pregnancy.
- A careful history, physical examination, and measurement of gonadotropins, prolactin, and TSH will identify the most common causes of amenorrhea.
- The most common cause of primary amenorrhea is constitutional delay.
- In androgen insensitivity syndrome, gonads should be removed after the end of puberty, but in cases of gonadal dysgenesis with a Y chromosome, gonads should be removed at the time of diagnosis because of high risk for malignancy.
- The most common causes of secondary amenorrhea are PCOS, hyperprolactinemia, hypothalamic amenorrhea, and ovarian failure.
- Signs of virilization should always prompt an evaluation for an androgen-secreting tumor.
- If the underlying cause of amenorrhea cannot be reversed, treatment should be aimed at alleviating the symptoms of chronic hypoestrogenemia, avoiding the long-term sequelae of hypoestrogenemia, and, if possible and desired, achieving fertility.

REFERENCES AND SUGGESTED READINGS

Baird DT. Amenorrhea. *Lancet* 1997;350:275–279.

Crowley WF Jr, Jameson JL Jr. Clinical counterpoint: gonadotropin-releasing hormone deficiency: perspectives from clinical investigation. *Endocr Rev* 1992;13:635.

Current evaluation of amenorrhea. The practice committee of the American Society of Reproductive medicine. *Fertil Steril* 2004;82[suppl 1]:33–39.

Groff TR, Shulkin BL, Utiger RD, et al. Amenorrhea, galactorrhea, hyperprolactinemia, and suprasellar pituitary enlargement as presenting features of primary hypothyroidism. *Obstet Gynecol* 1984;63:86S.

Hoek A, Schoemaker J, Drexhaga HA: Premature ovarian failure and ovarian autoimmunity. *Endocr Rev* 1997;18:107–134.

Marshall JC, et al. Hypothalamic dysfunction. *Mol Cell Endocrinol* 2001;183:29–32.

McIver B, Romanski SA, Nippoldt TB. Evaluation and management of amenorrhea. *Mayo Clin Proc* 1997;72:1161–1169.

Rosen MP, Cedars MI: Female reproductive endocrinology and infertility. In: *Greenspan's Basic and Clinical Endocrinology*, 8th ed. McGraw Hill; 2007:502–561.

Rosenfield RL. Clinical review 6: diagnosis and management of delayed puberty *J Clin Endocrinol Metab* 1990;70:559–562.

Rowe PJ, Comhaire FH, Hargreave TB, et al Female partner. In: *WHO Manual for the Standardized Investigation and Diagnosis of the Infertile Couple.* Cambridge: Press Syndicate of the University of Cambridge; 2000:40–67.

Santoro N, Filicori M, Crowley WF. Hypogonadotropic disorders in men and women: diagnosis and therapy with pulsatile gonadotropin-releasing hormone. *Endocr Rev* 1986;7:11.

Speroff L, Fritz MA. Amenorrhea. In: *Clinical Gynecologic Endocrinology and Infertility*, 7th ed. Philadelphia: Lippincott Williams and Wilkins; 2005:401–64.

Welt CK, Barbieri RL. Etiology, diagnosis and treatment of primary amenorrhea. *UpToDate*. Wellesley, MA: UpToDate; 2007.

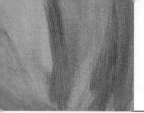

Gynecomastia

17

Runhua Hou

INTRODUCTION

Gynecomastia is a glandular enlargement of the male breast that is often asymmetrical or unilateral and may be tender. It is caused by excessive estrogen action or an increased estrogen–androgen ratio. True gynecomastia needs to be differentiated from breast cancer and **pseudogynecomastia,** which occurs commonly in obese men and is characterized by adipose tissue deposition without glandular proliferation. Male breast cancer is rare and is generally unilateral and eccentric in location rather than symmetric to the nipple, and may be associated with skin changes. Gynecomastia commonly occurs during the neonatal period, in puberty, and with aging or as a side effect of multiple medications. However, it can be the first sign of a serious pathologic condition associated with estrogen excess or androgen deficiency.

CAUSES

The common causes of gynecomastia are summarized in Table 17-1. In contrast to women, in men estrogen is the only hormone that promotes breast growth. Many disorders that result in gynecomastia are characterized by an imbalance between circulating inhibitory androgens and stimulating estrogens. Mechanisms include excessive estrogen or deficient androgen production, increased estrogen precursors available for peripheral conversion, androgen receptor blockade, and increased binding of androgen to sex-hormone binding globulin.

Physiologic Gynecomastia

Gynecomastia is common during infancy, in adolescence, and in middle-aged to older adult males. Transient gynecomastia occurs in 60% to 90% of newborns due to high levels of circulating estrogen during pregnancy, and it typically regresses within 2 to 3 weeks after birth. Pubertal gynecomastia typically occurs in adolescents between the ages of 13 and 14 years, and regresses within 18 months and is uncommon after age 17. It is the result of a transient imbalance of estrogen-androgen levels as estradiol concentrations rise to adult levels before testosterone concentrations during puberty. Gynecomastia of aging can occur in otherwise healthy older males in their 50s to 80s and is related to decreased testosterone synthesis or increased body fat leading to increased aromatization of testosterone to estradiol and of androstenedione to estrone.

Pathologic Gynecomastia

Pathologic gynecomastia can occur through several different mechanisms.

TABLE 17-1   CAUSES OF GYNECOMASTIA

Physiologic causes

Neonatal period

Puberty

Aging

Pathologic causes

Decreased production/action of androgens: Primary (Klinefelter's syndrome, trauma, viral orchitis) or secondary hypogonadism, enzymatic defects in testosterone synthesis, androgen resistance

Increased estrogen production: adrenal, testicular, or ectopic carcinoma producing estrogen or hCG, true hermaphroditism

Systemic illness: Chronic liver or kidney disease, thyrotoxicosis, malnutrition, Refeeding after starvation

Drugs: antiandrogens (spironolactone , finasteride), estrogens and their analogs, growth hormone, gonadotropins, calcium channel blockers, ACE inhibitors, amiodarone, digitoxin, tricyclic antidepressants, haloperidol, diazepam, omeprazole, cimetidine, ranitidine, alkylating agents, antiretroviral agents, methotrexate, imatinib, phenytoin, phenothiazines, ketoconazole, isoniazid, metoclopramide, heroin, marijuana, methadone, alcohol, amphetamines, androgens, and anabolic steroids

Idiopathic

ACE, angiotensin-converting enzyme; hCG, human chorionic gonadotropin.

Adapted from Wilson JD. Endocrine disorders of the breast. In: Braunwald E, et al., eds. *Harrison's Principles of Internal Medicine,* 15th ed. New York: McGraw-Hill; 2002:2170–2172.

Decreased Production and Effect of Androgens

Primary hypogonadism (reviewed in Chapter 19, Male Hypogonadism) can be due to testicular disorders such as trauma, infection, vascular insufficiency, infiltrative disorders or congenital abnormalities such as Klinefelter's syndrome, enzymatic defects in the testosterone biosynthesis pathway, or androgen resistance. The deficiency in testosterone production leads to a compensatory increase in LH release and enhanced aromatization of testosterone to estradiol, resulting in relative estrogen excess. Secondary hypogonadism can also be associated with gynecomastia, although this is less common. In secondary hypogonadism, the pituitary gland fails to produce LH, leading to decreased testosterone secretion, but the adrenal cortex continues to produce estrogen precursors that are aromatized in extraglandular tissues. The net effect is an estrogen–androgen imbalance. In addition to being caused by low testosterone levels, gynecomastia could also occur as a result of ineffective testosterone action due to defects in or absence of the intracellular androgen receptor in androgen target tissues. In androgen insensitivity syndromes, genotypic male patients appear as phenotypic females with breasts that resemble those of a normal woman.

Increased Production of Estrogen

Some tumors secrete estrogen, and patients develop gynecomastia as a result. Examples include Leydig and Sertoli cell tumors and feminizing adrenocortical carcinomas. Patients with true hermaphroditism may have gynecomastia, owing to increased estrogen production from the ovarian component of their gonads. Germ cell tumors of the testes or bronchogenic carcinomas can secrete human chorionic gonadotropin (hCG), which in turn stimulates Leydig cell aromatase activity and leads to increased conversion of androgen precursors to estrone and estradiol, resulting in gynecomastia.

Drugs

Drugs can cause gynecomastia via several mechanisms (Table 17.1). Estrogen and its analogs and gonadotropins directly increase estrogenic activity in the plasma. Antiandrogens, such as spironolactone (Aldactone), can block androgen receptors, thereby altering the androgen-to-estrogen ratio. Some drugs, such as alkylating agents and ketoconazole (Nizoral), can suppress testosterone biosynthesis. Finally, the mechanisms through which certain drugs induce gynecomastia remain to be determined. Examples in this category include tricyclic antidepressants, diazepam (Valium), and antiretroviral agents.

Systemic Illnesses

Roughly two-thirds of patients with cirrhosis have gynecomastia. Increased production of androstenedione from the adrenals as well as enhanced aromatization to estrone and estradiol are possible mechanisms. Up to 50% of patients with end-stage renal disease on hemodialysis may have gynecomastia as a result of Leydig cell dysfunction, leading to decreased testosterone levels. Gynecomastia has also been associated with malnutrition, refeeding syndrome, and thyrotoxicosis.

MANAGEMENT

Diagnosis

A careful history and physical examination should be obtained in all patients. The etiology of gynecomastia can be determined in the majority of the patients. Key elements in the **history** include a detailed medication list, the timing of the onset, presence of pain, and symptoms of systemic illnesses such as liver disease, renal disease, or thyrotoxicosis. The **physical examination** should focus on the breast and testicular examination and an assessment for virilization.

If the patient is taking medications associated with gynecomastia, discontinuation of the offending drugs with resultant symptomatic improvement generally confirms the diagnosis.

In peripubertal boys with normal physical and genital examinations, reevaluation at 6 months is appropriate. Further testing can be carried out if there is no improvement.

In elderly men, it is important to differentiate between gynecomastia and pseudogynecomastia by examination of the areolar tissue. True gynecomastia is characterized by a symmetric ridge of glandular tissue, is rubbery-to-firm in consistency, and contains a fibrous-like cord. Pseudogynecomastia presents no discrete mass.

A more conservative approach with periodic follow-up is appropriate if gynecomastia is asymptomatic and discovered during routine examination in a patient with no underlying disease and not taking medications associated with gynecomastia. In patients with symptoms or signs of liver disease, renal disease, or thyrotoxicosis, further laboratory diagnosis of these specific etiologies should be pursued.

If the gynecomastia is of recent onset, rapid growth, tender tissue, or occurs in a lean patient, a more extensive evaluation is warranted. If there is a firm or hard breast mass, a biopsy should be performed to rule out breast cancer. If testes are small, a karyotype analysis would be appropriate to rule out Klinefelter's syndrome. A workup of testicular tumor should be pursued if testes are asymmetric. Gynecomastia associated with features of androgen deficiency should be investigated for potential treatable causes such as a pituitary tumor.

Laboratory Evaluation

Testosterone, estradiol, LH, and hCG levels are measured to differentiate among various etiologies.

- Plasma **LH** and **testosterone** levels. An elevated LH and low testosterone are seen in primary hypogonadism. If both LH and testosterone levels are low, secondary hypogonadism is likely, provided prolactin levels are normal. If prolactin is elevated in this setting, it implies that hyperprolactinemia is the cause of the consequent hypogonadism. An elevation of both LH and testosterone levels characterizes androgen resistance in the presence of normal thyroid function.
- An elevated **β-hCG** level suggests an hCG-secreting neoplasm. Further evaluation should include testicular ultrasound to rule out testicular germ cell tumors. If the patient has a normal testicular ultrasound, then a chest radiograph or abdominal computed tomography (CT) scan is necessary to localize an extragonadal germ cell tumor or bronchogenic carcinoma.
- An elevated **estradiol** level should be investigated with testicular ultrasound to rule out a Leydig or Sertoli cell tumor. If the ultrasound is normal, an adrenal CT scan or magnetic resonance imaging (MRI) is indicated to rule out an adrenal neoplasm. 24-Hour urinary 17-ketosteroids levels are elevated in adrenocortical carcinoma. If the adrenal imaging studies are negative, workup should focus on causes of increased extraglandular aromatase activity.
- If none of the above workup is revealing, a diagnosis of **idiopathic gynecomastia** may be entertained.

Treatment

The approach to treatment depends on the etiology of the gynecomastia. Observation, surgery, and medical therapy are appropriate for different conditions. When an underlying cause for gynecomastia is identified, treatment of that condition typically resolves the gynecomastia. For example, hormone-replacement therapy improves gynecomastia in hypogonadal males. Drug-induced gynecomastia resolves after the offending drugs have been removed. Observation is appropriate when pubertal gynecomastia is suspected. **Surgery** is indicated when there are severe psychological and/or cosmetic problems; continued growth, tenderness, malignancy; or if the underlying cause cannot be corrected. In addition to avoidance of an offending agent, several **medications** including androgens, antiestrogens, and aromatase inhibitors can be helpful in reducing, although not eliminating, symptoms. Tamoxifen 10 mg orally twice a day or danazol 400 mg orally daily is commonly used in reducing pain and breast size. More than 50% of patients taking tamoxifen have breast-size reduction, whereas 40% of the patients on danazol have improvement in gynecomastia. Unfortunately, the use of these agents is associated with adverse effects such as headache, nausea, impotence and loss of libido, and the breast reduction effects tend to relapse after the mediation has been discontinued.

KEY POINTS TO REMEMBER

- Gynecomastia is caused by an imbalance between circulating levels of androgens and estrogens.
- A careful drug history should be obtained in all patients presenting with gynecomastia.

(continued)

KEY POINTS TO REMEMBER *(Continued)*

- A thorough physical examination includes careful palpation of the breast tissue for masses or tenderness; evaluation of testicular volume and masses; and evaluation for systemic illness such as cirrhosis, renal failure, and thyrotoxicosis.
- Further laboratory tests may include plasma LH, testosterone, β-hCG, and estradiol levels.
- Testicular ultrasound and adrenal CT or MRI may be needed to rule out neoplasm.
- A diagnosis of idiopathic gynecomastia should be entertained only after other causes have been ruled out.
- Correction of the underlying cause generally results in resolution of gynecomastia.

REFERENCES AND SUGGESTED READINGS

Bhasin S, Jameson JL. Disorders of the testes and male reproductive systems. In: Jameson JL, et al, eds. *Harrison's Endocrinology,* New York: McGraw-Hill; 2006:185–186.

Braunstein GD, Glassman H. Gynecomastia. In: Bardin CW, ed. *Current Therapy in Endocrinology and Metabolism,* 6th ed. Philadelphia: Mosby; 1997.

Braunstein GD. Gynecomastia. *N Engl J Med* 1993;328:490.

Carlson HE. Gynecomastia. *N Engl J Med* 1980;303:795.

Freeman RM, Lawton RL, Fearing MO. Gynecomastia: an endocrinologic complication of hemodialysis. *Ann Intern Med* 1968;69:67.

Gordon GG, Olivo J, Fereidoon R, et al. Conversion of androgens to estrogen in cirrhosis of the liver. *J Clin Endocrinol Metab* 1975;40:1018.

Parker LN, Gray DR, Lai MK, et al. Treatment of gynecomastia with tamoxifen: a double-blind crossover study. *Metabolism* 1986;35:705.

Staiman VR, Lowe FC. Tamoxifen for flutamide/finasteride-induced gynecomastia. *Urology* 1997;50:929.

Waterfall NB, Glaser MG. A study of the effects of radiation on prevention of gynecomastia due to estrogen therapy. *Clin Oncol* 1979;5:257.

Wilson JD. Endocrine disorders of the breast. In: Braunwald E, et al., eds. *Harrison's Principles of Internal Medicine,* 15th ed. New York: McGraw-Hill; 2002:2170–2172.

Hirsutism

Runhua Hou

INTRODUCTION

Hirsutism is the development of androgen-dependent terminal body hair in a woman in places where terminal hair is normally not found, such as the face, chest, back, and abdomen. It is caused by increased androgen production by the ovaries, adrenal glands or, rarely, increased target-organ production of androgen. It affects 5% to 10% of women of reproductive age and is commonly accompanied by other cutaneous manifestations such as acne and male-pattern balding. Although it may be a normal variant of hair growth, it can also be the first sign of a serious androgen disorder. Polycystic ovary syndrome (PCOS) and idiopathic hirsutism are the most common causes of hirsutism. However, ominous causes such as adrenal or ovarian neoplasms need to be considered if hirsutism is accompanied by virilization manifested by deepening of the voice, increased muscle mass, clitoromegaly, and breast atrophy.

Hair Follicle Growth and Differentiation

Androgen is important for terminal hair and sebaceous gland development, and it mediates differentiation of pilosebaceous units into either a terminal hair follicle or a sebaceous gland. Androgens transform vellus hair into terminal hair. Vellus hairs are fine, soft, and nonpigmented. Terminal hairs are long, coarse, and pigmented. Although excessive androgen underlies most cases of hirsutism, the amount of androgen does not always correlate with the extent of hair growth. Local factors and variability in end-organ sensitivity to circulating androgens also affect hair growth; therefore, hirsutism can occur in the presence of normal androgen levels.

Race, ethnic background, and family history of the patient should be considered in determining the definition of "normal" hair growth. In general, dark-haired individuals tend to be more hirsute than blonde or fair individuals. Women of Mediterranean origin tend to have more hair, whereas Native American and Asian women have less hair in androgen-dependent areas. However, changes in pattern or rate of growth irrespective of ethnicity should prompt further evaluation.

True hirsutism needs to be differentiated from **hypertrichosis,** a condition in which there is an increase in total body hair, for example, androgen-independent vellus hair in nonsexual areas. Hypertrichosis is commonly associated with some metabolic disorders and adverse effects of some medications and does not represent true hirsutism.

CAUSES

Common etiologies of hirsutism are listed in Table 18-1.

TABLE 18-1   CAUSES OF HIRSUTISM

Common causes

Polycystic ovary syndrome (PCOS)

Idiopathic

Other causes (less common)

Ovarian

Ovarian neoplasms

Insulin resistance syndromes

Adrenal

Classic and nonclassic congenital adrenal hyperplasia

Adrenal neoplasms

Premature adrenarche

Drugs

Oral contraceptives containing androgenic progestins

Cyclosporine, minoxidil, diazoxide, androgens, phenytoin

Other endocrine disorders

Hyperprolactinemia, Cushing's syndrome, acromegaly

Miscellaneous

Peripheral androgen overproduction

Obesity

idiopathic

Pregnancy-related hyperandrogenism

Adapted from Ehrmann D. Hirsutism and virilization. In: Jameson JL, et al., eds. *Harrison's Endocrinology,* New York: McGraw-Hill; 2006:185–186.

Polycystic Ovary Syndrome

PCOS is the most common cause of hyperandrogenism in women of reproductive age. The criteria for diagnosis are menstrual irregularity and clinical or biochemical evidence of hyperandrogenism. The onset of menstrual irregularity is usually in the peripubertal period. The clinical features, diagnosis, and management of PCOS are discussed in Chapter 20, Polycystic Ovary Syndrome (PCOS).

Idiopathic Hirsutism

Idiopathic hirsutism refers to hirsute women with regular menses, normal serum androgen levels, and no identifiable underlying disorder. It may represent a mild form of PCOS, but the absence of irregular menses distinguishes this disorder from PCOS.

Ovarian Causes

An androgen-secreting tumor of the ovary usually occurs later in life and progresses rapidly. Sertoli-Leydig cell tumors, hilus-cell tumors, and granulosa-theca cell tumors are a few examples. Other ovarian causes of hyperandrogenism include syndromes of severe insulin resistance that are accompanied by hyperinsulinemia. Insulin can promote ovarian hyperandrogenism by interacting with insulin-like growth factor 1 receptors in theca cells. In addition, insulin decreases sex hormone–binding globulin (SHBG) concentration, and thereby increases the free testosterone level.

Adrenal Causes

Adrenal neoplasms secrete testosterone, dehydroepiandrosterone sulfate (DHEA-S), dehydroepiandrosterone (DHEA), and cortisol (Cushing's syndrome), and they are rare causes of hirsutism. Congenital adrenal hyperplasia (CAH) usually presents at birth or in early infancy, but late-onset forms of CAH present at puberty with hirsutism and menstrual irregularity, or as primary amenorrhea without manifestations of cortisol deficiency. This nonclassic form of CAH is usually due to 21-hydroxylase deficiency, and results in excessive production of 17-hydroxyprogesterone and androstenedione, which in turn leads to hirsutism and, sometimes, menstrual irregularity.

Other Causes

Many medications are associated with hirsutism (Table 18-1); therefore, a careful drug history should be obtained in all patients evaluated for hirsutism. Rarely, women with hyperprolactinemia can have hirsutism. It is unclear whether hyperprolactinemia alone is adequate for inducing hirsutism or if hyperprolactinemia is a result of increased estrone commonly seen in PCOS.

PRESENTATION

Most women with hirsutism have the idiopathic form or PCOS. Nonetheless, it is important to exclude rare and more serious causes such as ovarian or adrenal neoplasms.

Some important clinical features that suggest these other causes include:

- Virilization
- Abrupt onset or progressive worsening of symptoms
- Late onset (third decade or later)—PCOS typically manifests around puberty
- Moderately or significantly elevated DHEA-S and free testosterone in a young woman

History

The history should include the age of onset of symptoms, rate of progression, and associated features such as acne or frontal balding, symptoms of virilization, abnormal menstrual cycles, and weight, drug, and family history. The most important points are the rate of progression and symptoms of virilization. Rapid progression and symptoms of virilization are usually ominous and may indicate ovarian or adrenal neoplasms. Irregular menses usually indicates an ovarian cause of hyperandrogenism. Galactorrhea may indicate hyperprolactinemia. Weight gain, striae, hypertension, and easy bruising suggest Cushing's syndrome.

Physical Examination

Physical examination should include measurement of height, weight, and blood pressure, and calculation of body mass index. An objective assessment of hair distribution and quality of hair should be documented. A simple scoring scale can be used, such as the modified scale of Ferriman and Gallwey in which a scoring system of 0 to 4 is used for each of the nine androgen-dependent sites. Skin should be examined for acne, seborrhea, temporal balding, acanthosis nigricans, striae, thinning, or bruising. Signs of virilization such as deepening of the voice, increased muscle mass, and clitoromegaly should be carefully sought.

Laboratory Data

Women with regular ovulatory menses and mild hirsutism can be followed without any further testing. More extensive testing is indicated if moderate to severe hirsutism occurs. The following laboratory tests are often used in the evaluation of hirsutism.

Serum Testosterone

Serum testosterone can be measured either as total or free testosterone and it provides the best overall estimate of androgen production in hirsute women. Free testosterone, the biologically active form is typically higher in women with androgen excess because of an androgen-induced decrease in SHBG concentrations. Therefore, free testosterone is more sensitive, but it is only accurate when measured with equilibrium dialysis or calculated using total testosterone and SHBG. Clinically, total testosterone typically provides an adequate estimate of androgen excess and is widely available and better standardized. Serum total testosterone is often high (>150 ng/dL) in androgen-secreting tumors. Patients with PCOS or idiopathic hirsutism typically have normal or slightly above normal levels of testosterone.

Dehydroepiandrosterone Sulfate

Women with androgen-secreting adrenal tumors typically have DHEA-S levels >700 mcg/dL. This test is usually indicated when signs of virilization are present, the symptoms are more abrupt in nature, and serum testosterone levels are elevated.

Serum Prolactin

Prolactin should be measured in women with hirsutism and irregular menstrual cycles to rule out prolactin-secreting pituitary adenoma.

17-Hydroxyprogesterone

Measurement of 17-hydroxyprogesterone is useful to differentiate between late-onset CAH and PCOS. If the early morning 17-hydroxyprogesterone is <200 ng/dL or if adrenocorticotropic hormone (ACTH)–stimulated 17-hydroxyprogesterone level is <1000 ng/dL, late-onset CAH is unlikely to be the diagnosis. Testing in women of Hispanic, Yugoslav, or Eastern European Jewish origin may have a higher yield due to increased prevalence. Because therapy with oral contraceptive and/or antiandrogens will often be effective for both CAH and PCOS, the diagnosis of CAH may not always be necessary. Nonetheless, CAH can respond to glucocorticoids, and in some instances testing for CAH is indicated (see Chapter 12, Congenital Adrenal Hyperplasia).

Dexamethasone Androgen Suppression Test

The dexamethasone androgen suppression test can be used to distinguish ovarian from adrenal androgen overproduction. A blood sample is obtained before and after administering dexamethasone (0.5 mg orally every 6 hours for 4 days). Suppression of free testosterone into the normal range suggests an adrenal etiology; failure of suppression indicates an ovarian cause of hyperandrogenism.

Cushing's Syndrome

Tests to rule out Cushing's syndrome may be warranted in the appropriate clinical setting (reviewed in Chapter 14, Cushing's Syndrome).

Further radiologic studies, such as pelvic ultrasound, abdominal CT, and MRI, are indicated only if a tumor is suspected due to the presence of markedly elevated androgen levels.

MANAGEMENT

For hirsutism caused by ovarian or adrenal tumors, treatment should be focused on correction of the underlying etiology. For hirsutism due to other causes, such as PCOS or idiopathic hirsutism, the treatment should be individualized according to patient preference as response to pharmacologic therapy is slow and may take several months. Typically, biochemical abnormalities resolve before clinical improvement. Reassurance may be sufficient in a woman with mild hirsutism and normal ovulatory menses. More specific therapy is indicated for more severe forms or if the patient requests therapy. Women who desire pregnancy should not be started on pharmacotherapy for hirsutism. Pregnancy should be excluded before initiation of antiandrogens, and **continued contraception is imperative for all patients taking antiandrogens, as these drugs are teratogenic.** The treatment specific for PCOS is discussed in Chapter 20, Polycystic Ovary Syndrome (PCOS).

Nonpharmacologic and Topical Treatments

Nonpharmacologic treatment should be considered in all patients, either as the only treatment or as an adjunct to drug therapy. Weight loss should be encouraged in obese women as it can lower androgen levels and improve hirsutism. Bleaching, waxing, shaving, depilatories, electrolysis, and laser are possible ways of removing the undesired hair. Laser treatment is expensive, but effective, as it removes hair permanently. It is especially useful in women with dark hair and light skin. Topical eflornithine (Vaniqa) applied twice daily has been used for removal of facial hair; however, it must be used indefinitely to prevent hair re-growth. Women with androgenic alopecia may be treated with topical minoxidil 2% solution applied chronically twice daily to a dry scalp.

Oral Contraceptives

Combination estrogen–progestin oral contraceptives are the best first-line agents in patients who do not desire pregnancy. Treatment should be initiated by a combination preparation that contains ethinyl estradiol in conjunction with a progestin with little or no androgenic activity such as desogestrel or norgestimate. Oral contraceptives cause a suppression of luteinizing hormone (LH) release leading to decreased ovarian androgen production, which, in turn, increases SHBG levels and lowers the free testosterone level. Oral contraceptives also decrease adrenal DHEA-S production by reducing adrenocorticotropic hormone (ACTH) level.

Antiandrogens

Antiandrogens are more effective when added to oral contraceptives than when used alone. Spironolactone (Aldactone) (100–200 mg orally daily) can decrease the effect of androgens by blocking the androgen receptor. When used in combination with an oral contraceptive, both androgen levels and action are decreased. Finasteride (Propecia), 5 mg orally daily, competitively inhibits 5-α-reductase and can also be used to treat hirsutism. Flutamide (Eulexin), 250 mg orally daily, is a potent nonsteroidal antiandrogen that effectively treats hirsutism, but concerns for liver dysfunction limits its use. When used in combination with an oral contraceptive, it appears to be more effective than spironolactone in improving hirsutism, acne, and male pattern baldness. It has not yet been approved in the United States for use in hirsutism, although it is available in Europe. Because of the teratogenic potential of antiandrogens, they can be used only when women are using effective contraception.

Glucocorticoids

Glucocorticoids are an option for patients with CAH, as adrenal androgens are sensitive to the suppressive effects of glucocorticoids. Dexamethasone (0.2–0.5 mg) or prednisone

(5–10 mg) should be taken at the bedtime to suppress the nocturnal surge of ACTH (see Chapter 12, Adult Congenital Adrenal Hyperplasia).

Gonadotropin-Releasing Hormone Agonists

Gonadotropin-releasing hormone (GnRH) agonists inhibit ovarian androgen production by inhibiting gonadotropins. The ensuing estrogen deficiency can be treated with a combination estrogen-progestin pill. The GnRH agonist–oral contraceptive combination is less effective and more expensive than the antiandrogen–contraceptive combination.

KEY POINTS TO REMEMBER

- The most common causes of hirsutism are PCOS and idiopathic hirsutism.
- Rapid progression and signs of virilization may indicate ovarian or adrenal neoplasms.
- Women who desire pregnancy should not be treated with medications for hirsutism.
- Nonpharmacotherapy should be considered in all patients.
- Combination estrogen–progestin oral contraceptives are the best first-line agents for patients who do not desire pregnancy.
- Antiandrogens are more effective when added to oral contraceptives than when used alone.

REFERENCES AND SUGGESTED READINGS

Azziz R, Dewailly D, Owerbach D. Nonclassic adrenal hyperplasia: current concepts. *J Clin Endocrinol Metab* 1994;78:810.

Derksen J, Nagesser SK, Meinders AE, et al. Identification of virilizing adrenal tumors in hirsute women. *N Engl J Med* 1994;331:968.

Ehrmann D. Hirsutism and virilization. In: Jameson JL, et al., eds. *Harrison's Endocrinology,* New York: McGraw-Hill; 2006:185–186.

Ehrmann DA, Barnes RB, Rosenfield RL. Hyperandrogenism, hirsutism and polycystic ovary syndrome. In: DeGroot LJ, Jameson JL, eds. *Endocrinology,* 4th ed. Philadelphia: WB Saunders, 2001:2122–2137.

Ehrmann DA. Hirsutism and virilization. In: Braunwald E, et al., eds. *Harrison's Principles of Internal Medicine,* 15th ed. New York: McGraw-Hill; 2001:297–301.

Hatch R, Rosenfield RL, Kim MH, et al. Hirsutism: implications, etiology, and management. *Am J Obstet Gynecol* 1981;140:815.

Kirschner MA, Samojlik E, Silber D. A comparison of androgen production and clearance in hirsute and obese women. *J Steroid Biochem* 1983;19:607.

Matteri RK, Stanczyk FZ, Gentzschein EE, et al. Androgen sulfate and glucuronide conjugates in nonhirsute and hirsute women with polycystic ovarian syndrome. *Am J Obstet Gynecol* 1989;161:1704.

Pazos F, Escobar-Morreale HF, Balsa J. Prospective randomized study comparing the long-acting gonadotropin-releasing hormone agonist triptorelin, flutamide, and cyproterone acetate, used in combination with an oral contraceptive, in the treatment of hirsutism. *Fertil Steril* 1999;71:122.

Taylor AE, Barbieri RL. Treatment of hirsutism. In: Rose BD, ed. *UpToDate.* Wellesley: UpToDate; 2003.

Zawadzki JK, Dunaif A. Diagnostic criteria for polycystic ovary syndrome: towards a rational approach. In: Dunaif A, ed. *Polycystic Ovary Syndrome, Current Issues in Endocrinology and Metabolism,* 4th ed. Boston: Blackwell Scientific Publications; 1992.

Male Hypogonadism

Sheri Nishimoto

19

INTRODUCTION

Male hypogonadism refers to impairment of the two major functions of the testis; either decreased testosterone or sperm production, or both. It can be further classified into primary or secondary hypogonadism. In primary hypogonadism, the abnormality is caused by the failure of the testis (hypergonadotropic hypogonadism), and the secondary form results from defects at the hypothalamic–pituitary level (hypogonadotrophic hypogonadism). Rarely, hypogonadism can be due to defects at the receptor level, seen in androgen-resistance syndromes, which are characterized by resistance to the effects of testosterone. Symptoms depend primarily on the age of the male patient at the time of onset of the disease. The production of an adequate amount of testosterone is necessary for the development of external genitalia and secondary sexual characteristics in children and adolescents. In adults, androgen production is necessary for the maintenance of lean body mass, bone mass, libido, sexual function, and spermatogenesis.

Men with a total testosterone level less than ~300 ng/dL often develop symptoms and signs of hypogonadism that can have long-term clinical effects.

Overview of Male Gonadal Function

An overview of the male gonadal axis is outlined in Figure 19-1. The testis functions as part of the hypothalamic–pituitary–gonadal axis. A hypothalamic pulse generator resides in the arcuate nucleus, which releases gonadotropin-releasing hormone (GnRH) into the hypothalamic–pituitary portal system. In response to these pulses of GnRH, the anterior pituitary secretes the gonadotropins—follicle-stimulating hormone (FSH) and luteinizing hormone (LH)—which in turn stimulate gonadal activity. LH and FSH control testosterone production by Leydig cells and spermatozoa production by seminiferous tubules. GnRH, LH, and FSH secretion is controlled by the negative feedback from the testis by testosterone and inhibin B.

Testosterone is the major product of Leydig cells. LH stimulates the testis in a pulsatile manner, resulting from the pulsatile GnRH secretion by the hypothalamus. An adult testis produces approximately 7 mg of testosterone daily. FSH is necessary for seminiferous tubule growth.

FSH and LH control seminiferous tubule production of sperm. The action of LH is through local secretion of testosterone. Both FSH and testosterone are required to stimulate spermatogenesis quantitatively. LH secretion is negatively regulated by testosterone, estradiol, and dihydrotestosterone (DHT). FSH is under the negative influence of inhibin B and testosterone. They are stimulated in a pulsatile fashion by GnRH (see Fig. 19-1).

Sixty percent to 70% of **testosterone** is transported in plasma bound to sex hormone–binding globulin (SHBG), 2% is free, and the remainder is bound to albumin. Both free testosterone and albumin-bound testosterone are bioavailable. Circulating

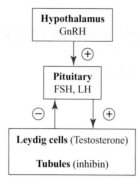

FIGURE 19-1. The male gonadal axis. FSH, follicle-stimulating hormone; GnRH, gonadotropin-releasing hormone; LH, luteinizing hormone.

SHBG levels (and, therefore, total testosterone) can be increased in cirrhosis, hyperthyroidism, HIV infection, estrogen use, and anticonvulsant use. Reduction in SHBG level is associated with aging, obesity, low protein states (nephrotic syndrome), hypothyroidism, hyperinsulinism, and glucocorticoid use. Testosterone levels are high in the morning and reach nadir in the afternoon. This diurnal rhythm is lost in older men.

Approximately 6% to 8% of testosterone is converted to more potent DHT by 5-α-reductase in prostate, testis, liver, kidney, and skin. A small proportion (0.2%) of testosterone is converted to estradiol by aromatase. The actions of testosterone are the combined effects of testosterone, plus its active androgenic (DHT) and estrogenic (estradiol) metabolites. The testosterone-receptor complex is responsible for gonadotropin regulation, stimulation of spermatogenesis, and virilization of the Wolffian ducts, whereas the DHT-receptor complex mediates virilization of the external genitalia during embryogenesis and most of the virilization that occurs at male puberty. Estradiol inhibits gonadotropin secretion and promotes epiphyseal maturation in the adolescent male.

Hypogonadism may occur if the hypothalamic–pituitary–gonadal axis is interrupted at any level. Primary hypogonadism results if the testis does not produce the amount of sex steroid sufficient to suppress secretion of LH and FSH at normal levels. Secondary hypogonadism may result from failure of the hypothalamic GnRH pulse generator or from inability of the pituitary to respond with secretion of LH and FSH. Most commonly, secondary hypogonadism is observed as one aspect of multiple pituitary hormone deficiencies resulting from malformations or lesions of the pituitary that are acquired postnatally.

Epidemiology

In the United States, 4 to 5 million men have hypogonadism. In longitudinal studies, as men advance in age, total testosterone declines. Serum testosterone declines at ~1% to 2% a year after age 30. It is estimated that 30% to 40% of men older than 65 years of age, and 79% to 80% of men older than age 80 have hypogonadism.

CAUSES

Primary Hypogonadism

Primary hypogonadism is more common than the secondary form and is more likely to be associated with a decrease in sperm production than in a decrease in testosterone production.

In addition, primary hypogonadism is more likely to be associated with gynecomastia. Supernormal serum FSH and LH levels stimulate testicular aromatase to increase the conversion of testosterone to estradiol, resulting in elevated levels of estradiol relative to testosterone.

Developmental Defects

Klinefelter's syndrome is the most common congenital defect causing male hypogonadism (1 in 1000 males). Clinical features include small, firm testis; varying degrees of impaired sexual development; azoospermia; gynecomastia; and elevated gonadotrophins. The underlying defect is the presence of an extra X chromosome, 47,XXY being the most common. Diagnosis is confirmed by karyotype analysis.

The 46,XY/XO karyotype (mosaic for loss of Y chromosome) leads to a syndrome characterized by short stature and features typical of Turner's syndrome. The gonads vary from streak to normal testes; as a result, the sexual phenotype varies from complete female to complete male. If the patient has both a streak gonad and a dysgenetic testis ("mixed gonadal dysgenesis"), the risk of gonadoblastoma is about 20%. Gonadectomy should, therefore, be performed in these patients.

A congenital decrease in testosterone synthesis and secretion can result from mutations of the genes that encode enzymes necessary for testosterone biosynthesis. These mutations may result in decreased testosterone secretion, beginning in the first trimester of pregnancy, and in incomplete virilization.

Acquired Disease

Mumps is the most common infection affecting the testis and leads to infertility and reduced testosterone level.

Radiation affects both spermatogenesis and testosterone production. Impaired testosterone production is caused by reduced blood flow to testis. The extent of damage to Leydig cells is directly related to dose of radiation and, inversely, to age.

Drugs, such as ketoconazole (Nizoral), spironolactone (Aldactone), and cyproterone, interfere with testosterone synthesis. Enzyme-inducing drugs, such as phenytoin (Dilantin) and carbamazepine (Carbatrol), can lower the bioavailable testosterone, raise SHBG and LH levels, and decrease metabolic clearance. Ethanol ingestion can reduce testosterone levels by inhibiting the synthesis of testosterone and by impairing the hypothalamic–pituitary axis. Cyclophosphamide and other alkylating agents can induce infertility. Spironolactone, cyproterone, cimetidine, and omeprazole compete for the androgen receptor and can cause gynecomastia and impotence.

Systemic illnesses, such as renal failure (testicular failure, hyperprolactinemia), liver failure (both testicular failure and inhibition of the hypothalamic–pituitary axis), sickle cell disease, chronic illness, thyrotoxicosis, HIV, and immune disorders can lead to hypergonadotrophic hypogonadism.

Secondary Hypogonadism

Congenital Disorders

Congenital abnormalities causing decreased gonadotrophins are rare. Idiopathic hypogonadotropic hypogonadism (IHH) is a heterogeneous disorder caused by isolated GnRH deficiency. Affected individuals are males presenting as teenagers because of deficient sexual maturation. They have a normal male phenotype at birth because maternal human chorionic gonadotropin (hCG) stimulates normal sexual differentiation in the first trimester. However, they have impaired phallic development characterized by microphallus at birth owing to lack of testosterone production in the final trimester. Clinical features include delayed bone age (typically not beyond 11–12 years in males), osteopenia, eunuchoid body proportions, gynecomastia, and delayed puberty. These patients have low testosterone and LH levels. Male patients with testes ≥4 cm have incomplete IHH, but those with testes <4 cm have complete IHH. Gonadotropin and testosterone values cannot differentiate the two disorders. The diagnosis must be differentiated from delay of puberty and cannot be given until patients are >18 years of age. Pulsatile GnRH treatment induces full pubertal development.

Karyotype analysis is not recommended unless multiple congenital anomalies are present, or if there is a suspicion of Prader-Willi syndrome (deletion of 15q11–q13). IHH has been associated with mutation in KAL1 (X-linked recessive), GNRHR (autosomal recessive), and FGFR1 (autosomal dominant).

Kallmann's syndrome is characterized by hypogonadotropic hypogonadism and hyposmia with or without other nongonadal anomalies. Some patients with the X-linked form have a deletion of the *KAL* gene located on short arm of the X chromosome, which prevents migration of GnRH neurons to the brain from the olfactory placode during embryogenesis. Patients may also have midfacial clefting, renal agenesis, and neurologic abnormalities (deafness, cerebellar dysfunction, mental retardation, eye abnormalities).

Secondary hypogonadism can also occur in Laurence-Moon syndrome and Bardet-Biedl syndrome. The *DAX1* gene is associated with X-linked adrenal hypoplasia congenita (hypogonadotropic hypogonadism and adrenal insufficiency).

Androgen receptor dysfunction causes incomplete virilization in 46,XY males, who have bilateral testes and normal testosterone production. The diagnosis should be considered in girls with inguinal or labial masses, women with primary amenorrhea, adolescent girls who become virilized and develop clitoromegaly, adolescent boys who have persistent gynecomastia and fail to undergo puberty, adult males with undervirilization or infertility associated with azoospermia or severe oligospermia.

In addition, hypogonadotropic hypogonadism can be caused by impaired development of the pituitary gland. Mutations in the *PROP1* gene have resulted in absence of several pituitary hormones, including growth hormone, thyroid-stimulating hormone, prolactin, and gonadotropins. *PROP1* encodes a protein expressed in the embryonic pituitary, which is necessary for function of *POU1F1*, which codes for a pituitary transcription factor. *HESX1* gene mutations result in septooptic dysplasia, which may include poor development of the pituitary.

Acquired Disorders

Any disease that affects the hypothalamic–pituitary axis by one of the following mechanisms leads to hypogonadotropic hypogonadism.

- Hypothalamus—impairs GnRH secretion
- Pituitary stalk—inhibits GnRH from reaching the pituitary gland
- Pituitary gland—directly impairs LH and FSH secretion

Mass lesions of the pituitary or of the hypothalamus preferentially affect gonadotropins. In many patients with space-occupying lesions, adrenocorticotropic hormone (ACTH) and TSH are unaffected. Gonadotropin deficiency may result from a space-occupying lesion of the sella, either by destroying the pituitary gland or by interrupting the nerve fibers that bring GnRH to the hypophyseal circulation. Patients present with headaches, visual disturbances, and variable manifestations of hypopituitarism. ACTH-producing tumors can cause impotence, decreased libido, and infertility. Testosterone levels are low, and GnRH-stimulated LH concentrations are suppressed. Prolactinoma affects the pulsatile GnRH secretion and subsequently causes hypogonadism. Men have low testosterone levels and attenuated pulsatile LH secretion. Treatment with dopamine agonists can normalize prolactin levels and restore sexual function.

Infiltrative diseases such as Langerhans' cell histiocytosis and sarcoidosis may involve the hypothalamus and pituitary gland, and cause hypogonadism. Hemochromatosis can cause selective gonadotropin deficiency owing to deposition of iron in the pituitary cells. Leydig cell tumors and adrenal tumors produce estradiol, leading to gynecomastia and gonadotropin deficiency. hCG secreted by choriocarcinoma can increase estradiol levels and suppress gonadotropins.

Trauma severing the pituitary stalk, postinfectious lesions of the central nervous system (CNS), vascular abnormalities of the CNS, critical illness, chronic narcotic administration, exogenous steroids, brain irradiation, and pituitary apoplexy are some other causes of secondary hypogonadism.

Excessive exercise can cause hypothalamic hypogonadism in men as it does in women with hypothalamic amenorrhea.

Differential Diagnosis

Patients with other diseases may present with similar signs and symptoms. Patients with headaches, visual problems, galactorrhea, papilledema, or optic disc pallor should raise concern for a pituitary tumor. Malaise, fatigue, anorexia and weight loss are seen in hypopituitarism.

PRESENTATION

Clinical features depend on whether the impairment involves spermatogenesis or testosterone secretion, or both. It also depends on the time of onset of the defect. Impaired spermatogenesis typically leads to reduced sperm count and testicular size.

- Reduced testosterone production during the first trimester of pregnancy leads to partial virilization—ranging from severe deficiency that leads to posterior labial fusion to mild deficiency resulting in hypospadias. Complete lack of testosterone during this period results in female external genitalia (both clitoris and labia).
- If the defect occurs during the third trimester, it leads to micropenis and cryptorchidism.
- If testosterone production is inhibited before puberty, males will fail to initiate (average age 14) or complete puberty (completed in 3–4 years).
- Postpubertal deficit leads to decreased libido, muscle mass, hair growth, energy, mood, concentration, hematocrit, and bone mass. Decreased libido and fatigue are most readily experienced, whereas other symptoms take years to manifest. Long-standing hypogonadism in males manifests with decreased facial hair growth (female hair distribution) and development of fine wrinkles at the corners of the mouth and eyes.
- Hypogonadism has been associated with several co-morbid conditions, including metabolic syndrome, diabetes, dyslipidemia, sleep apnea, and erectile dysfunction.

History

History should include developmental milestones, with emphasis on sexual development, current symptoms, and information pertaining to possible causes. History of ambiguous genitalia; micropenis; cryptorchidism; failed or delayed puberty; or decrease in libido, sexual function, and/or energy gives clues regarding time of onset of the hypogonadism. Inquiry should be made into the rapidity of onset and progression of the symptoms, presence or absence of early morning erections, and changes in voice, muscle strength, or hair growth. History of headache, visual problems, symptoms suggestive of kidney or liver disease, depression, thyroid disease, drug abuse, chemotherapy, radiation therapy, anosmia, ethanol abuse, and medication history can yield important clues regarding the etiology of the disease. Patients should also be screened for sleep apnea symptoms. It is unknown if obstructive sleep apnea precedes testosterone deficiency or is a clinical manifestation of it.

Physical Examination

A complete physical examination should be done to look for the presence of eunuchoid proportions (a lower body segment [floor to pubis] that is more than 2 cm longer than upper body segment [pubis to crown], and an arm span that is more than 2 cm longer than height), other developmental anomalies, visual problems, abnormal hair distribution, and gynecomastia. Examination of the external genitalia should include measuring testicular size (normal, 4–7 cm) and volume (normal, 15–30 mL) and Tanner stage for adolescents. Consistency of the testicle should also be noted. Typically, firm testes are associated with Klinefelter's syndrome owing to hyalinization or fibrosis. Small, rubbery testes are characteristically found in prepubertal males, whereas postpubertal testicular atrophy results in a soft or mushy consistency.

Physical findings are not always present in adults, as some secondary sexual characteristics, such as reduced muscle mass, may take years to develop. In such instances, appropriate laboratory evaluation may be helpful.

MANAGEMENT

Diagnosis

Diagnosis is based on a thorough history, physical examination, and laboratory data. The general scheme for assessment of hypogonadism is outlined in Figure 19-2. Initial laboratory evaluation should include (preferably morning between 8 AM and 10 AM) testosterone, FSH, and LH levels. Presence of low testosterone with elevated FSH and LH denotes primary hypogonadism, whereas low testosterone and low or normal FSH and LH levels indicate secondary hypogonadism.

A man with total testosterone levels below 300 ng/dL is likely hypogonadal. Levels between 200 and 400 ng/dL should be repeated with the measurement of free testosterone. Diurnal variations in the levels of testosterone need to be considered when interpreting results. As men age, the circadian rhythm is lost; consequently, advanced age sampling time may be less important. Measuring free testosterone becomes important when an abnormality affecting SHBG levels is suspected.

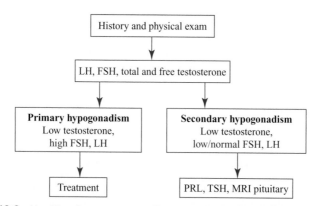

FIGURE 19-2. Algorithm for assessment of hypogonadism. FSH, follicle-stimulating hormone; LH, luteinizing hormone; PRL, prolactin; TSH, thyroid-stimulating hormone.

Semen analysis is the best means of analyzing sperm count and is typically ordered for men who desire fertility. It should be performed after 1 to 3 days of sexual abstinence and examined within 2 hours of specimen collection. Sperm are analyzed for number, motility, and morphology. Typically, normal semen analysis parameters are $>20 \times 10^6$ sperm per mL, $>50\%$ progressive motility, and $>30\%$ normal morphology (lower limits are permissible for patients desiring artificial reproductive technology). Abnormal results might be caused by recent fever, trauma, or drug exposure that can transiently impair spermatogenesis. Subnormal sperm count and a normal serum testosterone concentration associated with a supranormal serum FSH and normal LH concentration indicates that the seminiferous tubules have been damaged, whereas testosterone production by the Leydig cells is still normal.

If secondary hypogonadism is suspected, a prolactin level, thyroid-stimulating hormone (TSH), free thyroxine (T_4), and cortisol (8-AM level or cosyntropin stimulation testing) should be performed. Magnetic resonance imaging (MRI) is indicated if a low testosterone level and low LH or elevated prolactin level is found. If other pituitary hormones are abnormal or if visual field abnormalities or other neurologic abnormalities are present, an MRI of the pituitary gland must be ordered to rule out a lesion. If an MRI is contraindicated, although of inferior quality, a head computed tomography (CT) scan with and without contrast can be performed. Primary hypothyroidism can cause hyperprolactinemia and hypogonadism (due to elevated thyrotropin-releasing hormone [TRH]).

Treatment

Testosterone should be administered only to a man who is hypogonadal, as evidenced by symptoms and signs consistent with androgen deficiency and a distinctly subnormal serum testosterone concentration. Increasing the serum testosterone in a man who has symptoms suggestive of hypogonadism but has normal testosterone concentrations will not relieve those symptoms.

Treatment for both primary and secondary hypogonadism consists of replacing testosterone. The following are initial dose and preparation recommendations.

- Testosterone enanthate/cypionate intramuscular injections, 200 mg every 2 weeks
- Transdermal testosterone (Androderm), 5 mg patch daily
- Scrotal patch, 6 mg patch daily (hair needs to shaved and adhesive may not last 24 hours)
- Testosterone gel (Androgel or Testim), 2.5 to 5 g applied topically to upper arm each day
- Buccal tablet (Striant), 30 mg twice daily

Generally, the gels are the most costly, whereas patches and injectable esters are the least costly. The possibility of skin transfer of the gel to a female partner is unlikely.

Patients with secondary hypogonadism desiring fertility are treated with pulsatile GnRH or gonadotropins with hCG (human chorionic gonadotropin). Spermatogenesis can also be stimulated by GnRH in men who have secondary hypogonadism from hypothalamic disease. Replacement of GnRH in a physiologic manner will cause secretion of LH and FSH, which in turn will stimulate the testes to produce testosterone and sperm. hCG stimulates the testes to make testosterone and is especially useful in stimulating both testosterone and sperm production. FSH is typically not used, since it is extremely costly and LH and hCG alone can stimulate spermatogenesis. Use of gonadotropins in conjunction with artificial reproductive technologies are also a consideration.

Prognosis

Normalizing testosterone levels leads to improvement in symptoms and normal virilization in men. Dramatic improvements in muscle mass and bone density can be seen in the first year of treatment. Typically by 24 months men with osteoporosis reach and maintain normal bone mineral density. Increases in lean body mass, prostate volume, erythropoiesis, energy, and sexual function occur within the first 6 months.

Follow-up

Serum testosterone measurements are helpful to assess the adequacy of treatment and should be checked 1 to 2 months after initiating treatment. They should be measured midway between injections in patients receiving injectable testosterone. The dosage should be adjusted to maintain total testosterone levels in the mid-normal range (600 to 750 ng/dL). In patients treated with a testosterone patch, levels should be checked 3 to 12 hours after application. With use of the gel or buccal tablets, serum levels of testosterone can be measured at any time and should be in the normal range (400–900 ng/dL). In postpubertal men, it is reasonable to treat with the minimum amount of testosterone that alleviates symptoms of decreased libido, impaired sexual function, and energy levels. In primary hypogonadism, normalization of serum LH can be used as a surrogate marker to determine the adequacy of therapy.

A minimum of 3 months of treatment should be attempted to see if there is a clinical improvement.

Complications

Transdermal testosterone patches can be associated with skin rash and itching and may require application of corticosteroid cream. Men treated with testosterone injections will have wide swings of plasma testosterone levels and can develop emotional and physiologic effects. These include breast tenderness, hyperactivity at peak levels, and at the nadir fatigue, depression, or anger. Thus it is advisable to start at lower doses, especially in older men and then titrating upward to reduce mood fluctuations. Buccal preparations can cause gingival irritation, taste perversion, and bitter taste.

Patients receiving testosterone should be monitored for potential side effects including: benign prostatic hyperplasia, prostate cancer, erythrocytosis, and the development or worsening of sleep apnea. Other minor effects are acne/oily skin and reduced sperm production/infertility. Digital rectal examination (DRE) and measurement of prostate-specific antigen (PSA) should be performed in men 50 years or older before initiation of testosterone therapy and annually thereafter. The patient should be promptly referred for a prostate biopsy if a nodule is palpated by DRE or if the PSA is elevated, and discontinuation of therapy may be warranted. The hemoglobin and hematocrit should be monitored after 3 months, and then yearly to screen for the development of erythrocytosis.

SPECIAL TOPICS

Emerging Treatments

- An intramuscular formulation of testosterone, undecanoate (Nebido), given every 12 weeks is completing phase III pharmacokinetic studies. Serum testosterone concentration is maintained within the normal range.
- An implantable pellet system (Tesopel) can result in physiologic testosterone levels with little fluctuations over 4 to 6 months, but requires a minor surgical procedure with potential risks of infection and extrusion of the pellet.

KEY POINTS TO REMEMBER

- Male hypogonadism is divided into primary (caused by the failure of the testis) and secondary (resulting from defects at the hypothalamic–pituitary level) causes.
- Primary hypogonadism is associated with a low testosterone level but high FSH and LH levels.
- Secondary hypogonadism is associated with a low testosterone level, as well as low or normal FSH and LH levels.
- Reduced testosterone production during the prepubertal period results in micropenis and incomplete pubertal development.
- Reduced testosterone production during the postpubertal period leads to decreased libido, muscle mass, hair growth, energy, mood, libido, hematocrit, and bone mass.
- Treatment for both causes of hypogonadism consists of testosterone replacement, with the goal of achieving normal serum testosterone levels and alleviating symptoms.
- DRE and PSA testing should be performed before initiating testosterone therapy and annually thereafter.

REFERENCES AND SUGGESTED READINGS

Bhasin, S, et al. Testosterone replacement increases fat-free mass and muscle size in hypogonadal men. *J Clin Endocrinol Metab* 1997;82:407.

Boulous P-MG, Legros JJ, Mueleman EJ, et al. Testosterone replacement in symptomatic late-onset hypogonadism: clinical and metabolic responses in a randomized-placebo controlled study. #519-3. Clinical Trials Symposium ENDO 2007, Toronto, Canada.

Burris AS, Gonadotropin therapy in men with isolated hypogonadotropic hypogonadism: the response to human chorionic gonadotropin is predicted by initial testicular size. *J Clin Endocrinol Metab* 1988;66:1144–1151.

Christensen AK. Leydig cells. In: Hamilton DW, Greep RO, eds. *Handbook of Physiology*.

Feldman HA, et al. Age trends in the level of serum testosterone and other hormones in middle-aged men: longitudinal results from the Massachusetts Male Aging Study. *J Clin Endocrinol Metab* 2002;87:589–598.

Finkel DM, Phillips JL, Snyder PJ, et al. Stimulation of spermatogenesis by gonadotropins in men with hypogonadotropic hypogonadism. *N Engl J Med* 1985;313:651–655.

Finkelstein JS, Klibonski A, Neer RM, et al. Osteoporosis in men with idiopathic hypogonadotropic hypogonadism. *Ann Intern Med* 1987;106:354–361.

Gabrilove JL, Sharma DC, Wotiz HH, et al. Feminizing adrenocortical tumors in the male: a review of 52 cases. *Medicine (Baltimore)* 1965;44:37–79.

Harman SM, Metter EJ, Tobin JD, et al. Longitudinal effects of aging on serum total and free testosterone levels in healthy men. Baltimore Study of Male Aging. *J Clin Endocrinol Metab* 2001:86:724–731.

Hearle L. Nebido: a long-acting injectable testosterone for the treatment of male hypogonadism. *Expert Opin Pharmacother* 2005;6:1751–1759.

Kuhn JM, Mahoudeau JA, Billaud L, et al. Evaluation of diagnostic criteria for Leydig cell tumors in adult men revealed by gynecomastia. *Clin Endocrinol* 1987;26:407–416.

Layman, LC. Hypogonadotropic hypogonadism. *Endocrinol Metab Clin North Am* 2007;37:283–296.

Luton JP, Thieblot P, Valcke JC, et al. Reversible gonadotropin deficiency in male Cushing's disease. *J Clin Endocrinol Metab* 1977;45:488–495.

MacAdams MR, White RH, Chipps BE, et al. Reduction of serum testosterone levels during chronic glucocorticoid therapy. *Ann Intern Med* 1986;104:648–651.

Maya-Nunez G, Zentero JC, Ulloa-Aguirre A, et al. A recurrent missense mutation in the KAL gene in patients with X-linked Kallmann's syndrome. *J Clin Endocrinol Metab* 1998;83:1650–1653.

Morley JE, Kaise FR, Perry HM, et al. Longitudinal changes in testosterone, luteinizing hormone, and follicle-stimulating hormones in healthy older men. *Metabolism* 1997;46:410–413.

Rolf C, Knie U, Lemmitz G, et al. Interpersonal testosterone transfer after topical application of a newly developed testosterone gel preparation. *Clin Endocrinol (Oxf)* 2002;56:637.

Russell DW, Wilson JD. Steroid 5 alpha-reductase: two genes/two enzymes. *Annu Rev Biochem* 1994;63:25–61.

Schubert M, Minnemann T, Hubler D, et al. Intramuscular testosterone undecanoate: pharmacokinetic aspects of a novel testosterone formulation during long-term treatment of men with hypogonadism. *J Clin Endocrinol Metab* 2004;89:5429.

Sherins RJ, Loriaux DL. Studies on the role of sex steroids in the feedback control of FSH concentrations in men. *J Clin Endocrinol Metab* 1973;36:886–893.

Snyder PJ. Clinical features, diagnosis and treatment of male hypogonadism in adults. In: Rose BD, ed. *UpToDate*. Wellesley, MA: UpToDate, 2003.

Spratt DI, Finkelstein JS, O'Dea LS, et al. Long-term administration of gonadotropin-releasing hormone in men with idiopathic hypogonadotropic hypogonadism: a model for studies of the hormone's physiological effects. *Ann Intern Med* 1986;105:848–855.

Stepanas AV, Samaan NA, Shultz PN, et al. Endocrine studies in testicular tumor patients with and without gynecomastia: a report of 45 cases. *Cancer* 1978;41:369–376.

Von Schoultz B, Carlstrom K. On the regulation of sex-hormone binding globulin: a challenge of an old dogma and outlines of an alternative mechanism. *J Steroid Biochem Mol Biol* 1989;32:327–334.

Wu FC, Bulter GE, Kelnar CJ, et al. Patterns of pulsatile luteinizing hormone and follicle-stimulating hormone secretion in prepubertal (midchildhood) boys and girls and patients with idiopathic hypogonadotrophic hypogonadism (Kallmann's syndrome): a study using an ultrasensitive time-resolved immunofluorometric assay. *J Clin Endocrinol Metab* 1991;72: 1229–1237.

Polycystic Ovary Syndrome (PCOS)

20

Paraskevi Mentzelopoulos

INTRODUCTION

Polycystic ovary syndrome (PCOS) is the *most common endocrine disorder in women of reproductive age (7%–10%)* and a major cause of infertility. PCOS was first described in 1935 by Stein and Levinthal as a syndrome of signs and symptoms including oligomenorrhea, hirsutism, and enlarged ovaries and obesity, varying in severity from subject to subject. The pathophysiologic characteristics of the syndrome remain unclear, and its definition continues to be a topic of controversy.

Definition

In 1990, the National Institutes of Health (NIH) Conference on PCOS proposed the following diagnostic criteria:

- Chronic anovulation **and**
- Clinical (acne, hirsutism) or biochemical (elevated androgen level) evidence of hyperandrogenism.

Both features were required to make the diagnosis of PCOS. More recently, revised criteria have been proposed by the Rotterdam PCOS Consensus Workshop Group in 2003. According to these revised criteria, two of three of the following are sufficient for establishing the diagnosis of PCOS:

- Oligo- or anovulation
- Clinical and/or biochemical evidence of hyperandrogenism
- Polycystic ovaries. Ultrasound criteria that were considered specific and sensitive in defining PCOS were given (see Diagnosis).

Exclusion of other etiologies of female hyperandrogenism, such as androgen-secreting tumors, Cushing's syndrome, nonclassic congenital adrenal hyperplasia (CAH), *is essential for diagnosis with **both** the 1990 and the 2003 Diagnostic criteria.*

Pathophysiology

The etiology of PCOS remains unknown. A prominent characteristic of the syndrome is that reproductive (hyperandrogenemia, anovulation) and metabolic (insulin resistance, obesity) disorders coexist to the degree that it is unclear which are primary. No single etiologic factor can account for the whole spectrum of abnormalities seen in PCOS.

Increased frequency of hypothalamic release of gonadotropin-releasing hormone (GnRH) is found in women with PCOS. It is unclear if this defect in GnRH pulse generation is a primary or secondary abnormality. Increasing frequency of GnRH favors the secretion of luteinizing hormone (LH) versus follicle-stimulating hormone (FSH) from the anterior pituitary, so that LH pulses also increase in frequency and amplitude. An elevated LH-to-FSH ratio can be seen in most women with PCOS. The ovary in PCOS responds to the LH stimulation with a preferential increase in the production of androgen versus estrogen. Low circulating progestin levels (as a result of oligo-ovulation) and elevated androgen levels create a feedback that further potentiates inappropriate hypothalamic–pituitary gonadotropin secretion and leads to a vicious cycle. Estradiol levels are typically normal to low, but estrone levels are significantly elevated. This is because of conversion of androstenedione to estrone in adipose tissue, which further stimulates LH and suppresses FSH.

The observation that hyperinsulinemia is a feature of PCOS was first made in 1980. Before this, the observation was made that women with syndromes of extreme insulin resistance also had hyperandrogenemia and anovulation. Insulin and insulin-like growth factor 1 (IFG-1) can impact several of the pathways that contribute to the pathogenesis of PCOS. They prime theca cells for LH-stimulated androgen synthesis. Insulin decreases the synthesis of SHBG (sex hormone–binding globulin), the effect of which would be to increase androgen bioactivity. A direct role of insulin in the production of adrenal androgens and in the hypothalamic–pituitary–gonadal axis disorder has been proposed.

Evidence suggests that PCOS is heritable, but the pathogenesis of the syndrome points to a complex, multigenic disorder. Candidate genes that may be responsible for alterations in ovarian, hypothalamic, and insulin receptor function have been the focus of linkage and case-control studies. It has also been suggested that prenatal androgenization of the female fetus induced by genetic and environmental factors, or the interaction of both, may program differentiating target tissues toward the development of PCOS phenotype in adult life.

PRESENTATION

Clinical Presentation

PCOS is characterized by clinical and/or biochemical hyperandrogenism and by chronic anovulation. Most of the features of the syndrome develop at the onset of puberty, and the severity varies from mild hirsutism to amenorrhea and infertility. Infertility may be the presenting complaint.

Androgen Excess

Androgen excess can result in hirsutism, acne, seborrhea, and androgenic alopecia (male pattern baldness). Hirsutism is characterized by excess terminal pigmented hair in a male pattern of distribution, and commonly occurs on the chin, upper lip, periareolar area, and the lower abdomen. Assessment of hyperandrogenism is dependent on a number of factors, including the observer, race of the patient, and use of cosmetic hair-removal agents. Alopecia is rare in PCOS.

Signs of virilization, such as deepening of voice, increased muscle mass, and clitoromegaly, are rarely seen with PCOS and, if present, should prompt evaluation for an androgen-secreting tumor.

Menstrual Irregularities

Menstrual dysfunction is a defining characteristic of PCOS and may manifest in several different forms. It is usually associated with chronic oligo- or anovulation. Women with PCOS usually have adequate estrogen but are deficient in progesterone. This results in endometrial hyperplasia and dysfunctional uterine bleeding caused by chronic estrogenic stimulation, which increases the risk for endometrial cancer. Less commonly, women with PCOS present with secondary amenorrhea (~24%); these women have lower estrogen levels and higher testosterone and free androgens levels and respond less favorably to treatment.

Infertility

Women with PCOS may ovulate intermittently and, therefore, take longer to conceive. If pregnancy does occur, there is an increased risk for pregnancy-induced hypertension, preeclampsia, gestational diabetes, pregnancy loss, and preterm labor. A subset of women with PCOS has persistent anovulation and infertility.

Obesity

Central visceral obesity (android type) affects 40% to 50% of women with PCOS. Interestingly, the mean body mass index (BMI) in women with PCOS in the United States is 35 to 40, but in Europe and other countries it is 25 to 28 or less.

Obesity is not considered a triggering event in the development of the syndrome but is an independent risk factor for reproductive and metabolic complications. The android body phenotype (increased waist-to-hip ratio) that is associated with higher risk for insulin resistance and development of type 2 diabetes has been noted in both obese and lean women with PCOS.

Hyperinsulinemia/Insulin Resistance

Hyperinsulinemia and insulin resistance can be present even in the absence of obesity, but these conditions are exacerbated by the presence of it. Severe insulin resistance is usually appreciated clinically by the presence of acanthosis nigricans, but many women may have a mild form with slightly elevated fasting serum insulin levels. Reducing insulin resistance by weight loss or pharmacologic means (metformin [Glucophage], thiazolidinediones) can be associated with increased ovulation and lower androgen levels, thereby suggesting an important role for insulin resistance in the pathogenesis of this disorder.

MANAGEMENT

Diagnosis

PCOS belongs in a category of diseases that are characterized by normogonadotropic, normoestrogenic hyperandrogenic anovulation and **is a diagnosis of exclusion.** All women who meet diagnostic criteria for PCOS should undergo screening to exclude other common reasons for anovulation, such as hyperprolactinemia and hypothyroidism, and to exclude other etiologies of female hyperandrogenism, including androgen-secreting tumors (adrenal or ovarian), nonclassic CAH, or Cushing's syndrome. Use of exogenous androgens or medications that can cause a similar picture, like some antipsychotic agents, should be excluded by a careful history. PCOS is diagnosed according to clinical criteria (Table 20-1).

Laboratory Evaluation
The laboratory workup is aimed at excluding other disorders. An androgen-secreting neoplasm can be suspected if there is an abrupt onset of signs of virilization, hirsutism, and amenorrhea. Typically, patients with adrenal tumors have markedly elevated **testosterone** (>200 ng/dL) and dehydroepiandrosterone sulfate (**DHEA-S**) (>600 mcg/dL) levels. Serum LH is usually suppressed. A random **17-hydroxyprogesterone level** of <200 ng/dL excludes nonclassic CAH. For further workup of nonclassic CAH, refer to Chapter 12, Adult Congenital Adrenal Hyperplasia. Overnight **1-mg dexamethasone suppression** of morning cortisol to <1.2 ng/mL rules out Cushing's syndrome.

TABLE 20-1	CLINICAL AND BIOCHEMICAL FEATURES OF PCOS

1. **Clinical signs of hyperandrogenism**
   –Acne
   –Alopecia
   –Hirsutism
2. **Menstrual irregularities associated with chronic oligo- or anovulation**
3. **Polycystic ovaries**
4. **Other causes of hyperandrogenemia must be excluded**
5. **Associated features (not required for diagnosis)**
   –Hypothalamic–pituitary abnormalities (elevated LH/FSH ratio >2)
   –Insulin resistance and obesity

FSH, follicle-stimulating hormone; LH, luteinizing hormone.

Hyperprolactinemia and hypothyroidism are not usually associated with hyperandrogenemia, but a serum **prolactin** and **TSH** level should be checked in any woman with menstrual irregularity. **There is no universally accepted definition for PCOS based on hormonal criteria,** but the following biochemical abnormalities are usually seen:

- Roughly 80% of the women with PCOS have an elevated serum androgen level, with increases in both total and free testosterone levels in the upper normal to twofold higher range.
- Because of decreased production of hepatic SHBG, the total testosterone may be in the normal range despite the free testosterone being elevated. DHEA-S levels are sometimes mildly elevated.
- Elevated LH and normal FSH, resulting in an elevated LH/FSH ratio that may be >2 is usually seen, but gonadotropin values are not useful in confirming the diagnosis. LH levels could be useful as a secondary parameter, especially in lean women with amenorrhea.
- Serum estrone levels can be increased (with normal serum estradiol levels).
- Mild elevations in prolactin can be seen in women with PCOS.
- Impaired glucose tolerance (and even frank diabetes) is found in 30% to 40% of women after a 2-hour glucose tolerance test. Fasting blood glucose levels may be normal. The 2003 guidelines suggest to screen obese women (BMI, >27 kg/m^2) with PCOS with an oral glucose tolerance test (OGTT).
- Dyslipidemia. The prevalence of atherogenic lipid profile [high very-low-density lipoprotein (VLDL), high low-density lipoprotein (LDL), and low high-density lipoprotein (HDL)] is increased in women with PCOS after adjusting for BMI. Low HDL levels are associated with obesity and high LDL levels with hyperandrogenemia.

Ultrasound Characteristics

The specific ultrasound characteristics proposed by the 2003 consensus are (a) presence of 12 or more follicles in each ovary measuring 2 to 9 mm in diameter and (b) increased ovarian volume (>10 mL) and stroma. Only one ovary with these criteria is sufficient. **The subjective appearance of polycystic ovaries should not be substituted for this definition.** These ultrasound criteria do *not apply to women on oral contraceptive pills (OCPs)*. If there is evidence of a dominant follicle (>10 mm), the scan should be repeated.

TREATMENT

The treatment of women with PCOS should be individualized to the patient and can involve both nonpharmacologic and pharmacologic approaches. There are several treatment options for each of the manifestations of PCOS. Most manifestations can be reversed by improving insulin resistance, either by weight loss or by pharmacologic therapy. Typically, response to therapy is slow, with clinical changes lagging behind biochemical improvement by several months. **Pregnancy should be excluded before initiation of pharmacologic therapy with oral contraceptives or antiandrogens.** Table 20-2 lists different treatment options for the main complaints of women with PCOS.

Nonpharmacologic Treatment

Weight Loss/Life Style Modifications

Weight loss should be the first-line therapeutic option in all women who are overweight or obese and who are diagnosed with PCOS. Weight loss of >5% of body weight has been

TABLE 20-2	TREATMENT OPTIONS FOR THE MOST COMMON FEATURES OF PCOS

1. **Oligo- or amenorrhea**

   (A) Overweight and obese patients

   –Lifestyle modifications to achieve weight loss for at least 6 months is the first-line option

   –If this fails, oral contraceptives with low-dose estrogen and an antiandrogenic or low androgenic potential progestin with metformin

   (B) Lean patients

   –Oral contraceptives or periodic progesterone withdrawal +/− metformin (if there are clinical signs of insulin resistance)

2. **Hirsutism**

   (A) Mechanical/topical treatments:

   –Plucking, shaving, laser

   –Eflornithine hydrochloride 13.9% (Vaniqa cream)

   (B) Decrease testosterone production:

   –If overweight, obese: lifestyle modification/weight loss first

   –If lean: oral contraceptives with antiandrogenic progestin

   –Metformin (indirectly, by decreasing insulin levels)

   (C) Decrease testosterone action:

   –Spironolactone

   –Increase in SHBG (exercise, decrease in insulin level by weight loss or insulin sensitizers)

3. **Infertility**

   (A) Overweight and obese patients: life style changes and weight loss first

   (B) Metformin

   (C) Clomiphene citrate with or without metformin for 6–9 cycles

   (D) Injectable gonadotropins or in vitro fertilization

shown to decrease testosterone levels, improve hirsutism, increase SHBG, improve menstruation and ovulation, and increase pregnancy rates if it is maintained for at least 12 months.

Hirsutism
Hirsutism can be treated by removal of hair by bleaching, waxing, shaving, electrolysis, or laser treatment.

Pharmacologic Treatment

Oral Contraceptives
OCPs are the standard therapy for patients with PCOS who do not desire pregnancy. OCPs are not a treatment for PCOS, but rather an interruption of the vicious cycle of hyperandrogenemia and oligomenorrhea. They allow the resumption of normal menses and prevent the chronic, unopposed, estrogenic stimulation of the endometrium. They lower androgen levels by 50% to 60%. Hirsutism and acne respond well to estrogen therapy. Pregnancy should be excluded before initiating treatment. Typically, treatment should be initiated by a combination preparation that contains ethinyl estradiol in conjunction with a progestin with low androgenic activity such as norgestimate or a progestin with antiandrogenic effects like drospirenone or cyproterone acetate (the latter is not available in the United States). Controversy exists about the long-term use of OCPs in this group of women who may be at increased risk for developing metabolic and cardiovascular complications. Estrogens impair carbohydrate tolerance in a dose-dependent manner, as do androgens and progestins with greater androgenic activity. The choice of oral contraceptive should be individualized for each patient based on the degree of insulin resistance, degree of androgenicity, anthropometric characteristics, and presence of other risk factors for metabolic and cardiovascular complications. Women must stop smoking prior to beginning OCPs, owing to the increased risk of thromboembolic disease. A careful history must be taken for contraindications for OCP therapy.

In women who do not desire (or cannot take) oral contraceptive therapy, oral intermittent progestin therapy with a 7- to 10-day course of medroxyprogesterone acetate (Provera) once every 1 to 3 months can be considered. Although this therapy can offer endometrial protection, it does not reduce the effects of hyperandrogenism such as hirsutism and acne.

Antiandrogens
Antiandrogens can be used in conjunction with oral contraceptives to derive further benefit in cases for which hirsutism is the primary complaint. Spironolactone (Aldactone) (50–100 mg twice daily) decreases the effect of androgens by blocking the androgen receptor. When used alone, it has minimal effects on free testosterone levels. When used in combination with an oral contraceptive, both androgen levels (via estrogen) and androgen action (via spironolactone) are decreased. Finasteride (Propecia), which blocks conversion of testosterone to dihydrotestosterone, can also be used to treat hirsutism. Because of the teratogenic potential of antiandrogens, they must be used only when women are treated with effective contraception.

Enflornithine hydrochloride 13.9% cream (Vaniqa), which slows hair growth, can be used to treat facial hirsutism. It is usually not covered by insurance. Topical minoxidil can be used for male pattern hair loss.

Insulin Sensitizers
The use of medications that improve insulin sensitivity was initially based on the observation that interventions that improve insulin resistance, such as weight loss, reduce androgen levels and induce ovulation. The clinical response to insulin-lowering therapies does not seem to be related to the magnitude of insulin resistance.

Although it is not approved by the Food and Drug Administration (FDA) for the treatment of PCOS, metformin is an effective treatment, especially for women who are anovulatory and desire pregnancy. Metformin decreases testosterone levels and fasting insulin and glucose levels. The rate of improvement in menses/ovulation ranges from 40% to 90% in different studies. Metformin can be used in pregnancy (category B). Effective doses of metformin are between 1500 and 2000 mg/day, although randomized studies have not been done.

Thiazolindiones are another class of drugs that improve insulin sensitivity. All the initial studies in women with PCOS were done with troglitazone and showed ovulatory rates >40%. Troglitazone has since been removed from the market due to serious hepatotoxicity. Newer agents (rosiglitazone, pioglitazone) have been used in studies and have shown similar effects in increasing insulin sensitivity, decreasing testosterone levels, and inducing ovulation. These agents should not be used in women who desire pregnancy, because they are contraindicated in pregnancy (category C). In addition, very recent data suggest the possibility of increased cardiovascular mortality with rosiglitazone, an important consideration for this group of patients who may already be at increased risk for cardiovascular disease.

Weight Loss Agents

More recently, studies in women with PCOS have used agents like Orlistat to achieve weight loss and have shown reduction of testosterone levels in addition to weight loss.

Infertility

When fertility is desired, oral contraceptives and antiandrogens cannot be used. It is important to complete a basic infertility evaluation of the couple, including a semen analysis of the man, to rule out other contributing factors. Weight loss and insulin sensitizers, such as metformin, may induce ovulatory cycles and permit pregnancy. Clomiphene citrate (Clomid) is a triphenylethylene-derived nonsteroidal agent that is theorized to function at the level of the hypothalamus as an antiandrogen to restore gonadotropin secretion. It is superior to metformin in achieving conception, but there is a relatively high rate of multiple pregnancies. Combination of clomiphene with metformin may increase pregnancy rates. If pregnancy is not achieved after 6 to 9 months of clomiphene with or without metformin, the patient should be referred to a fertility specialist for use of injectable gonadotropins or in vitro fertilization.

An increased incidence of spontaneous miscarriage is associated with PCOS. Treatment with metformin may reduce the rate of miscarriage. Women with PCOS have significant reproductive morbidity, as mentioned previously.

SPECIAL CONSIDERATIONS

Long-Term Risks

The long-term metabolic and cardiovascular disease risks associated with PCOS heighten the importance of proper diagnosis. The prevalence of impaired glucose tolerance and type 2 diabetes is increased in women with PCOS (3–7 times higher risk of developing diabetes).

This association is seen in both obese and lean women with PCOS. Women with a family history of type 2 diabetes are at even greater risk for development of diabetes. Hypertension is not common in young women with PCOS, but studies have shown that a longer or irregular menstrual cycle length can lead to a twofold increase in risk for hypertension in women with PCOS. The prevalence of hypertension increases dramatically by the time of perimenopause. Women with PCOS also have an increased risk for dyslipidemia and have been shown to have abnormal vascular function, higher rates of coagulopathy, and increased markers of inflammation. Whether women with PCOS and the metabolic syndrome are at increased cardiovascular risk remains a question for future investigation, although predictions of a sevenfold relative risk for myocardial infarction have been made.

Unopposed estrogenic stimulation of the uterus may increase the likelihood of endometrial hyperplasia and endometrial carcinoma.

Sleep apnea also occurs at a higher incidence in women with PCOS.

KEY POINTS TO REMEMBER

- Minimum criteria to diagnose PCOS are two of three of the following: oligo- or anovulation, clinical or biochemical evidence of hyperandrogenism, or polycystic ovaries. **PCOS is a diagnosis of exclusion**, and other treatable conditions associated with hyperandrogenism should first be excluded (androgen-producing tumors, nonclassic CAH, Cushing's syndrome).
- PCOS is the most common endocrinopathy in women of reproductive age.
- Other conditions associated with PCOS may include the metabolic syndrome, glucose intolerance or type 2 diabetes, dyslipidemia, hypertension, sleep apnea, and infertility. Obesity increases the risk for these long-term complications.
- The chronic estrogenic stimulation seen in PCOS results in endometrial hyperplasia and dysfunctional uterine bleeding and may lead to endometrial carcinoma.
- The first-line treatment for overweight and obese patients with PCOS should be weight loss and life style modifications.
- The mainstay for treatment of olimenorrhea/amenorrhea includes a combination oral contraceptive preparation that contains low-dose ethinyl estradiol, in conjunction with a progestin with low androgenic activity or even antiandrogenic activity.
- An antiandrogen may be added for additional benefit in controlling hirsutism when this is the main complaint.
- Insulin sensitizers can reduce insulin and androgen levels and increase ovulatory cycles.
- Clomiphene citrate has been shown to be superior to metformin in achieving conception but has a risk of multiple pregnancies.
- Women with PCOS are at high risk for developing gestational diabetes, pregnancy-induced hypertension, preeclampsia, and preterm labor.

REFERENCES AND SUGGESTED READINGS

Azziz R, Hincapie LA, Knochenhauer ES, et al. Screening for 21 hydroxylase deficient non classical adrenal hyperplasia among hyperandrogenic women: a prospective study. *Fertil Steril* 1999;72:915–925.

Baillargeon JP, McClish DK, Essah PA, et al. Association between the current use of low dose oral contraceptives and cardiovascular arterial disease: a metaanalysis. *J Clin Endocrinol Metab* 2005;90:3863–3870.

Boosma CM, Eijkemans MJ, Hughes EG, et al. A meta analysis of pregnancy outcomes in women with PCOS, *Hum Reprod Update* 2006;12:673–683.

Burghen GA, Givens JR, Kitabchi AE, et al. Correlation of hyperandrogenism with hyperinsulinemia in PCOS. *J Clin Endocrinol Metab* 1980;50:113–116.

Coulam CB, Anneger JF, Kranz JS. Chronic anovulation syndrome and associated neoplasia. *Obstet Gynecol* 1983;61:403.

Dahlgren E, Janson PO, Johansson S, et al. PCOS and the risk for myocardial infarction evaluated from a risk factor model based on a prospective study of women. *Acta Obstet Gynecol Scand* 1992;71: 599–604.

DeLeo V, La Marca A, Petraglia F. Insulin lowering agents in the management of PCOS. *Endocr Rev* 2003;24:633–667.

Derksen J, Nagesser SK, Meinders AE. Identification of virilizing adrenal tumors in hirsute women. *N Engl J Med* 1994;331:968.

Ehrmann DA. Medical progress: polycystic ovary syndrome. *N Engl J Med* 2005;352: 1223–1236.

Jayagopal V, Kilpatrick ES, Holding S, et al. Orlistat is as beneficial as metformin in the treatment of PCOS. *J Clin Endocrinol Metab* 2005;90:729–733.

Legro RS, Barnhart HX, Schlaff WD, et al. Clomiphene, metformin, or both for infertility in the polycystic ovary syndrome. *N Engl J Med* 2007;356:551–566.

Legro RS, Kunselmal AR, Dodson WC, et al. Prevalence and predictors of the risk for type 2 diabetes and impaired glucose tolerance in PCOS: a prospective study in 254 affected women. *J Clin Endocrinol Metab* 1999;84:165–169.

Legro RS. A 27 y.o. woman with a diagnosis of PCOS. *JAMA* 2007;297:509–519.

Nader S, Diamanti-Kandarakis E. PCOS, oral contraceptives and metabolic issues: new perspectives and a unifying hypothesis. *Hum Reprod* 2007;22:317–322.

Nam Menke M, Strauss J. Genetics of PCOS. *Clin Obstet Gynecol* 2007;50:188-204.

Nestler JE, Jakubowicz DJ, Evans WS, et al. Effects of metformin on spontaneous and clomiphene-induced ovulation in the polycystic ovary syndrome. *N Engl J Med* 1998;338:1876.

Pasquali R, Antenucci D, Casimirri F, et al. Clinical and hormonal characteristics of obese amenorrheic hyperandrogenic women before and after weight loss. *J Clin Endocrinol Metab* 1989;68:173.

Srikanthan P, Korenman S, Davis S. PCOS: The next cardiovascular dilemma in women? *Endocrinol Metab Clin North Am* 2006;35:611–631.

Stein I, Leventhal M. Amenorrhea associated with bilateral polycystic ovaries. *Am J Obstet Gynecol* 1935;29:181.

The Rotterdam ESHRE/ASRM-sponsored PCOS consensus workshop group. Revised 2003 consensus on diagnostic criteria and long-term health risks related to polycystic ovary syndrome (PCOS). *Hum Reprod* 2004;19:41–47.

Xita N, Tsatsoulis Review: Fetal programming of PCOS by androgen excess: evidence from experimental, clinical and genetic association studies. *J Clin Endocrinol Metab* 2006;91:1660–1666.

Hypercalcemia

Kent Ishihara

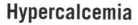

21

INTRODUCTION

Hypercalcemia is defined as an excessive amount of calcium in the blood. Depending on the population being studied, hypercalcemia affects up to 0.1% to 2.6% of hospitalized patients, with malignancy and primary hyperparathyroidism (PHP) accounting for 50% to 90% of all cases. In the hospital setting, malignancy is the leading cause of hypercalcemia, and it often has a more acute presentation. PHP is the leading cause of hypercalcemia in the outpatient setting and is often asymptomatic. Therefore, the chronicity of the disease is often a clue to the underlying process—the longer the patient has been noted to be hypercalcemic, the less likely it is caused by a malignancy. Conversely, the more rapidly progressive the hypercalcemia, the more likely it is due to a malignancy.

CAUSES

Disorders causing hypercalcemia are most easily classified according to parathyroid hormone (PTH) levels: (a) PTH-dependent (elevated or inappropriately normal PTH) and (b) PTH-independent (low PTH) (Table 21-1).

Parathyroid Hormone–Dependent Hypercalcemia

Hypercalcemia associated with an inappropriately normal or elevated PTH level is considered to be PTH-dependent. In other words, PTH is the driving force for the elevated calcium levels.

Discussed in more detail in Chapter 22, Hyperparathyroidism, elevations in PTH cause an increase in serum calcium by three separate mechanisms.

- Elevated $1,25(OH)_2D$ leads to an increase in calcium absorption from the gut.
- There is an increase in calcium reabsorption from bone.
- There is an increase in renal calcium reabsorption.

Primary Hyperparathyroidism

The most common cause of PTH-dependent hypercalcemia is primary hyperparathyroidism. Typically, primary hyperparathyroidism is caused by a parathyroid adenoma; however, four-gland hyperplasia and carcinoma are also seen, and may be part of a familial syndrome, such as the multiple endocrine neoplasia (MEN) syndromes. PHP is associated with an elevated PTH in the setting of hypercalcemia. In its earliest stage, "incipient" PHP may occur with a normal calcium level, but secondary hyperparathyroidism (most commonly from vitamin D deficiency or chronic kidney disease) must first be excluded. Hypophosphatemia and an elevated urine calcium excretion are also typically present.

TABLE 21-1 DIFFERENTIAL DIAGNOSIS OF HYPERCALCEMIA

Parathyroid Hormone–Dependent
Primary hyperparathyroidism
Tertiary hyperparathyroidism
Familial hypocalciuric hypercalcemia
MEN syndromes
Lithium therapy
Parathyroid Hormone–Independent
　Malignancy related
　　Secretion of parathyroid hormone–related peptide
　　Osteoclastic activation
　　Secretion of vitamin D
　　Unknown mechanisms
　Vitamin D related
　　Granulomatous disease
　　Infectious (mycobacterial, fungal, etc.)
　　Noninfectious (sarcoidosis, eosinophilic granuloma, Wegener's
　　　granulomatosis, etc.)
　　Vitamin D intoxication
　　Williams' syndrome
　Miscellaneous endocrine
　　Hyperthyroidism
　　Pheochromocytoma
　　Adrenal insufficiency
　　Islet cell tumors
　Miscellaneous
　　Immobilization
　　Milk-alkali syndrome
　　Other medications/intoxications

MEN, multiple endocrine neoplasia.

Complications include nephrolithiasis and a reduction in cortical bone density leading to osteoporosis.

Familial Hypocalciuric Hypercalcemia
Far less common than primary hyperparathyroidism, familial hypocalciuric hypercalcemia (FHH) is caused by a calcium sensor defect that increases the set point for serum calcium homeostasis (see also Chapter 22, Hyperparathyroidism). In this autosomal-dominant disorder, PTH secretion is inhibited only at supernormal concentrations of calcium in the blood. Elevations in calcium and PTH are usually only mild, urine calcium excretion is typically low, and complications are unusual. A previous history of normal calcium levels effectively rules out FHH, since it is a lifelong condition.

Lithium

Lithium therapy may also lead to hypercalcemia in 15% to 60% of patients by an unknown mechanism that shifts the set point for calcium sensing in a manner similar to the defect in FHH. Therefore, these patients are usually asymptomatic, with only mild elevations of calcium and PTH, urine calcium excretion is typically low, and complications are unusual. Hypercalcemia often resolves after withdrawal of lithium.

Parathyroid Hormone–Independent Hypercalcemia

Malignancy-Associated Hypercalcemia

Hypercalcemia is the most common life-threatening metabolic disorder associated with malignant neoplasia, occurring in an estimated 10% to 20% of all adults with cancer. It also occurs in children with cancer, but with a frequency of only 0.5% to 1% (www.cancer.gov 2007). The frequency of hypercalcemia in various malignancies is found in Table 21-2.

The syndrome of humoral hypercalcemia of malignancy (HHM) is the most common cause of malignancy-associated hypercalcemia. HHM is mediated by PTH-related peptide (PTHrP), a peptide with amino-terminus homology to PTH and a similar biologic activity. Commonly seen in patients with squamous carcinomas and cancers of the kidney, ovary, and bladder, HHM is also a frequent complication in patients with lymphomas associated with human T-cell lymphoma/leukemia virus 1 (HTLV-1). HHM can be differentiated from PHP by finding an elevated PTHrP level in the setting of an elevated calcium level with a suppressed PTH. In addition, unlike in PHP, $1,25(OH)_2D$ levels and intestinal calcium absorption are typically low. The mechanisms underlying these differences have not been elucidated, since nearly identical alterations in bone and kidney physiology occur when either PTHrP or PTH are infused into humans.

TABLE 21-2	FREQUENCY OF HYPERCALCEMIA IN VARIOUS MALIGNANCIES

More common
Breast cancer with bone metastases
Squamous cell cancers (particularly lung)
Multiple myeloma
T- and B-cell lymphomas
Hodgkin's disease
Pancreatic islet cell tumors
Cholangiocarcinoma
Common
Adenocarcinomas (lung, renal, pancreatic, ovarian)
Uncommon
Breast cancer without bone metastases
Small cell lung cancer
Colon cancer
Uterine cancer
Occult malignancy

Less commonly, malignancy-associated hypercalcemia may develop in the presence of skeletal involvement from a primary hematologic neoplasm (e.g., multiple myeloma, leukemia, and lymphoma) or skeletal metastases from a solid tumor (e.g., breast cancer) causing local osteolysis. Hypercalcemia in these patients was originally thought to be caused by direct physical destruction of bone by malignant cells; however, there is growing evidence that this process is mediated indirectly through the activation of osteoclasts. The exact paracrine factors or cytokines involved have not been determined. In breast cancer, PTHrP produced locally may also act to induce osteoclastic bone resorption, despite low serum levels of the hormone. Clinically, these patients can be differentiated from both PHP and HHM by the finding of a low PTH and PTHrP in the setting of hypercalcemia. These patients also typically have low 1,25(OH)$_2$D levels and an elevated fractional excretion of calcium.

Ectopic PTH secretion from carcinomas of the lung, thymus, ovary, and undifferentiated neuroendocrine tumors are an extremely rare cause of malignancy-associated hypercalcemia. Also described are lymphomas causing hypercalcemia through increased synthesis of 1,25(OH)$_2$D.

Milk-Alkali Syndrome

The milk-alkali syndrome was first described in the 1920s when the treatment for peptic ulcer disease involved the use of dairy products and alkaline powders. Today, it is often seen in patients taking excessive amounts of calcium-containing antacids or dietary supplements for osteoporosis, and is now the third most common cause of hypercalcemia. Acute, subacute, and chronic presentations of this syndrome all include hypercalcemia, alkalosis, and renal failure. Hypercalcemia is associated with a suppressed PTH; however, a rebound hyperparathyroidism with an elevated PTH can be found if the PTH is determined after aggressive volume repletion leading to mild hypocalcemia. Typically, >5 g of calcium per day are required to produce the syndrome, but is dependent on individual patient susceptibility (intestinal absorption and renal clearance of calcium). Once hypercalcemia develops, it tends to cause volume depletion through emesis and increased renal excretion of sodium and water. Volume depletion then leads to a contraction alkalosis by increasing bicarbonate reabsorption in the proximal tubule of the kidney, and hypercalcemia exacerbates this alkalosis by suppressing PTH, which normally inhibits bicarbonate reabsorption in the proximal tubule. Alkalosis itself selectively enhances calcium reabsorption in the distal nephron, thereby exacerbating the hypercalcemia. With continued ingestion of calcium and absorbable alkali, the cycle perpetuates itself. The entire syndrome tends to resolve after discontinuation of calcium supplementation, but in the chronic form, renal failure may persist.

Vitamin D–Related Hypercalcemia

Hypercalcemia can be caused by excessive ingestion of vitamin D, or enhanced conversion of 25(OH)D to 1,25(OH)$_2$D. Chronic ingestion of more than 50,000 to 100,000 IU/day of ergocalciferol (vitamin D$_2$) or cholecalciferol (vitamin D$_3$) is required to produce significant hypercalcemia in normal individuals. Because vitamin D is highly fat soluble, intoxication may persist for weeks. Excessive or accidental ingestion of 1,25(OH)$_2$D (calcitriol) can also lead to hypercalcemia, but should resolve within days after discontinuation.

Granulomatous diseases may cause hypercalcemia through increased conversion of 25(OH)D to 1,25(OH)$_2$D by macrophages, which is insensitive to feedback regulation by calcium or PTH. Hypercalcemia develops in 10% to 20% of patients with sarcoidosis and has also been associated with lymphomas; Wegener's granulomatosis; berylliosis; eosinophilic granuloma; Crohn's disease; acute granulomatous pneumonia; hepatic granulomatosis; talc granulomatosis; silicone granulomatosis; Bacille Calmette-Guérin (BCG) therapy; lipoid pneumonia; and several infectious causes, including tuberculosis, histoplasmosis, candidiasis, coccidioidomycosis, and cat scratch fever.

Thyroid Disease

Hypercalcemia has been estimated to occur in 17% to 50% of patients with hyperthyroidism. The elevation in blood calcium is typically mild and is thought to be caused by an increase in bone turnover. Typically, PTH levels are suppressed, but they may be normal. Likewise, levels of $1,25(OH)_2D$ are also typically suppressed but may be normal. The hypercalcemia typically resolves with treatment of the underlying thyroid disorder, although β-blockers may be of some benefit in the acute setting.

Pheochromocytoma

Hypercalcemia is an infrequent complication of pheochromocytoma, and may be associated with primary hyperparathyroidism as part of MEN2A. In addition, pheochromocytoma has also been associated with PTH-independent hypercalcemia mediated by PTHrP.

Adrenal Insufficiency

Adrenal insufficiency has been associated with hypercalcemia. Primary adrenal failure has been implicated more commonly, but there are case reports in secondary adrenal failure as well. The exact pathophysiology is not known, but hypercalcemia is thought to be caused by a decrease in intravascular volume and relative hemoconcentration of serum albumin and bound calcium.

Islet Cell Tumors of the Pancreas

Islet cell tumors of the pancreas have been associated with hypercalcemia, usually in association with MEN1. However, some tumors have been found to secrete PTHrP. In others, secretion of vasoactive intestinal peptide have been found to cause hypercalcemia through unknown mechanisms, but are often associated with the WDHA syndrome—*w*atery *d*iarrhea, *h*ypokalemia, and *a*chlorhydria.

Immobilization

Prolonged immobilization typically causes bone resorption with hypercalciuria that, in rare cases, may also cause hypercalcemia. Hypercalcemia due to immobilization is more common in children and adolescents, but has also been described in burn patients, patients with spinal cord injuries or other severe neurologic deficits, and patients with underlying high bone-turnover states (e.g., Paget's disease). The mechanism by which this occurs is not entirely known, but is thought to be due to increased osteoclast and decreased osteoblast activity. Laboratory findings include hypercalciuria, elevated PTH, and low $1,25(OH)_2D$ levels. Resumption of normal physical activity typically corrects the hypercalcemia.

Vitamin A

Excessive intake of vitamin A (>50,000–100,000 IU daily) is a rare cause of hypercalcemia. Retinoic acid derivatives used in the treatment of malignancies have also been reported as a cause of hypercalcemia. The mechanism by which this occurs is not known, but it is thought to be caused by increased bone resorption. PTH is suppressed, and the diagnosis is confirmed with an elevated serum vitamin A level. Because vitamin A is highly fat soluble, hypercalcemia may take months to resolve after discontinuation of the supplement.

Aluminum Intoxication

In the past, aluminum intoxication was a significant problem in patients with chronic kidney disease treated with hemodialysis. These patients were at increased risk for hypercalcemia because aluminum accumulation in bone resulted in diminished osteoblastic activity and reduced calcium incorporation into the skeleton. When treated with calcitriol, enhanced gut absorption of calcium along with calcium in the dialysate increases the amount of bioavailable calcium flux into the body without an active reservoir to store the extra calcium, thereby resulting in hypercalcemia.

Medications

Many medications have been associated with hypercalcemia. Thiazide diuretics, in particular, are frequently implicated as a cause of hypercalcemia. However, hypercalcemia due to thiazides is typically only mild and transient (1–2 weeks) unless some other high bone-turnover state is present, such as primary hyperparathyroidism. Otherwise, PTH levels are usually normal, and the hypercalcemia is thought to arise primarily from a reduction in renal calcium excretion, although other mechanisms may also be involved.

Additional medications that have been reported to cause hypercalcemia include estrogens used in the treatment of breast cancer with bony metastases, growth hormones in intensive care unit patients, ganciclovir in renal transplantation, omeprazole in acute interstitial nephritis, 8-Cl-cAMP chemotherapy, manganese toxicity, foscarnet, hepatitis B vaccination, and theophylline.

PRESENTATION

The symptoms and signs of hypercalcemia often correlate with the age of the patient; the underlying disease process; concurrent comorbidities; and the degree, duration, and rate of development of hypercalcemia. Patients who are older or who have significant comorbidities are more likely to be sensitive to the effects of hypercalcemia. Likewise, hypercalcemia associated with malignancies or infectious disorders may present with symptoms of the underlying disease, which may overlap with mild symptoms of hypercalcemia. In general, levels <12 mg/dL are asymptomatic; levels >15 mg/dL cause severe symptoms such as coma and cardiac arrest. However, longstanding or slowly developing hypercalcemia may be well tolerated, whereas, rapidly progressing hypercalcemia is more likely to be symptomatic. The old saying "stones, bones, (psychiatric) moans, and (abdominal) groans" is a useful tool for remembering the most common symptoms.

Renal

Polyuria and polydipsia may develop as chronically elevated calcium levels cause nephrogenic diabetes insipidus. Nephrolithiasis is associated with longstanding hypercalcemia, most commonly in the setting of primary hyperparathyroidism. Renal insufficiency secondary to chronic hypercalcemic nephropathy may be irreversible.

Skeletal

Skeletal manifestations of hypercalcemia depend on the underlying pathophysiology. Patients with hyperparathyroidism may develop osteoporosis or osteitis fibrosa cystica. Patients with an underlying malignancy may present with bony pain due to metastases or pathologic fractures. In addition, patients may develop metastatic calcification of the myocardium and soft tissues.

Neurologic

Neuropsychiatric symptoms are common, but are usually very subtle. Patients with chronic, mild hypercalcemia complain of fatigue, difficulty concentrating, depression, and anxiety. Some may complain of headaches, emotional lability, and irritability. With more severe hypercalcemia, patients may present with weakness, personality changes, confusion, hallucinations, psychosis, and even coma.

Gastrointestinal

Constipation is the most common gastrointestinal complaint associated with hypercalcemia. Other symptoms include nausea, vomiting, and anorexia. There may also be some association with pancreatitis and peptic ulcer disease.

Cardiac

Hypercalcemia may be associated with hypertension and, rarely, with bradyarrhythmias. Ventricular arrhythmias have also been reported, but without proven causality. Electrocardiographic findings may include a shortened QT_c interval and first-degree atrioventricular block. With severe hypercalcemia, ST-segment elevation mimicking myocardial infarction has been described, typically with a "scooped" appearance followed by indistinct T waves.

MANAGEMENT

Workup

The initial workup of hypercalcemia is fairly straightforward. A careful history should be obtained, assessing for potential symptoms of hypercalcemia and looking for any potential medications, ingestions, or exposures that could explain the disease. A basic biochemical workup should begin with a complete metabolic panel and intact PTH to determine whether the hypercalcemia is PTH-dependent or PTH-independent. An ionized calcium level may be helpful, although ionized calcium levels are sensitive to changes in pH and heparin contamination, and, therefore, may not always be reliable. If the PTH is elevated, 25(OH)D should also be measured, since vitamin D deficiency is extremely common and may cause secondary hyperparathyroidism. However, vitamin D deficiency per se should not cause hypercalcemia. Magnesium and phosphorus levels may also provide clues to the diagnosis, but are usually not particularly helpful. PTHrP can be measured if a malignancy is suspected and PTH levels are low. Of note, PTHrP does not cross-react with the PTH assay and should not falsely elevate these levels.

Treatment

Acute Management of Hypercalcemia

- **Serum Calcium Levels <12 mg/dL.** Mild hypercalcemia <12 mg/dL is usually asymptomatic and does not require urgent therapy, although patients should be monitored closely for the development of symptoms or worsening hypercalcemia. Treatment should focus on the underlying cause of the hypercalcemia.
- **Serum Calcium Levels >12 mg/dL.** With levels >12 mg/dL, emergent treatment may become necessary, especially if the patient is symptomatic or has markedly elevated calcium levels. Most of the acute management of hypercalcemia focuses on increasing the urinary excretion of calcium. Patients should be aggressively hydrated with normal saline over 24 to 48 hours to lower the serum calcium concentration by as much as 3 to 9 mg/dL, depending on the initial degree of hypercalcemia. Only after the patient has become volume replete and when volume overload may become an issue (e.g., in elderly patients or those with underlying cardiac dysfunction), the addition of a loop diuretic may enhance calcium excretion. It is important to note that aggressive diuresis in a volume-depleted patient may worsen the hypercalcemia by exacerbating the volume loss. In addition, precautions should be taken to prevent potassium and magnesium depletion. Thiazide diuretics are contraindicated, as they increase renal reabsorption of calcium. Patients who are oliguric or anuric, or those with severe symptomatology, may require urgent hemodialysis against a low calcium bath.

Salmon calcitonin (4 U/kg subcutaneously or intramuscularly every 12 hours, increased up to 6–8 U/kg every 6 hours) has few adverse effects and can be used in conjunction with volume expansion and diuresis during the acute treatment of hypercalcemia, since it also acts rapidly (usually within 4–6 hours) to lower serum calcium. However, it is a relatively weak agent, only lowering serum calcium concentrations by 1 to 2 mg/dL, and tachyphylaxis often develops within the first 48 hours.

Combination therapy with longer acting agents to block bone resorption should also be considered early in the acute management based on the severity of the hypercalcemia and the underlying disease process. Many of these therapies do not become effective for several days, and maintaining saline hydration and forced diuresis may be difficult.

Long-Term Management of Severe Hypercalcemia

Further therapy to alleviate hypercalcemia focuses on the underlying cause of the disorder.

Primary Hyperparathyroidism

Discussed in more detail in Chapter 22, Hyperparathyroidism, when primary hyperparathyroidism is severe or symptomatic, it should be treated with parathyroidectomy by an experienced surgeon. Cinacalcet (Sensipar) is a calcimimetic that has proven efficacy in patients with secondary hyperparathyroidism or parathyroid carcinoma, and may be of benefit in patients who are unable or unwilling to undergo parathyroidectomy.

Malignancy-associated Hypercalcemia

Bisphosphonates are analogs of pyrophosphate that are concentrated in areas of high bone turnover and inhibit both calcification and osteoclastic bone resorption. Many different bisphosphonates are available and effective for the treatment of malignancy-associated hypercalcemia; however, the second-generation bisphosphonates (e.g., pamidronate and zoledronic acid) are the most potent. The previous standard of therapy for moderate-to-severe hypercalcemia was pamidronate (Aredia) given as a single 60 to 90 mg intravenous infusion over 4 hours, with a second dose given after at least 7 days if there was only a partial response or if hypercalcemia returned during that time. Recently, zoledronic acid (Zometa) has become the bisphosphonate of choice, due to its greater potency and short infusion time (4-mg intravenous infusion over 15 minutes). Like pamidronate, a second dose can be given after at least 7 days if there is only a partial response or if hypercalcemia returns during that time. All of the bisphosphonates are well tolerated, and side effects are usually mild and transient. Fever is the most common reaction to intravenous administration. Renal toxicity is the most common serious side effect, so renal function should be monitored closely. Osteonecrosis of the jaw is an extremely rare complication of bisphosphonate therapy, but should be considered when treating patients who have had a recent dental procedure or who will be having one in the near future.

Gallium nitrate has also been shown to be efficacious in the treatment of malignancy-associated hypercalcemia, including PTHrP-mediated hypercalcemia, in which the bisphosphonates may have limited efficacy. At least one study has shown improved response rates and similar tolerability to pamidronate, but no direct comparisons have been made with zoledronic acid. Furthermore, treatment may be limited by the need for a continuous infusion over 5 days, and if there is a potential for renal toxicity.

Hypercalcemia in hematologic malignancies associated with increased production of $1,25(OH)_2D$ may be treated effectively with moderately high-dose glucocorticoids (e.g., prednisone 40–60 mg daily). Glucocorticoids increase urinary calcium excretion and decrease intestinal calcium absorption, but may also have direct antitumor effects. Calcium levels usually fall within 48 hours, with a peak response in 7 to 10 days.

Granulomatous Diseases

Glucocorticoids are also effective in the management of patients with granulomatous diseases, in which macrophages increase conversion of $25(OH)D$ to $1,25(OH)_2D$. Low to moderate doses of glucocorticoids (prednisone 10–40 mg/day) may be effective in normalizing calcium levels, but higher doses may be needed. Hydroxychloroquine (Plaquenil) and ketoconazole may be useful alternatives or adjuncts to glucocorticoid therapy.

Other Causes of Hypercalcemia

Hypercalcemia due to medication or supplement overdose should first be treated by withdrawing the offending medication. Corticosteroids are the definitive therapy for hypercalcemia due to adrenal insufficiency. They are also highly effective in treating hypercalcemia caused by excess vitamin A or vitamin D. Ketoconazole acts as an inhibitor of the cytochrome P-450 hydroxylation of 25(OH)D to 1,25(OH)$_2$D, and may also be effective in treating hypercalcemia caused by vitamin D intoxication.

KEY POINTS TO REMEMBER

- The majority of cases are caused by primary hyperparathyroidism and malignancy, but other treatable causes should also be sought when the diagnosis is not straightforward.
- Symptoms of hypercalcemia are usually subtle, but more severe manifestations may be summarized by the classic memory aid "stones, bones, moans, and groans."
- The history (especially the chronicity and severity) and PTH levels often provide the most helpful clues for establishing the cause of hypercalcemia.
- Acute management for severe hypercalcemia begins with aggressive intravenous volume expansion; additional medications should also be considered early.
- Long-term management focuses on the underling etiology of the hypercalcemia.

REFERENCES AND SUGGESTED READINGS

Adams JS. Vitamin D metabolite-mediated hypercalcemia. *Endocrinol Metab Clin North Am* 1989;18:765–778.

Beall DP, Scofield RH. Milk-alkali syndrome associated with calcium carbonate consumption. Report of 7 patients with parathyroid hormone levels and an estimate of prevalence among patients hospitalized with hypercalcemia. *Medicine (Baltimore)* 1995;74:89–96.

Bhalla K, Ennis DM, Ennis ED. Hypercalcemia caused by iatrogenic hypervitaminosis A. *J Am Diet Assoc* 2005;105:119–121.

Bilezikian JP, Silverberg SJ. Clinical practice: asymptomatic primary hyperparathyroidism. *N Engl J Med* 2004;350:1746–1751.

Brickman AS. Disorders of calcitropic hormones in adults. In: Lavin N, ed. *Manual of Endocrinology and Metabolism*, 3rd ed. Philadelphia: Lippincott Williams & Wilkins; 2002:293–324.

Caruso JB, Patel RM, Julka K, et al. Health-behavior induced disease: return of the milk-alkali syndrome. *J Gen Intern Med.* 2007;22(7):1053–1055.

Christensson T, Hellstrom K, Wengle B. Hypercalcemia and primary hyperparathyroidism. Prevalence in patients receiving thiazides as detected in a health screen. *Arch Intern Med* 1977;137:1138–1142.

Dent DM, Miller JL, Klaff L, et al. The incidence and causes of hypercalcaemia. *Postgrad Med J* 1987;63:745–750.

Farford B, Presutti RJ, Moraghan TJ. Nonsurgical management of primary hyperparathyroidism. *Mayo Clin Proc* 2007;82:351–355.

Finkelstein JS, Potts JT. Medical management of hypercalcemia. In: DeGroot LJ, Jameson JL, eds. *Endocrinology*, 5th ed. Philadelphia: Elsevier; 2006:1567–1577.

Fisken RA, Heath DA, Somers S, et al. Hypercalcaemia in hospital patients. Clinical and diagnostic aspects. *Lancet* 1981;1:202–207.

Harrop JS, Bailey JE, Woodhead JS. Incidence of hypercalcaemia and primary hyperparathyroidism in relation to the biochemical profile. *J Clin Pathol* 1982;35: 395–400.

Inzucchi SE. Understanding hypercalcemia. Its metabolic basis, signs, and symptoms. *Postgrad Med* 2004 Apr;115:69–70, 73–76.

Iqbal AA, Burgess EH, Gallina DL, et al. Hypercalcemia in hyperthyroidism: patterns of serum calcium, parathyroid hormone, and 1,25-dihydroxyvitamin D3 levels during management of thyrotoxicosis. *Endocr Pract* 2003;9:517–521.

Jacobs TP, Bilezikian JP. Clinical review: rare causes of hypercalcemia. *J Clin Endocrinol Metab* 2005;90:6316–6322.

Katahira M, Yamada T, Kawai M. A case of Cushing syndrome with both secondary hypothyroidism and hypercalcemia due to postoperative adrenal insufficiency. *Endocr J* 2004;51:105–113.

Khandwala HM, Van Uum S. Reversible hypercalcemia and hyperparathyroidism associated with lithium therapy: case report and review of literature. *Endocr Pract* 2006;12:54–58.

Littmann L, Taylor L 3rd, Brearley WD Jr. ST-segment elevation: a common finding in severe hypercalcemia. *J Electrocardiol* 2007;40:60–62.

Mao C, Carter P, Schaefer P, et al. Malignant islet cell tumor associated with hypercalcemia. *Surgery* 1995;117:37–40.

Mohamadi M, Bivins L, Becker KL. Effect of thiazides on serum calcium. *Clin Pharmacol Ther* 1979;26:390–394.

Muls E, Bouillon R, Boelaert J, et al. Etiology of hypercalcemia in a patient with Addison's disease. *Calcif Tissue Int* 1982;34:523–526.

Newman EM, Bouvet M, Borgehi S, et al.. Causes of hypercalcemia in a population of military veterans in the United States. *Endocr Pract* 2006;12:535–541.

Nordt SP, Williams SR, Clark RF. Pharmacologic misadventure resulting in hypercalcemia from vitamin D intoxication. *J Emerg Med* 2002;22:302–303.

Potts TJ, Jameson JL. Diseases of the parathyroid gland and other hyper- and hypocalcemic disorders. In: Jameson JL, ed., *Harrison's Endocrinology*. New York: McGraw-Hill; 2006:431–464.

Saito T, Tojo K, Yamamoto H, et al. Isolated adrenocorticotropin deficiency presenting with impaired renin-angiotensin-aldosterone system and suppressed parathyroid hormone-vitamin D axis. *Intern Med* 2002;41:561–565.

Sam R, Vaseemuddin M, Siddique A, et al. Hypercalcemia in patients in the burn intensive care unit. *J Burn Care Res* 2007;28(5):742–746.

Silverberg SJ, Bilezikian JP. Primary hyperparathyroidism. In: DeGroot LJ, Jameson JL, eds. *Endocrinology*, 5th ed. Philadelphia: Elsevier; 2006:1533–1554.

Stewart AF, Broadus A. Malignancy-associated hypercalcemia. In: DeGroot LJ, Jameson JL, eds. *Endocrinology*, 5th ed. Philadelphia: Elsevier, 2006:1555–1565.

Takeuchi Y, Fukumoto S, Nakayama K, et al. Parathyroid hormone-related protein induced coupled increases in bone formation and resorption markers for 7 years in a patient with malignant islet cell tumors. *J Bone Miner Res* 2002;17:753–757.

Tokuda Y, Maezato K, Stein GH. The causes of hypercalcemia in Okinawan patients: an international comparison. *Intern Med* 2007;46:23–28.

Wermers RA, Khosla S, Atkinson EJ, et al. Incidence of primary hyperparathyroidism in Rochester, Minnesota, 1993–2001: an update on the changing epidemiology of the disease. *J Bone Miner Res* 2006;21:171–177.

Wermers RA, Khosla S, Atkinson EJ, et al. The rise and fall of primary hyperparathyroidism: a population-based study in Rochester, Minnesota, 1965–1992. *Ann Intern Med* 1997;126:433–440.

Yamaguchi K, Abe K, Adachi I, et al. Clinical and hormonal aspects of the watery diarrhea-hypokalemia-achlorhydria (WDHA) syndrome due to vasoactive intestinal polypeptide (VIP)-producing tumor. *Endocrinol Jpn* 1980;27(Suppl 1):79–86.

Yoshioka M, Sakazume M, Fukagawa M, et al. A case of the watery diarrhea-hypokalemia-achlorhydria syndrome: successful preoperative treatment of watery diarrhea with a somatostatin analogue. *Jpn J Clin Oncol* 1989;19:294–298.

Hyperparathyroidism

Kent Ishihara

INTRODUCTION

Hyperparathyroidism is defined as the elevated production of parathyroid hormone by the parathyroid glands. Primary hyperparathyroidism (PHP) occurs when one or more of the parathyroid glands produce an excessive amount of parathyroid hormone for the amount of calcium present in the blood. Secondary hyperparathyroidism is a normal elevation in the production of parathyroid hormone that occurs in response to a derangement in calcium homeostasis that would otherwise lead to hypocalcemia, such as renal failure or vitamin D deficiency. Tertiary hyperparathyroidism develops in the setting of severe secondary hyperparathyroidism when hypertrophied parathyroid glands continue to produce an excessive amount of parathyroid hormone, even after correction of the underlying derangement in calcium homeostasis. This is most commonly seen in the setting of renal transplantation for chronic kidney disease (CKD).

PHP is one of the most common causes of hypercalcemia, especially in the outpatient setting. With the development of automated serum chemistry analyzers in the mid-1970s, asymptomatic hypercalcemia became a common incidental finding and the reported incidence of PHP increased. However, a more recent analysis suggests that the incidence is now lower than before screening was started. Nevertheless, PHP is a relatively common disease that affects about 1% of the adult population. Women with the disease outnumber men by as much as 3:1, and the disease most commonly presents after age 45. An increased incidence of malignancies (breast cancer, nonmelanoma skin cancer, renal parenchymal cancer, and endocrine malignancies) has been reported in patients with PHP, but the reason for the association is not known. An association with thyroid malignancies has also been reported; however, it is not clear if the reported incidence is higher simply because of increased detection during the evaluation and management of PHP. Overall, the effect of mild PHP on mortality is still being debated, with several reports suggesting that mild PHP is associated with an increased mortality, and others suggesting that there is no difference. On the other hand, there seems to be a more firmly established association between moderate to severe PHP and all-cause mortality, particularly from cardiovascular disease and malignancies. Increasing calcium levels have also been shown to be an independent risk factor for death.

CAUSES

Parathyroid hormone (PTH) is typically secreted by the parathyroid gland as an 84–amino acid peptide often referred to as "intact PTH." The single most important regulator of PTH secretion is the level of serum ionized calcium, which acts through the calcium-sensing receptor (CaSR) to produce rapid (within seconds) and relatively large responses in PTH secretion to small changes in calcium. The synthesis and processing of PTH within the parathyroid gland also adapt quickly to changes in calcium levels, and parathyroid hyperplasia may develop in response to more chronic hypocalcemia. Phosphate and vitamin D levels are also important in the regulation of PTH, with higher levels of phosphate and lower levels of $1,25(OH)_2D$, increasing synthesis and secretion of PTH. Lower levels of $25(OH)D$ also increase levels of PTH. The effects of PTH are mediated primarily through the PTH-1 receptor, a transmembrane G protein–coupled receptor found in the kidneys, intestine, and bone.

PTH causes an increase in serum calcium through three mechanisms:

- Prolonged secretion of PTH leads to increased bone resorption and decreased bone mass. The process by which this occurs has not been fully elucidated, but involves the activation of osteoclasts, likely through paracrine signaling from osteoblasts. Paradoxically, when given intermittently, PTH leads to increased bone mass through an unknown mechanism.
- In the kidney, PTH acts to increase calcium and decrease phosphate reabsorption. PTH-dependent reabsorption of calcium occurs in the distal convoluted tubule. Phosphate reabsorption is reduced by PTH in the proximal tubule.
- PTH acts to increase the activity of 1α-hydroxylase in proximal tubular cells, increasing the level of $1,25(OH)_2D$ over several hours, and ultimately leading to increased absorption of calcium and phosphate by the small intestine.

Primary Hyperparathyroidism

PHP is the inappropriate secretion of PTH from one or more of the parathyroid glands that leads to hypercalcemia. Expression of the CaSR may be downregulated in these abnormal glands, shifting calcium homeostasis to a higher set point, but maintaining responsiveness to feedback regulation. A single benign parathyroid adenoma is found in 80% to 90% of cases. There are several genetic abnormalities that may contribute to the development of parathyroid hyperplasia, including sporadic mutations in the multiple endocrine neoplasia 1 (*MEN1*) gene that occur in 12% to 16% of single adenomas. Four-gland hyperplasia is seen in approximately 6% of cases. Parathyroid carcinoma is reported to occur in 0.5% to 5% of cases, but seems to be rare and is probably in the lower half of that range. Carcinomas may have characteristic pathologic findings, but are often only distinguished from adenomas by the degree of invasion or the presence of lymph node metastases.

Familial hyperparathyroidism is rare and most commonly associated with MEN1 and MEN2A. Described in Chapter 33, Multiple Endocrine Neoplasia Syndromes, MEN1 is caused by a defect in a tumor suppressor gene inherited in an autosomal-dominant fashion. It is most commonly associated with parathyroid hyperplasia, pancreatic tumors, and pituitary adenomas, although it may also be associated with other tumors. Hypercalcemia can be found in approximately 95% of those with MEN1, typically developing around age 25 years as the earliest manifestation of the syndrome. Although it may be associated with a single parathyroid adenoma at presentation, it almost always involves multiglandular hyperplasia.

MEN2 is inherited in an autosomal-dominant fashion and is associated with defects in the *RET* proto-oncogene. It is characterized chiefly by medullary thyroid cancer, which occurs with complete penetrance, and pheochromocytoma. Approximately 25% to 35% of patients develop asymmetric parathyroid hyperplasia in MEN2A.

Less commonly primary hyperparathyroidism may be caused by familial isolated hyperparathyroidism or is part of the hyperparathyroidism–jaw tumor syndrome.

Familial hypocalciuric hypercalcemia (FHH) is an autosomal-dominant disorder that is caused by heterogeneous mutations of the CaSR that shift the set point for calcium to a higher level. FHH is typically asymptomatic and is thought to be a rare disorder with estimates of prevalence as low as 1 in 78,000, and as high as 1 in 15,625 in Scotland and 1 in 31,250 in Australia. Nevertheless, since the biochemical abnormalities in FHH overlap with those of primary hyperparathyroidism, the diagnosis must be considered; otherwise, a patient may undergo an unnecessary parathyroidectomy that is rarely curative in this disorder. Lithium therapy can produce alterations in calcium metabolism that mimic the changes in FHH and resolve when lithium is withdrawn, see Chapter 21, Hypercalcemia.

Secondary and Tertiary Hyperparathyroidism

Secondary hyperparathyroidism is an appropriate increase in the production of PTH by the parathyroid glands. Although it is most commonly associated with CKD, it can occur in any derangement of calcium homeostasis that may lead to hypocalcemia, hyperphosphatemia, or a deficiency in vitamin D. Vitamin D deficiency is an often-overlooked cause of secondary hyperparathyroidism that may be misdiagnosed as "incipient" primary hyperparathyroidism (normal calcium, elevated PTH).

Secondary hyperparathyroidism develops in virtually all patients with CKD. The initial inciting factor is not clear, but both decreased production of $1,25(OH)_2D$ and diminished phosphorous excretion by the diseased kidneys are soon involved. Even in the early stages of renal impairment, production of $1,25(OH)_2D$ may be decreased, leading to a decline in calcium absorption in the gut as well as in the distal convoluted tubules of the kidneys. Diminished phosphate clearance by the kidneys leads to hyperphosphatemia, with excess phosphate forming complexes with free ionized calcium ions to cause hypocalcemia. In addition, hyperphosphatemia impairs renal 1α-hydroxylase, lowering $1,25(OH)_2D$ production, and directly stimulates PTH synthesis and secretion by the parathyroid gland. Uremia may also produce changes associated with PTH-resistance in bone. All of these changes contribute to the physiologic increase in PTH synthesis and secretion in order to maintain normal calcium and phosphorous homeostasis.

Under chronic stimulation to produce PTH, the parathyroid glands will hypertrophy over time and, in some patients, will become resistant to normal feedback mechanisms and autonomously produce PTH. Tertiary hyperparathyroidism is said to be present when these autonomously elevated PTH levels are associated with hypercalcemia. This is most commonly seen after renal transplantation for end-stage renal disease that is complicated by severe secondary hyperparathyroidism.

PRESENTATION

PHP is now most often discovered incidentally, but it may present with nephrolithiasis, decreased bone mass, or typical symptoms of hypercalcemia (see Chapter 21, Hypercalcemia). Many patients are asymptomatic at diagnosis, but many have nonspecific symptoms such as weakness, fatigue, neuromuscular dysfunction, and neuropsychiatric disturbances that may improve after parathyroidectomy. Nephrolithiasis is the most common renal manifestation of PHP and occurs in approximately 15% to 20% of patients. Other renal manifestations include hypercalciuria, nephrocalcinosis, renal tubular dysfunction, and chronic renal insufficiency. The skeletal manifestation of classic, severe PHP is osteitis fibrosa cystica, which presents with typical radiographic features, including a "salt-and-pepper" appearance of the skull, bone cysts, and brown tumors of the long bones. However, this condition is now seen in less than 2% of patients with PHP. The most common skeletal finding is decreased bone mass in a distribution reflecting PTH's catabolic effects on cortical bone and anabolic effects on cancellous bone (greatest loss at the distal one-third radius > hip > spine). More generalized loss of bone mass can occur in PHP, and the risk of fractures seems to be increased, except perhaps at the hip.

Secondary hyperparathyroidism due to severe vitamin D deficiency may present with osteomalacia because of abnormal mineralization of bone. Uremic bone disease, also termed renal osteodystrophy, is the usual presentation—and most feared complication—of secondary hyperparathyroidism due to chronic renal failure. As with PHP, uremic bone disease typically manifests itself as osteitis fibrosis cystica; however, it can also be manifest as osteomalacia and dialysis-related amyloidosis. Patients with a chronically elevated calcium–phosphate product are also at an increased risk of calciphylaxis—a painful ischemic necrosis of the skin and soft tissues.

MANAGEMENT

Workup

The diagnostic workup of hyperparathyroidism is fairly straightforward and is discussed in more detail in Chapter 21, Hypercalcemia. Primary hyperparathyroidism is suspected if an elevated PTH level is found in the setting of hypercalcemia. There are essentially only two other considerations in the differential diagnosis for a persistently elevated calcium and PTH level—FHH and lithium therapy. Lithium use can easily be determined by the history. On the other hand, differentiating patients with PHP from patients with FHH can be very difficult.

The presentation of FHH is typically benign, and rates of nephrolithiasis are no different from those in the general population. Patients with FHH typically have calcium levels that are high normal or mildly elevated, and PTH levels are typically inappropriately normal to mildly elevated (almost always <100 pg/mL) in the absence of concomitant vitamin D deficiency. The most useful factor in differentiating PHP from FHH is a previous calcium level. Because FHH is a lifelong autosomal-dominant condition, an elevated calcium level early in life is highly suggestive of the disease, and any previously normal calcium level essentially rules out the disease. Likewise, a strong family history of benign hypercalcemia is suggestive of FHH. If none of that information is known or available to the patient, further information may be helpful. FHH is typically associated with a low 24-hour urine calcium excretion (usually <100 mg/day) as compared to PHP, which often is associated with elevated calcium excretion. Calcium excretion may be more accurately determined by the ratio of calcium clearance (Cl_{Ca}) to creatinine clearance (Cl_{Cr}). This can be calculated from the following formula:

$$Cl_{Ca}/Cl_{Cr} = (Ca_u \times Cr_s)/(Cr_u \times Ca_s)$$

where Ca_u and Cr_u represent values of creatinine and calcium from a 24-hour urine collection and Cr_s and Ca_s are spot serum values. A value of <0.01 is suggestive of FHH, and a value >0.02 essentially rules out the condition, but there is a lot of overlap between urine calcium excretion in PHP and FHH. (Of note, vitamin D deficiency can theoretically falsely lower urine calcium excretion in PHP, and replacing vitamin D may provide a more accurate assessment of urine calcium excretion. However, there is some evidence to suggest that vitamin D status may not significantly affect urine calcium excretion in patients with PHP. Likewise, a thiazide diuretic will decrease urine calcium excretion and may need to be discontinued if the diagnosis is in question. Usually the calcium effects of the thiazide will disappear after a few days, but there are reports of continued effects up to a few months in some patients.)

Levels of phosphorus can be very low in PHP, but they can also be mildly low in FHH, and can be normal in either condition. To make things even more complicated, there have been a number of different mutations found in the CaSR that produce different phenotypic expressions of the disease with variable severity in its manifestations and complications. Therefore, if the diagnosis is still in question, sequencing of the CaSR is now commercially available and may be helpful.

For the case of the patient who is found to have an elevated PTH in the setting of a normal calcium level, the differential diagnosis includes "incipient" PHP (thought to be the earliest stage of PHP), FHH, and secondary hyperparathyroidism. Secondary hyperparathyroidism is most often due to vitamin D deficiency or renal failure. Therefore, levels of blood urea nitrogen (BUN), creatinine, and 25(OH)D should be determined. The 25(OH)D level should typically be replaced to a value >30 ng/mL to ensure adequate replacement. It is generally safe to replace vitamin D in patients with mild primary hyperparathyroidism, with little change in calcium levels and some improvement in PTH levels in most patients. However, calcium levels should be monitored at least every 2 to 4 weeks initially, since a rare patient may develop worsening hypercalcemia.

Malignancies are also a common cause of hypercalcemia, but only rarely do they produce hypercalcemia through ectopic production of PTH. In most cases, hypercalcemia of malignancy is caused by PTH–related peptide (PTHrP), which is not detected by the common commercially available assays for PTH.

Treatment

Primary Hyperparathyroidism

The natural history of PHP suggests that in many cases it is a benign, nonprogressive disorder. Therefore, once a diagnosis of PHP has been established, the next step is to determine whether treatment will be necessary.

Surgical Therapy. The only curative treatment for PHP is parathyroidectomy and is recommended for all patients with symptomatic disease. However, in asymptomatic patients, the difficulty is in determining which patients are most appropriate for surgery versus watchful waiting. Consensus guidelines formulated in 1991 and updated in 2002 suggest that surgery is indicated under the following conditions:

- Age <50 years
- Serum calcium >1 mg/dL above the upper limit of normal
- Patients for whom medical follow-up is either not possible or not desirable
- Marked hypercalciuria (>400 mg daily excretion)
- Reduction in bone mineral density at any site to a T score less than –2.5
- Decrease in ClCr to 70% of normal

Once a decision is made to proceed with surgery, preoperative imaging may be helpful in determining the surgical approach. High-resolution neck ultrasonography and ^{99m}Tc-sestamibi have emerged as the most useful imaging techniques for locating a single parathyroid adenoma or multigland disease prior to surgery in patients with PHP. Ultrasonography has been reported to have a sensitivity of 72% to 89% in detecting solitary adenomas, but has poor sensitivity for detecting multigland disease. An advantage of ultrasonography is the ability to fully image the thyroid gland and help characterize any thyroid nodules that also may require surgical management. The sensitivity of ^{99m}Tc-sestamibi is similar to ultrasound and is reported to be 68% to 95% in detecting single adenomas, but like ultrasound, has poor sensitivity for detecting multigland disease. In addition, because ^{99m}Tc-sestamibi is also taken up by thyroid tissue, false positives may occur. An advantage of scintigraphy is that it can detect ectopic glands outside the neck. Therefore, some favor a combined approach to preoperative evaluation, which has been shown to more accurately predict solitary adenomas than either approach alone. Computed tomography (CT) and magnetic resonance imaging (MRI) are less commonly used for localization of parathyroid adenomas and are usually reserved for failed parathyroidectomy or recurrent disease.

The appropriate surgical procedure depends on the underlying cause of the disease. If a single adenoma is suspected by history or preoperative localization, the diseased gland can be removed by a minimally invasive approach. Because the half-life of immunoreactive parathyroid hormone (iPTH) is very short, intraoperative measurements can be very helpful in determining the success of the operation as each abnormal gland is removed. If imaging demonstrates a likely single adenoma, the surgeon can resect the suspected gland and monitor iPTH levels to ensure that the adenoma was appropriately removed. In these cases, extensive dissection and inspection of all four glands and the thymus can be avoided. In those suspected to have multigland disease, a more traditional bilateral approach is often used. If hyperplasia of all four glands is found, all parathyroid tissue is removed except for a small remnant that is left in situ or transplanted to the nondominant forearm. Typically, a small amount of tissue is cryopreserved in the event that the transplanted tissue fails.

Common complications of parathyroid surgery include the so-called "hungry bone syndrome," in which profound hypocalcemia develops, requiring parenteral calcium supplementation. Rates of postsurgical hypocalcemia may be higher in those with hyperplasia than in those with a single adenoma. Persistent hypoparathyroidism may also occur, mainly in those who have had surgery for parathyroid hyperplasia. Recurrent laryngeal nerve injury occurs in 1% to 2% of surgeries. In general, improved outcomes correlate directly with the experience of the surgeon.

Nonsurgical Therapy.　In those patients who do not meet the recommended guidelines for surgical intervention, and in those who either refuse surgery or for those who are poor surgical candidates, medical management may be appropriate. Adequate hydration should be ensured, as should a moderate calcium intake (~1000 mg/day). Thiazide diuretics and other drugs that can exacerbate hypercalcemia should probably be avoided. However, there is limited evidence to suggest that the addition or discontinuation of a thiazide diuretic in patients with mild hyperparathyroidism may not significantly change the degree of hypercalcemia in most patients, and, theoretically, the ability of thiazides to decrease urinary calcium excretion may be beneficial. Therefore, if the degree of calcium elevation is only mild, and the patient is already on a thiazide diuretic for hypertension, it may not be necessary to discontinue this medication. On the other hand, adding a thiazide in a patient with primary hyperparathyroidism is not recommended, since there are rare case reports of severe elevations of hypercalcemia when the thiazide is added. The calcium level should be followed at least semi-annually, and creatinine measurements and bone density should be monitored annually.

Additional medical therapy may be helpful in preventing complications from untreated primary hyperparathyroidism. Oral phosphate decreases gut uptake of calcium, inhibits bone reabsorption of calcium, and inhibits production of calcitriol. However, supplementation of phosphorus is generally not recommended, since long-term use may cause ectopic calcifications and may increase PTH levels. The bisphosphonates are effective treatments for osteoporosis and have shown promise in preventing the loss of bone mass associated with PHP. Alendronate is the most promising of the bisphosphonates, and has been shown to increase bone mineral density at the lumbar spine, and less consistently at the hip, without any significant change in calcium, PTH, or urinary calcium excretion in patients with PHP. Older bisphosphonates (etidronate and clodronate) have not been proven to be efficacious, and newer bisphosphonates still require further study. Estrogens have been shown to lower serum and urinary calcium levels and decrease bone resorption in postmenopausal women with mild PHP; however, the use of estrogens for PHP has fallen out of favor owing to the recently reported adverse effects of hormone replacement therapy, and the need for higher-than-usual doses of estrogen for maximal effect. Raloxifene is a selective estrogen-receptor modulator that has also been shown in preliminary studies to reduce serum and urine calcium levels as well as markers of bone resorption in postmenopausal women with PHP. A promising new class of medications known as calcimimetics (e.g., cinacalcet hydrochloride) has been shown to lower PTH and calcium levels in patients with hyperparathyroidism by increasing the sensitivity of the CaSR to calcium. Preliminary studies in primary hyperparathyroidism are promising, but currently cinacalcet is approved by the Food and Drug Administration (FDA) only for the treatment of secondary hyperparathyroidism in patients with CKD on dialysis and for patients with parathyroid carcinomas. Finally, percutaneous ethanol ablation of parathyroid adenomas has been recently advocated as a possible alternative treatment for patients with PHP.

Secondary Hyperparathyroidism

Secondary hyperparathyroidism caused by vitamin D deficiency is relatively easy to correct. In general, vitamin D stores should be repleted until the 25(OH)D level is >30 ng/mL. The standard treatment is ergocalciferol (D2) 50,000 IU weekly or monthly, depending on the severity of the deficiency. Approximately 500,000 total IU are required for full replacement of a severely deficient patient. Cholecaliferol (D3) can also be used for replacement, and may have slightly more favorable pharmacodynamic properties, but has not been as readily available as ergocalciferol.

Management of secondary hyperparathyroidism due to CKD can be far more challenging. The goal of therapy is to maintain PTH levels in the acceptable range based on the stage of CKD, in order to prevent both renal osteodystrophy (high-turnover bone disease) due to hyperparathyroidism and adynamic (low turnover) bone disease due to overly suppressed PTH levels.

The initial goal is to decrease the calcium–phosphorus product to <55 mg^2/dL^2, primarily by decreasing dietary uptake of phosphorus from the gut. In patients with CKD, the goal for daily intake of phosphorus is <800 to 1000 mg/day, and consultation with a dietitian may be necessary to help patients achieve this goal. Ultimately, most patients will require therapy with phosphorus-binding agents. The aluminum-containing agents that were once typically used have been linked to osteomalacia and encephalopathy and are now avoided. Currently, the mainstays of therapy are calcium-based binders such as calcium carbonate and calcium acetate. Calcium acetate has the benefit of binding more phosphorus with less calcium being absorbed per milligram of elemental calcium than calcium carbonate. To minimize calcium absorption, the dose should be limited to <2000 mg/day and titrated to the lowest dose needed to maintain a PO$_4$ level between 2.7 and 5.5 mg/dL (depending on the stage of CKD).

Once the levels of calcium and phosphorus are in an acceptable range, vitamin D therapy may be necessary to lower PTH levels into the target range. Calcitriol or one of its analogs can be used to stabilize or reduce PTH levels to an acceptable range. In addition to lowering PTH levels, vitamin D increases absorption of calcium and phosphorus from the gut and may increase the serum calcium–phosphate product, placing the patient at risk for calciphylaxis and hypercalcemia. Therefore, the serum levels of phosphorus and calcium should be controlled before beginning vitamin D therapy. Newer analogs of vitamin D (doxercalciferol and paricalcitol) may have less calcemic and phosphatemic effects, but have not been proven to be more effective than calcitriol.

Calcimimetics are a promising new therapy for hyperparathyroidism and have recently been approved by the FDA for the treatment of secondary hyperparathyroidism in patients on dialysis. Cinacalcet (Sensipar) is the first available calcimimetic and has been shown to produce a dose-dependent reduction in PTH as well as a decrease in the calcium–phosphate product. Reductions in the risk for parathyroidectomy, fracture, and cardiovascular hospitalizations have also been found in early studies. The initial dose of cinacalcet is 30 mg/day, and incremental dose increases can be made every 2 to 4 weeks to 60, 90, and 180 mg/day until goals are achieved. Serum calcium and phosphorus should be measured within 1 week and at frequent intervals during dose titration to monitor for hypocalcemia. Intact PTH can be measured 1 to 4 weeks after initiation of therapy or a change in dose.

Finally, surgical parathyroidectomy may become necessary in those with severe hyperparathyroidism (persistent serum levels >800 pg/mL) associated with hypercalcemia and/or hyperphosphatemia that are refractory to medical therapy.

KEY POINTS TO REMEMBER

- PHP and malignancy represent the two most common causes of hypercalcemia.
- Diagnosis of hyperparathyroidism is made by detecting a persistently elevated or normal PTH in the setting of hypercalcemia.
- PHP must be distinguished from FHH and secondary hyperparathyroidism.
- Vitamin D deficiency can complicate the diagnosis of primary hyperparathyroidism.
- Secondary hyperparathyroidism due to CKD can be challenging to manage.
- Definitive therapy for PHP is surgical, and specific guidelines exist to determine who should be referred for surgery.

REFERENCES AND SUGGESTED READINGS

Andersson P, Rydberg E, Willenheimer R. Primary hyperparathyroidism and heart disease—a review. *Eur Heart J* 2004;25:1776–1787.

Bilezikian JP, Potts JT Jr, Fuleihan Gel-H, et al. Summary statement from a workshop on asymptomatic primary hyperparathyroidism: a perspective for the 21st century. *J Clin Endocrinol Metab* 2002;87:5353–5361.

Bilezikian JP, Silverberg SJ. Clinical practice. Asymptomatic primary hyperparathyroidism. *N Engl J Med* 2004;350:1746–1751.

Bilezikian JP. Primary hyperparathyroidism: when to observe and when to operate. *Endocrinol Metab Clin North Am* 2000;29:465–478.

Bussey AD, Bruder JM. Urinary calcium excretion in primary hyperparathyroidism: relationship to 25-hydroxyvitamin D status. *Endocr Pract* 2005;11:37–42.

Consensus Conference on the Management of Asymptomatic Primary Hyperparathyroidism. *Ann Intern Med* 1991;114:593–597.

de Francisco AL. Secondary hyperparathyroidism: review of the disease and its treatment. *Clin Ther* 2004;26:1976–1993.

Farford B, Presutti RJ, Moraghan TJ. Nonsurgical management of primary hyperparathyroidism. *Mayo Clin Proc* 2007;82:351–355.

Farquhar CW, Spathis GS, Barron JL, et al. Failure of thiazide diuretics to increase plasma calcium in mild primary hyperparathyroidism. *Postgrad Med J* 1990;66:714–716.

Fuleihan GE. Clinical manifestations of primary hyperparathyroidism. *UpToDate* v15.1 2007.

Grey A, Lucas J, Horne A, et al. Vitamin D repletion in patients with primary hyperparathyroidism and coexistent vitamin D insufficiency. *J Clin Endocrinol Metab* 2005;90:2122–2126.

Gunn IR, Gaffney D. Clinical and laboratory features of calcium-sensing receptor disorders: a systematic review. *Ann Clin Biochem* 2004;41(Pt 6):441–458.

Hinnie J, Bell E, McKillop E, Gallacher S. The prevalence of familial hypocalciuric hypercalcemia. *Calcif Tissue Int* 2001;68:216–218.

Johnson NA, Tublin ME, Ogilvie JB. Parathyroid imaging: technique and role in the preoperative evaluation of primary hyperparathyroidism. *AJR Am J Roentgenol* 2007;188:1706–1715.

Juppner H, Gardella TJ, Brown EM, et al. Parathyroid hormone and parathyroid hormone-related peptide in the regulation of calcium homeostasis and bone development. In: DeGroot LJ, Jameson JL, eds. *Endocrinology*, 5th ed. Chapter 71. Philadelphia: Elsevier; 2006:1377–1417.

Lowe H, McMahon DJ, Rubin MR, et al. Normocalcemic primary hyperparathyroidism: further characterization of a new clinical phenotype. *J Clin Endocrinol Metab* 2007;92(8):3301–3305.

Marx SJ. Hyperparathyroid and hypoparathyroid disorders. *N Engl J Med* 2000;343: 1863–1875.

Nilsson IL, Zedenius J, Yin L, et al. The association between primary hyperparathyroidism and malignancy: nationwide cohort analysis on cancer incidence after parathyroidectomy. *Endocr Relat Cancer* 2007;14:135–140.

Noordzij M, Korevaar JC, Boeschoten EW, Dekker FW, Bos WJ, Krediet RT; Netherlands Cooperative Study on the Adequacy of Dialysis (NECOSAD) Study Group. The Kidney Disease Outcomes Quality Initiative (K/DOQI) Guideline for Bone Metabolism and Disease in CKD: association with mortality in dialysis patients. *Am J Kidney Dis* 2005;46:925–932.

Ogawa T, Kammori M, Tsuji E, et al. Preoperative evaluation of thyroid pathology in patients with primary hyperparathyroidism. *Thyroid* 2007;17:59–62.

Online Mendelian Inheritance in Man, OMIM (TM). McKusick-Nathans Institute of Genetic Medicine, Johns Hopkins University (Baltimore, MD) and National Center for Biotechnology Information, National Library of Medicine (Bethesda, MD), 2007. World Wide Web URL: http://www.ncbi.nlm.nih.gov/omim/.

Peacock M, Bilezikian JP, Klassen PS, et al. Cinacalcet hydrochloride maintains long-term normocalcemia in patients with primary hyperparathyroidism. *J Clin Endocrinol Metab* 2005;90:135–141.

Potts TJ, Jameson JL. Diseases of the parathyroid gland and other hyper- and hypocalcemic disorders. In: Jameson JL, ed., *Harrison's Endocrinology*. New York: McGraw-Hill; 2006:431–464.

Quarles LD, Cronin RE, Ringhofer B. Active vitamin D analogs and calcimimetics to control hyperparathyroidism in chronic renal failure. *UpToDate* v15.1. 2007.

Ruda JM, Hollenbeak CS, Stack BC Jr. A systematic review of the diagnosis and treatment of primary hyperparathyroidism from 1995–2003. *Otolaryngol Head Neck Surg* 2005;132:359–372.

Shoback DM, Bilezikian JP, Turner SA, et al. The calcimimetic cinacalcet normalizes serum calcium in subjects with primary hyperparathyroidism. *J Clin Endocrinol Metab* 2003;88:5644–5649.

Silverberg SJ, Bilezikian JP. Primary hyperparathyroidism. In: DeGroot LJ, Jameson JL, eds. *Endocrinology*, 5th ed. Philadelphia: Elsevier; 2006:1533–1554.

Silverberg SJ, Bilezikian JP. "Incipient" primary hyperparathyroidism: a "forme fruste" of an old disease. *J Clin Endocrinol Metab* 2003;88:5348–5352.

Silverberg SJ, Bilezikian JP. The diagnosis and management of asymptomatic primary hyperparathyroidism. *Nat Clin Pract Endocrinol Metab* 2006;2:494–503.

Silverberg SJ, et al. A 10-year course with or without parathyroid surgery. *N Engl J Med* 1999;341:1249–1255.

Strong P, Jewell S, Rinker J, et al. Thiazide therapy and severe hypercalcemia in a patient with hyperparathyroidism. *West J Med* 1991;154:338–340.

Wermers RA, et al. Survival after the diagnosis of hyperparathyroidism: a population-based study. *Am J Med* 1998;104:115–122.

Wermers RA, Khosla S, Atkinson EJ, et al. Incidence of primary hyperparathyroidism in Rochester, Minnesota, 1993–2001: an update on the changing epidemiology of the disease. *J Bone Miner Res* 2006;21:171–177.

Wesseling K, Coburn JW, Salusky ISB. The renal osteodystrophies. In: DeGroot LJ, Jameson JL, eds. *Endocrinology*, 5th ed. Philadelphia: Elsevier; 2006:1697–1718.

Wynne AG, van Heerden J, Carney JA, et al. Parathyroid carcinoma: clinical and pathologic features in 43 patients (review). *Medicine (Baltimore)* 1992;71: 197–205.

Hypocalcemia

Sheri Nishimoto

INTRODUCTION

Calcium homeostasis is essential for normal cell function, neural transmission, membrane stability, bone structure, blood coagulation, and intracellular signaling. Unrecognized or poorly treated hypocalcemic emergencies can lead to significant morbidity or mortality.

Hypocalcemia is defined as a decrease in the concentration of serum ionized calcium below 4.0 mg/dL or total serum calcium below 8.0 mg/dL with a normal serum albumin.

Generally, hypocalcemia is probably more common than hypercalcemia but receives less attention. In the inpatient setting, hypocalcemia is extremely common, and is estimated to occur in up to 88% of patients in an intensive care unit (ICU) and 26% of those admitted to a non-ICU ward (mostly due to acute/chronic renal failure, vitamin D deficiency, and magnesium deficiency).

CAUSES

Physiology

Approximately 99% of calcium is found in bone, and 1% is found in extracellular fluid. Of this 1%, 50% is in the free (active) ionized form, 40% is bound to protein (predominantly albumin), and 10% is complexed with anions (e.g., citrate).

Extracellular calcium levels are maintained at 8.7 to 10.4 mg/dL. Variations depend upon serum pH, protein and anion levels, and calcium-regulating hormone function. Approximately 500 mg of calcium are removed from the bones daily and replaced by an equal amount. Calcium absorbed by the intestines is matched by urinary calcium excretion. Despite these enormous fluxes of calcium, the levels of ionized calcium remain stable because of the rigid control of parathyroid hormone (PTH) and vitamin D levels.

Variations in calcium levels are recognized by the calcium-sensing receptor (CaSR), a 7-transmembrane receptor linked to G protein with a large extracellular amino-terminal region found in the cell membrane of the parathyroid cells. Binding of calcium to the CaSR induces activation of phospholipase C and inhibition of PTH secretion. A minor decrease in calcium stimulates the chief cells of the parathyroid gland to secrete PTH. CaSR is crucial in PTH secretion. PTH stimulates mobilization of calcium from bone via osteoclastic bone resorption and decreased renal calcium excretion by increasing distal tubular calcium reabsorption. Finally, PTH mediates 1,25-dihydroxyvitamin D intestinal calcium absorption.

Vitamin D is derived from dietary sources or from conversion from cholesterol precursors in the dermis by exposure to UV light. The typical light-skinned individual requires at least 10 minutes of sun exposure daily, and individuals with darker pigmentation may require longer exposure. Vitamin D_3 is converted to more potent 25-hydroxyvitamin

D by the liver and then, under regulation of PTH, to 1,25-dihydroxyvitamin D by the proximal renal tubular cells. Vitamin D stimulates intestinal absorption of calcium, regulates PTH release by the chief cells, and mediates PTH-stimulated bone resorption.

Hypocalcemia results from either increased loss of ionized calcium from the circulation (deposition in tissue, including bone, loss in urine, or increased binding of calcium in serum) or decreased entry of calcium into the circulation (gastrointestinal malabsorption, decreased bone reabsorption). The major factors that influence serum calcium are acutely, phosphate concentration; subacutely, serum PTH concentration; and chronically, vitamin D.

Differential Diagnosis

Broadly stated, there are four potential mechanisms of hypocalcemia:

- Insufficient supply of PTH
- Insufficient response to PTH
- Insufficient supply of vitamin D
- Insufficient response to vitamin D

PARATHYROID HORMONE DEFICIENCY/RESISTANCE

Hypoparathyroidism

Hypoparathyroidism is defined as an **inappropriately low secretion of PTH for a given ionized calcium**. Characteristic laboratory findings of hypoparathyroidism are hypocalcemia and hyperphosphatemia with normal renal function. Twenty-four hour urinary excretion of calcium is low, as is the blood calcitriol level.

Hypoparathyroidism may have a surgical, familial, autoimmune, or idiopathic origin. All varieties share the same symptoms, although hereditary hypoparathyroidism tends to have a gradual onset. **Surgical hypoparathyroidism** usually occurs on postoperative days 1 to 2 as a complication after surgery on the neck, although it may occur up to years after a procedure. It is caused by inadvertent injury to or removal of parathyroid tissue, and may be associated more with the experience of the surgeon than with the exact procedure performed. In the setting of parathyroidectomy, use of the intraoperative PTH value has been useful in predicting which patients are at risk for developing postoperative hypocalcemia. A >75% decline intraoperatively or postoperatively identifies patients at risk for development of symptomatic hypocalcemia. In addition, hypocalcemia in the postoperative setting may occur after multiple blood transfusions, as the citrate preservative in the blood chelates calcium.

Postoperative hypocalcemia may also be seen in the "hungry bone syndrome" after surgery for hyperparathyroidism, primary or secondary. It is caused by rapid precipitation of calcium-containing hydroxyapatite crystals in bone. This can also be seen in the setting of total thyroidectomy in patients with hyperthyroidism or in treatment of long-standing metabolic acidosis. A less-severe picture also is observed during the healing of rickets, after correction of thyrotoxicosis, and with tumors associated with bone formation (e.g., prostate, breast, leukemia). Hungry bone syndrome can be distinguished from hypoparathyroidism by the phosphorous level, which is low, and a PTH level that is appropriately elevated.

Hypoparathyroidism may also be associated with type 1 polyglandular syndrome, also known as **polyglandular autoimmune syndrome**. This disorder is either idiopathic, or acquired as an autosomal-recessive trait. It consists of the classic triad of hypoparathyroidism, adrenal insufficiency, and mucocutaneous candidiasis, two of which (diagnostic dyad) are required for diagnosis. Typical presentation is childhood candidiasis, followed several years later by hypoparathyroidism, and then adrenal insufficiency during adolescence. There is a wide clinical picture, and to date there are 58 known mutations of the *AIRE* (autoimmune regulator) gene, which is located on chromosome 21q22.3. (See Chapter 35, Autoimmune Polyendocrine Syndromes, for discussion of AIRE). The disease may also be associated with pernicious anemia, type 1 diabetes mellitus, and thyroiditis.

Idiopathic hypoparathyroidism typically presents in childhood but may present any time through the eighth decade of life. It has a 2:1 female predominance and may be associated with anti-PTH antibodies. About one-third of these patients also have antibodies to the parathyroid calcium sensor. The familial form of the disorder may be transmitted in an autosomal-dominant, recessive, or X-linked pattern.

Hypoparathyroidism may also result from agenesis or dysgenesis of the parathyroid glands. This is often associated with the **DiGeorge's syndrome**, in which malformation of the third and fourth branchial pouches causes absence of the thymus and parathyroid. The mnemonic used for the symptoms of DiGeorge syndrome is CATCH-22 (*c*ardiac anomalies, *a*bnormal facies, *t*hymic aplasia, *c*left palate, and *h*ypocalcemia seen with a deletion in chromosome *22*). Late-onset hypoparathyroidism can be observed in other congenital abnormalities or as part of a complex autoimmune disorder involving ovarian failure, adrenal failure, and parathyroid failure.

Hypoparathyroidism can be caused by direct destruction of the parathyroid glands in patients who are transfusion-dependent through iron deposition, copper deposition in Wilson's disease, and aluminum deposition in dialysis patients. Infiltration of the gland by metastatic carcinoma, granulomatous disease, or amyloidosis is a rare cause of hypoparathyroidism.

More recently, hypoparathyroidism can occur as a consequence of the use of calcimimetic agents, such as cinacalcet. These agents bind to the CaSR and lower the threshold for its activation by extracellular calcium. As a result, parathyroid hormone release from parathyroid cells decreases. Hypocalcemia has been described in up to 5% of these patients.

Pseudohypoparathyroidism

This cluster of inherited disorders is caused by **decreased end-organ responses to PTH**. The biochemical abnormalities mimic those of hypoparathyroidism (low calcium, high phosphorus); however, the PTH level is elevated. There are multiple possible defects in the PTH–receptor complex; therefore, there are several phenotypic presentations of the disease that have been described. Pseudohypoparathyroidism is classified into types 1 and 2. Type 1 is further subdivided into types 1A, 1B, and 1C.

The molecular basis of type 1 pseudohypoparathyroidism is a defect in the membrane-bound PTH-receptor/adenylate cyclase complex, which yields cyclic adenosine monophosphate (cAMP) as a secondary messenger in the cell. Patients with pseudohypoparathyroidism will not have a physiologic increase in cAMP in the urine after infusion of PTH.

Pseudohypoparathyroidism type 1A presents with the physical stigmata of **Albright's hereditary osteodystrophy** (AHO), which include short metatarsals and metacarpals, short stature, rounded facies, obesity, mental retardation, and heterotopic ossification. The disease is caused by a defect in Gs-alpha and leads to deficits in the cAMP cascade. The defect of the Gs-alpha protein is not confined to the effects of PTH but also affects other hormonal systems (e.g., resistance to glucagon, thyroid-stimulating hormone, gonadotropins) that use cAMP as a second messenger. The gene for the Gs-alpha protein is located on chromosome 20. Inheritance of the disease is autosomal dominant, and the expression of the gene is tissue specific and imprinted, with the maternal allele being expressed in the kidney. Therefore, if one inherits the defective allele from the mother, hypocalcemia is present. If the allele is inherited from the father, there is the physical appearance of AHO, but serum calcium homeostasis is maintained. This latter disorder is termed **pseudo-pseudohypoparathyroidism.**

Pseudohypoparathyroidism type 1B is characterized by a defective kidney response to PTH. The patients do not have AHO; instead, they often have skeletal findings consistent with hyperparathyroidism. These patients have normal Gs-alpha protein, with hormonal resistance to PTH—an impaired cAMP response to PTH, suggesting that the defect lies on the receptor. The level at which the receptor is affected is not yet clear.

Pseudohypoparathyroidism type 1C presents with resistance to multiple hormonal receptors but normal Gs-alpha protein expression.

Pseudohypoparathyroidism type 2 patients respond to PTH administration with an appropriate increase in urinary cAMP, but fail to increase urinary phosphate, suggesting that the defect is located downstream of the generation of cAMP. If the patient presents with hypocalcemia, hypophosphaturia, and elevated immunoreactive parathyroid hormone (iPTH) levels, first rule out vitamin D deficiency, which has a similar presentation. In patients with a vitamin D deficiency, all parameters return to normal after vitamin D administration. Pseudohypoparathyroidism type 2 is quite rare, with <50 cases having been described.

PTH resistance can be seen in severe hypomagnesemia. Initially, PTH resistance occurs when serum magnesium concentrations fall below 0.8 mEq/L (1 mg/dL or 0.4 mmol/L). Secondly, decreased PTH secretion occurs in patients with more severe hypomagnesemia. Malabsorption, diuretics, parenteral fluid administration, chronic alcoholism, and cisplatin therapy are the most common causes of hypomagnesemia. The associated hypocalcemia is resistant to administration of calcium and vitamin D. Restoration of the calcium levels can occur only after the magnesium deficiency is corrected. Levels of phosphorus are not elevated in patients with hypomagnesemia (as found in hypoparathyroidism), which probably is related to associated nutritional deficiencies. These patients present with low or inappropriately normal PTH levels in the presence of hypocalcemia.

Vitamin D Deficiency
Decreased production or activity of vitamin D more frequently causes hypocalcemia than disorders of PTH. Vitamin D deficiency is caused by several mechanisms: (a) decreased absorption of dietary calcium; (b) decreased renal reabsorption of calcium; and (c) resistance to the osteoclastic effects of PTH on bone. In vitamin D deficiency and hypocalcemia, the compensatory increase in PTH results in mild increases in serum calcium. However, this comes at the expense of serum phosphate, since PTH increases phosphaturia. These combined effects lead to a loss of bone mineralization and, if uncorrected, cause syndromes of **rickets** and **osteomalacia.** Rickets occurs in growing bone, typically in children, and results from abnormal calcification of cartilage at the physis. The typical presentation involves bowing of the limbs and cupping of the costochondral junctions (the rachitic rosary). Osteomalacia occurs after growth plates close and has a clinical appearance that is difficult to distinguish from osteoporosis. Patients frequently have hypophosphatemia.

Vitamin D deficiency may occur with **inadequate exposure to sun, inadequate dietary supply of vitamin D,** or **intestinal malabsorption of fatty acids.** Patients with inadequate sun exposure are often hospitalized or institutionalized, very young or very old, and may live in extremes of latitude. Patients of darker skin pigmentation have decreased conversion of vitamin D_2 to calcidiol for a given amount of sunlight. Dietary insufficiency may occur in those who live in areas where vitamin D supplementation of dairy products is not standard practice. In addition, an inadequate dietary intake may occur in the elderly or in breastfed infants of vegetarian mothers. Malabsorption may occur in patients with gastrojejunostomy, gastric resection, or celiac disease. These patients may have decreased calcitriol levels, but bone disease usually is dependent on other factors such as decreased sunlight exposure, malnutrition, or a postmenopausal state. Liver disease with decreased synthetic function can cause vitamin D deficiency from several sources: impaired 25-hydroxylation of vitamin D, decreased bile salts with malabsorption of vitamin D, decreased synthesis of vitamin D–binding protein, or other factors. Patients with chronic pancreatitis, pancreatic insufficiency, and steatorrhea have malabsorption of calcium and vitamin D.

There are two familial states of relative vitamin D deficiency. Patients with vitamin D–dependent rickets type 1, also known as **pseudovitamin D deficiency**, have a deficiency of 25(OH)D 1-hydroxylase. This condition is rare and is inherited in an autosomal recessive fashion typically manifesting prior to age 2. These patients have normal or elevated levels of 25(OH)D, and calcitriol administration can correct the defect. Vitamin D–dependent rickets type 2, also known as **hereditary calcitriol resistant rickets**, involves typical symptoms of rickets as well as alopecia. It is inherited as an autosomal recessive disease and is the result of a mutation in the vitamin D receptor gene. These patients have high serum levels of 1,25-hydroxyvitamin D and can be treated with high doses of calcium as well as calcitriol.

Miscellaneous Causes of Acute Hypocalcemia

There are several disorders that can result in acute hypocalcemia by overwhelming the normal mechanisms of control of calcium. One mechanism is acute hyperphosphatemia. Rapid release of phosphorous from injured muscle cells or dying tumor cells can quickly complex calcium in patients with rhabdomyolysis or tumor lysis. This can be compounded by the acute renal failure often associated with these conditions.

In addition, malignancy can cause hypocalcemia as a result of osteoblast activation in patients with blastic metastases from breast or prostate cancer via deposition of calcium in the lesions.

Chelation of calcium by citrate (anticoagulant in banked blood or plasma), lactate, gadolinium-based contrast material used in magnetic resonance imaging (MRI, gadodiamide and gadoversetamide), and ethylenediaminetetraacetic acid (EDTA) reduce serum ionized calcium concentrations, but not serum total calcium concentrations. Calcium is also chelated in acute pancreatitis, most likely due to the release of free fatty acids. The degree of hypocalcemia seen with pancreatitis can be a prognosticator, with lower levels predicting a worse prognosis.

Most patients in the ICU do not have an identifiable cause of hypocalcemia. Sepsis, especially if caused by gram-negative microorganisms, is associated with hypocalcemia, via endotoxins. Mortality rates increase among patients with sepsis and hypocalcemia.

Multiple medications cause hypocalcemia. Those that inhibit bone resorption include calcitonin, mithramycin, plicamycin, gallium nitrate, and estrogens. Cimetidine decreases gastric pH, slowing fat breakdown, which is necessary to complex calcium for gut absorption. Anticonvulsants may stimulate microsomal enzymes with resultant abnormal metabolism of vitamin D. Reports also show that phenytoin interferes with the intestinal absorption of vitamin D. Patients on anticonvulsant therapy may present with hypocalcemia, normal calcitriol levels, and increased PTH levels.

An increasing number of cancer patients are being treated with intravenous bisphosphonates for hypercalcemia or metastatic bone disease. In the setting of severe vitamin D deficiency, these patients can develop symptomatic hypocalcemia. This is most frequently reported with use of zoledronic acid, likely due to both its potency and frequency of use. Use of intravenous bisphosphonates is contraindicated in the setting of vitamin D deficiency; therefore, prior to use, a 25-OH vitamin D level should be obtained.

PRESENTATION

History

Symptomatic hypocalcemia depends upon the rate and magnitude of the fall in serum calcium.

- The most pronounced symptom is tetany. Patients typically complain of minor symptoms that include circumoral paresthesias, distal extremity numbness and tingling and carpopedal spasm—the classic example of which is the *main d'accoucheur* posture. This involves adduction of the thumb, flexion of the metacarpal joints, and flexion of the wrist. Patients may also develop potentially life-threatening laryngeal stridor due to laryngeal spasm.
- CNS manifestations of hypocalcemia include seizures, irritability, confusion, and delirium. Children with chronic hypocalcemia may have mental retardation, and adults may develop worsening dementia. Mental retardation is typically irreversible but dementia in adults can improve with correction in 50% of cases. Calcification of the basal ganglia may result in movement disorders.
- Cardiac manifestations include syncope, congestive heart failure, and angina, which occur in the acute setting.
- Chronic manifestations include cataracts, dry skin, coarse hair, brittle nails, psoriasis, chronic pruritus, and poor dentition.
- Related medical history may include pancreatitis, renal or liver failure, gastrointestinal disorders, and hyperthyroidism or hyperparathyroidism.
- Pertinent surgical history includes thyroid, parathyroid, or bowel surgeries, or recent neck trauma.
- To rule out pseudohypocalcemia, inquire about administration of radiocontrast, estrogen, loop diuretics, bisphosphonates, calcium supplements, antibiotics, and anti-epileptics.
- Family history of hypocalcemia may aid in the diagnosis of inherited conditions.

Physical Examination

The two classic physical examination findings include Chvostek's sign and Trousseau's sign. **Chvostek's sign** is elicited by tapping the facial nerve 2 cm in front of the tragus and observing for ipsilateral contraction of facial muscles. The sign is neither sensitive (27%) nor specific and may be seen in 25% of normal patients. If patients are undergoing parathyroidectomy, a Chvostek's sign should be elicited prior to surgery to determine the reliability of this sign. **Trousseau's sign** is elicited by inflating a blood pressure cuff to 20 mm Hg above the systolic blood pressure for 3 minutes and observing for *main d'accoucheur* posturing of the hand. It is reported to have a sensitivity of 66% and a false-positive rate of 4%.

Central nervous system manifestations include irritability, confusion, hallucinations, dementia, extrapyramidal manifestations, and seizures.

Potential cardiopulmonary findings include wheezing, stridor, bradycardia, rales, and an S$_3$ gallop. Acute hypocalcemia prolongs the QT interval, which may lead to ventricular dysrhythmias, and causes decreased myocardial contractility, leading to congestive heart failure (CHF), hypotension, and angina. Smooth muscle contraction may lead to laryngeal stridor, dysphagia, and bronchospasm.

Gastrointestinal symptoms include biliary colic, intestinal colic, and dysphagia from smooth muscle contractions. Diarrhea and/or gluten intolerance may be seen in cases of hypocalcemia that are due to malabsorption (e.g., from celiac sprue).

The primary dermatologic manifestation of hypocalcemia is impetigo herpetiformis, a form of acute pustular psoriasis associated with hypocalcemia in pregnancy. This appears as clusters of pinpoint pustules. Patients may also have less specific findings such as dry, flaky skin and brittle nails.

MANAGEMENT

Laboratory Evaluation

A patient with hypocalcemia should have a measurement of the serum albumin concentration.

To correct the total serum calcium in the setting of hypoalbuminemia, use the equation:

$$[4 - \text{serum albumin (g/dL)}] \times 0.8 + \text{serum } Ca^{2++} \text{ (mg/dL)} = \text{corrected } Ca^{2+}$$

Alternatively, one can measure serum ionized calcium directly. However, this test is less reliable with a single measurement. It can be falsely elevated with prolonged ischemia of the arm during acquisition of the serum sample.

Other tests should include measurement of serum phosphorus, intact PTH, magnesium, creatinine, and vitamin D metabolites. A low $25(OH)D$ level suggests vitamin D deficiency from poor nutritional intake, lack of sunlight, or malabsorption. Low levels of $1,25(OH)_2D$ in association with high PTH suggest impaired PTH sensitivity and failure to induce the $25(OH)D$ 1-hydroxylase, as observed in patients with chronic renal failure, Vitamin D–dependent Rickets-I, and pseudohypoparathyroidism.

Other Potential Studies

- The classic ECG finding of hypocalcemia includes prolongation of the QT interval. T-wave inversion may also occur, which does not revert with acute correction of the calcium.
- Skeletal x-rays: Rickets or osteomalacia presents with the pathognomonic Looser zones, better observed in the pubic ramus, upper femoral bone, and ribs.
- Urinary cAMP may help to differentiate hypoparathyroidism from pseudohypoparathyroidism types 1 and 2.

Treatment

The real treatment for hypocalcemia is appropriate **correction of the underlying condition**.

The indications for **emergent correction of hypocalcemia include severe symptomatic tetany, stridor, or seizures**. Calcium may be replaced with either calcium gluconate or calcium chloride as an intravenous bolus. A 10% calcium gluconate solution, 10 to 20 mL (1–2 standard ampules) may be given over 10 minutes; calcium chloride is equally effective. Care should be taken not to give the bolus more rapidly, as cardiac dysfunction may result, and patients should be monitored with a defibrillator or telemetry. The effect of this bolus is transient, and prolonged intravenous therapy should follow.

For urgent, but not emergent, replacement of calcium, 1 mg/kg/hour of elemental calcium may be given as an intravenous piggyback over several hours. Each 10-mL ampule of calcium gluconate contains 90 mg per 2.25 mmol of elemental calcium. As such, if 6 ampules of calcium gluconate are mixed in 500 mL of D_5W, a drip rate of 0.92 mL/kg/hour will provide 1 mg/kg/hour of elemental calcium. Because calcium is irritating, care should be given to ensure that the intravenous solution does not extravasate. In addition, bicarbonate and phosphate solutions cause calcium to precipitate and should not be run simultaneously. Serum calcium should be measured every 4 to 6 hours during intravenous infusion and the rate adjusted to maintain a serum calcium level of 8 to 9 mg/dL.

The goal of **chronic calcium replacement** therapy is to keep the calcium in the low range of normal. Approximately 1.5–3 g of elemental calcium should be given as a dietary supplement to ensure adequate intake. Supplementation should be given with meals to increase absorption and prevent hyperphosphatemia. There are multiple different preparations of oral calcium, in general, calcium carbonate is the cheapest, although absorption may be less than with other products.

Vitamin D supplementation is typically given as ergocalciferol (vitamin D_2). This preparation is the least expensive and has the longest half-life. The typical dose range for patients with hypoparathyroidism is on the order of 50,000 to 100,000 IU orally daily (1.25–2.5 mg/day). Serum 25(OH) vitamin D levels can be measured along with serum calcium levels to assess for adequacy of treatment. Vitamin D is extremely lipophilic and may require several weeks to reach a steady state with a new dose. Calcitriol, which has a shorter half-life (8 hours), may also be given with a typical starting does of 0.25 to 0.5 mcg orally daily.

Patients with hypoparathyroidism and pseudohypoparathyroidism can be managed initially with the oral administration of calcium supplements. In patients with severe hypoparathyroidism, vitamin D treatment may be required; however, PTH deficiency impairs the conversion of vitamin D to calcitriol. Therefore, the most efficient treatment is the addition of calcitriol.

Because the hypoparathyroid patient is dependent on renal excretion of calcium to maintain calcium homeostasis, careful attention should be paid to renal function. Any medication causing an acute decrease in glomerular filtration rate may cause symptomatic hypercalcemia. In addition, thiazide diuretics, by blocking calcium excretion, may lead to hypercalcemia in those taking chronic calcium or vitamin D replacement.

Patients with chronic hypocalcemia due to hypoparathyroidism may also be treated with Forteo, although expensive. Typically patients are treated with 20 mcg subcutaneously, twice a day, or up to 2 mcg/kg/day. In the post-parathyroidectomy setting it can be used to decrease hospitalization and expedite achievement of normocalcemia, which is most effective at 40 mcg, subcutaneously, twice daily.

Prognosis

The prognosis for correcting hypocalcemia is good if recognized and is dependent upon the etiology. Most symptoms can be alleviated. However, the eye damage or mental retardation that occurs in long-standing hypocalcemia cannot be reversed.

Complications

The goal of treatment of chronic hypocalcemia is a low-normal serum calcium level (8–8.5 mg/dL). If the calcium is kept below this level, the patient remains at risk for symptoms of hypocalcemia or cataracts. A higher calcium level may predispose patients to nephrolithiasis. In chronic hypocalcemia, the calcium–phosphate product (calculated by multiplying the calcium by the phosphate level) should be monitored. The goal is a product <60 to avoid calciphylaxis. In addition, a urine calcium-to-creatinine ratio should be periodically checked to evaluate for hypercalciuria. The ratio is determined by dividing spot urine calcium by spot urine creatinine. The ratio should be lower than 0.2; if it is higher, there is an increased risk of development of renal stones, particularly calcium phosphate stones. Patients treated with Forteo have a potential risk for development of osteosarcoma.

If hypercalcemia develops, vitamin D and calcium supplementation should be withheld until levels return to normal. The doses should be decreased. The effects of calcitriol typically last one week, but ergocalciferol can last more than one month.

KEY POINTS TO REMEMBER

- Pathophysiology of chronic hypocalcemia relates to a functional deficiency of either PTH or vitamin D.
- The most worrisome symptoms of acute hypocalcemia are neurologic (e.g., seizures) or neuromuscular (e.g., tetany).
- Acute management is with intravenous calcium supplementation.
- Chronic management is generally with vitamin D and oral calcium supplementation.

REFERENCES AND SUGGESTED READINGS

Becker KL, ed. *Principles and Practice of Endocrinology and Metabolism,* 2nd ed. Philadelphia: Lippincott; 1995:532–546.

Emerson J, Kost, G. Spurious hypocalcemia after Omniscan- or OptiMARK-enhanced magnetic resonance imaging: an algorithm for minimizing a false-positive laboratory value. *Arch Pathol Lab Med* 2004;128:1151–1156.

Favus MJ, ed. *Primer on the Metabolic Bone Diseases and Disorders of Mineral Metabolism,* 4th ed. Philadelphia: Lippincott Williams & Wilkins; 1999:226–240.

Mcleod Ik, Arciero C, Noordzij JP, et al. The use of rapid parathyroid hormone assay in predicting postoperative hypocalcemia after total or completion thyroidectomy. *Thyroid* 2006;16:259–265.

Perheentupa J. Autoimmune polyendocrinopathy-candidiasis-ectodermal dystrophy. *J Clin Endocrinol Metab* 2006;91:2843–2850.

Shoback D, et al. Mineral metabolism and metabolic bone disease. In: Greenspan FS, Gardner DG, eds. *Basic and Clinical Endocrinology.* New York: Lange Medical Books; 2001:273–333.

Simpson JA. The neurological manifestations of idiopathic hypoparathyroidism. *Brain* 1952;75:76–90.

Vanderark CR. Electrolytes and the electrocardiogram. *Cardiovasc Clin* 1973;5:269–294.

Vitamin D Deficiency

Carlos Bernal-Mizrachi, Ana Maria Arbelaez, and Sweety Bhandare

INTRODUCTION

Vitamin D is a nutrient and a pro-hormone largely regulated by environmental factors, including diet and exposure to the sun. There are several nutritional forms of vitamin D; the best known are vitamin D_3 (cholecalciferol), which is generated in the skin of animals, and vitamin D_2 (ergocalciferol), which is derived from plants. In this chapter, when we refer to vitamin D we imply vitamin D_2 or vitamin D_3. These parent compounds are biologically inert. To become physiologically active, vitamin D undergoes a first hydroxylation in the liver to 25(OH) vitamin D (25[OH]D), and then a second hydroxylation in the kidney to its active hormonal form $1\alpha,25(OH)_2D$.

The main role of vitamin D in the body is for calcium and phosphorous homeostasis, and deficiency of vitamin D is associated with negative balance of these minerals and osteomalacia. However, more extensive roles for vitamin D are suggested by the discovery of the vitamin D receptor (VDR) and the extrarenal production of active vitamin D in almost all tissues in the body. These observations have opened a new area of study in the physiologic and pharmacologic actions of vitamin D.

SYNTHESIS OF VITAMIN D

The skin is the main organ responsible for vitamin D production. Exposure to sunlight, especially ultraviolet B (UVB) photons between 290 and 315 nm, causes a photolysis of 7-dehydrocholesterol (DHC) in skin (7-DHC or provitamin D_3) to form previtamin D_3, which isomerizes into vitamin D_3. Vitamin D_3 binds to the vitamin D binding protein (DBP) and is transported in the circulation.

Vitamin D_3 synthesis in the skin is dependent on the number of UVB photons that penetrate the epidermis. A number of factors influence vitamin D synthesis in the skin, including time spent indoors, use of sunscreens due to greater awareness of skin cancer, latitude, season of the year, melanin content of the skin, and age-related decline in epidermal 7-DHC. For example, sunscreen with sun protection factor (SPF) of 8 reduces vitamin D_3 production by about 98%. The concentration of previtamin D in the skin reaches equilibrium in Caucasians within 20 minutes of UV exposure, but it takes 3 to 6 times longer for dark-skinned people to reach the equilibrium concentration. Lengthy sun exposure does not produce toxic levels of vitamin D_3 because sunlight itself induces photodegradation of previtamin D_3 and vitamin D_3, thereby regulating the total output in the circulation and preventing intoxication.

DIETARY INTAKE OF VITAMIN D

Vitamin D is fat soluble. It is principally absorbed in the proximal small intestine. Absorption of dietary vitamin D requires bile salts and an intact absorptive surface. Enterocytes absorb vitamin D by passive diffusion and then secrete it into the lymphatics in the form of chylomicrons. Endothelial lipoprotein lipase hydrolyzes triglycerides from chylomicrons producing chylomicron remnants that are rapidly cleared via the liver. Most of the vitamin D is metabolized in this fashion.

There are a few commonly consumed foods that are naturally good sources of vitamin D. Fish is the primary natural food source of dietary vitamin D_3; wild salmon (3.5 oz) provides 600 to 1000 IU. The same amount of mackerel, sardine, or tuna fish provides between 200 and 300 IU, whereas cod liver oil (1 tsp) provides between 600 and 1000 IU and egg yolks 20 IU of vitamins D_2 and D_3. Few sources of vitamin D_2 are regularly eaten; sun-dried shiitake mushrooms provide a good source of vitamin D_2. In the United States, the major dietary source is fortified foods. For example, a glass (8 oz) of fortified milk, orange juice, yogurt; 3 oz of fortified cheese; or a serving of fortified breakfast cereal each provides 100 IU vitamin D_3. Babies who are nourished exclusively by nursing must get vitamin D supplements or sun exposure to ensure adequate intake because breast milk is a very poor source of this vitamin.

The dietary intake of vitamin D varies from 90 IU/day to 212 to 392 IU/day for various populations in the United States assessed by The National Health Nutrition and Examination Survey (NHANES) III. Total-body sun exposure for 15 minutes easily provides 10,000 IU vitamin D per day for a Caucasian adult. This is 50 to 100 times the average food intake of vitamin D. Therefore, food intake is not a critical source to maintain vitamin D levels provided one has adequate sun exposure.

Metabolism of Vitamin D

Once vitamin D enters the circulation from the skin or from the lymph via the thoracic duct it is rapidly stored in fat or metabolized in the liver. The fat stores of vitamin D are used during the winter; however, obese individuals are only able to increase their blood levels of vitamin D by half when compared with individuals of normal weight. The **first step** in the metabolic activation of vitamin D is hydroxylation of carbon 25, which occurs primarily in the **liver**. Several hepatic cytochrome P-450s have been shown to 25-hydroxylate vitamin D compounds. CYP2R1, present in the liver and in testis, appears to be the critical 25-hydroxylase involved in both vitamin D_3 and vitamin D_2 metabolism. Mutations in the *CYP2R1* gene have been identified in patients with low 25(OH)D levels and rickets. **25(OH)D is the major circulating form** of vitamin D and has a half-life in human circulation of 10 days to 3 weeks. Hepatic 25-hydroxylation is poorly regulated. **Serum levels of 25(OH)D increase in proportion to cutaneous synthesis and dietary intake of vitamin D, and thus represent the best indicator of vitamin D status** (Fig. 24-1).

The **second step** in vitamin D activation is the formation of 1α,25-dihydroxyvitamin D $(1,25[OH]_2D)$ by 1α-hydroxylase, mainly in the **kidney**. The half-life of $1,25(OH)_2D$ in circulation of humans is approximately 4 to 6 hours. A congenital defect in renal tubular 1α-hydroxylase enzyme expression results in vitamin D–dependent rickets type I. Numerous cells and tissues including prostate, breast, colon, lung, placenta, pancreatic beta-cells, bone cells, activated immune cells, vascular wall and parathyroid cells express 1α-hydroxylase and are able to transform 25(OH)D to its active hormonal form. This increased local production of active vitamin D serves as an autocrine–paracrine factor, which is fundamental for cell-specific functions. The contribution of these extrarenal sources to circulating $1,25(OH)_2D$ levels is minimal and only occurs during pregnancy, chronic renal failure, sarcoidosis, tuberculosis, granulomatous disorders, and rheumatoid arthritis.

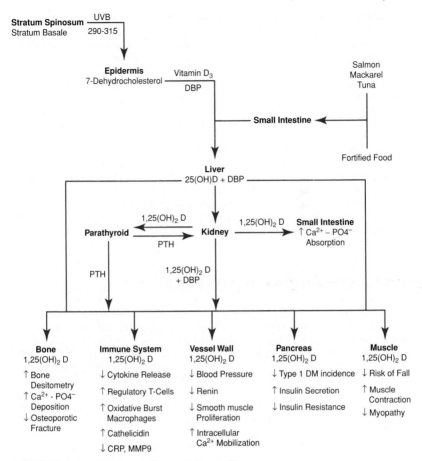

FIGURE 24-1. Synthesis and effects of Vitamin D.

Renal 1α-hydroxylase activity is highly regulated and functions to maintain serum calcium at normal levels. Low plasma calcium stimulates this enzyme by inducing parathyroid hormone (PTH) expression. Increased serum PTH enhances renal production of 1,25(OH)$_2$D directly by induction of 1α-hydroxylase expression and indirectly by the hypophosphatemia resulting from PTH-induced renal phosphate wasting. This compensatory event keeps the 1,25(OH)$_2$D hormone concentration nearly constant despite low levels of 25(OH)D. **Elevated 1,25(OH)$_2$D concentrations can mislead physicians into thinking that patients are vitamin D sufficient when they may be severely vitamin D deficient.**

Vitamin D is excreted principally in the bile. Although some of it is reabsorbed in the small intestine, the enterohepatic circulation of vitamin D is not considered to be an important mechanism to sustain adequate levels. Vitamin D is also catabolized to more water-soluble compounds, which are transported by DBP and albumin and excreted by the kidney.

Catabolism of both 25(OH)D and 1,25(OH)$_2$D is carried out by 24-hydroxylase, which catalyzes a series of oxidation steps resulting in side chain cleavage and inactivation.

The kidney is the major site of vitamin D catabolism. 1,24,25(OH)D or 24,25 (OH)D compounds are generated in the kidney under normal conditions; however, 24-hydroxylase is expressed throughout the body and attenuates the cellular responses induced by 1,25(OH)$_2$D. 1,25(OH)$_2$D controls its own degradation directly by stimulating the 24-hydroxylase activity or indirectly by reducing PTH levels.

In the plasma, vitamin D is transported bound to plasma proteins. More than 99% of circulating vitamin D metabolites are protein-bound, mostly to DBP, and minimally to albumin and lipoproteins. DBPs have the highest affinity for 25(OH)D and 24,25(OH)$_2$D and less affinity for 1,25(OH)$_2$D . The levels of 1,25(OH)$_2$D are normally 1000 times lower than those of 25(OH)D. DBP may be reduced by liver disease, nephrotic syndrome, or malnutrition. DBP may be increased during pregnancy and estrogen therapy. Despite changes in DBP, the circulating concentration of free vitamin D active hormone remains constant. Therefore, DBP works as a buffer, preventing deficiency of the active compound and/or intoxication. DBP also facilitates 25(OH)D entry into the proximal tubule cells by a receptor-mediated uptake of DBP in the brush border. Megalin facilitates the endocytosis of the DBP and 25(OH)D complex. Once inside, 25(OH)D is released and is converted into 1,25(OH)$_2$D in the mitochondria by 1α-hydroxylase.

MOLECULAR ACTIONS OF VITAMIN D

The VDR is expressed in almost all human tissues. 1,25(OH)$_2$D binds to the VDR, which acts as a ligand-activated transcription factor to regulate the expression of vitamin D–responsive genes. The VDR has a 100-fold affinity for 1,25(OH)$_2$D compared to 25(OH)D or other dihydroxy metabolites of vitamin D. Upon binding to VDR, vitamin D forms a heterodimeric complex with the retinoic acid X receptor (RXR), and the complex interacts vitamin D–responsive elements (VDRE) on DNA and promotes transcription of vitamin D–regulated genes. Specific mutations in the VDR gene cause vitamin D–dependent rickets type II due to 1,25(OH)$_2$D resistance. Some VDR genetic variants are associated with changes in mineral homeostasis, skeletal remodeling, and modulation of cell proliferation.

CLASSIFICATION OF VITAMIN D STATUS

Vitamin D status is usually estimated by measuring plasma 25(OH)D levels. Evidence that healthy outdoor workers, farmers, and lifeguards have 25(OH)D concentrations of 44 to 70 ng/mL suggest that an optimal healthy level is higher than the accepted levels reported to prevent rickets and osteomalacia. Establishment of new specific biomarkers such as intestinal calcium absorption, maximal PTH suppression, bone fracture prevention, and bone turnover have contributed to the development the following classification for vitamin D status. **An important concept is that most patients with suboptimal vitamin D levels are not hypocalcemic.**

- **Vitamin D Deficiency**—25(OH)D levels <10 ng/mL are associated with severe hyperparathyroidism, intestinal calcium malabsorption, rickets/osteomalacia, and myopathy.
- **Vitamin D Insufficiency**—25(OH)D levels 10 to 25 ng/mL are associated with mild hyperparathyroidism, low intestinal calcium absorption, reduced bone mineral density, and subclinical myopathy.
- **Hypovitaminosis D**—25(OH)D levels 26 to 30 ng/mL. PTH is slightly elevated.

- **Vitamin D Adequacy**—25(OH)D levels 30 to 40 ng/mL. To achieve maximal efficiency of vitamin D–dependent intestinal calcium transport, the serum 25(OH)D concentrations must be at least 30 ng/mL.
- **Vitamin D Toxicity**—25(OH)D levels >100 ng/mL. Toxicity manifests as hypercalcemia and its associated complications (described in subsequent text).

PREVALENCE

The prevalence of vitamin D deficiency appears widespread in all age groups. Latitude, time of day, season of the year, and race have a dramatic influence on the cutaneous production of vitamin D_3. In the southern United States during winter for men and women aged 30 to 59 years, vitamin D insufficiency (25[OH]D levels <25 ng/dL) varies from 12% among white males to 75% among African American women. In addition, vitamin D deficiency could be as high as 54% among homebound older adults; 84%, elderly black women; and 40%, pregnant African Americans and their neonates. The group at greatest risk includes African American men and women who live in the northern latitudes throughout the year.

ETIOLOGY OF VITAMIN D DEFICIENCY

- **Environmental Factors**
  - Premature birth
  - Pigmented skin
  - Low sunshine exposure
  - Breast-feeding
  - Use of sunscreen
  - Indoor activities
  - Obesity
  - Advanced age
  - Seasons
  - Latitudes further from the equator
- **Decreased Bioavailability**
  - Patients with decreased fat absorption (malabsorption) resulting from cystic fibrosis, celiac disease, Whipple's disease, Crohn's disease, gastric bypass surgery, or medications that reduce cholesterol absorption.
  - Obese individuals have increased vitamin D deposits in fat but decreased bioavailability availability for other tissues.
- **Increased Catabolism**
  - Patients taking anticonvulsants, glucocorticoids, highly active anti-retroviral therapy (HAART) (therapy for acquired immunodeficiency syndrome [AIDS]), and transplant antirejection medications.
  - **Decreased synthesis of 25(OH)D:** There is an inverse correlation between 25(OH)D levels and the severity of liver cirrhosis. Vitamin D deficiency has been found in approximately 66% of patients with Child–Turcotte–Pugh class B or C and in up to 96% of patients awaiting liver transplantation.
  - **Increased urinary loss of 25(OH)D:** Patients with nephrotic syndrome caused by loss of 25(OH)D bound to DBP in urine.
  - **Decreased synthesis of 1,25(OH)₂D:** This is characteristic of patients with chronic kidney disease (CKD). Decreased synthesis in the early stages is caused by hyperphosphatemia that decreases 1α-hydroxylase activity, whereas in late stages it is caused by tubular destruction and reduced substrate (25[OH]D) availability. In addition to low 1,25(OH)₂D, 25(OH)D deficiency is present in 70% to 80% in CKD patients in stages 3 and 4.

- **Rickets**
  - Heritable disorders: vitamin D–dependent rickets types I, II, III; X-linked hypophosphatemic rickets; autosomal dominant hypophosphatemic rickets; autosomal-recessive hypophosphatemic rickets.
  - Acquired disorders: tumor-induced osteomalacia.
- **Increased conversion of 25(OH)D to 1,25(OH)$_2$D**
  - Primary Hyperparathyroidism. PTH-induced tubular 1α-hydroxylase accelerates the conversion of 25(OH)D to 1,25(OH)$_2$D. Vitamin D insufficiency is reported in 53% of patients with primary hyperparathyroidism, and severe vitamin D deficiency (25(OH)D <12 ng/mL) is present in 27% of those patients.
  - Granulomatous disorders such as sarcoidosis, tuberculosis, and lymphomas. Cytokines induce macrophage 1α-hydroxylase, thereby converting 25(OH)D to its active hormonal form.
- **Accelerated metabolism**
  - Hyperthyroidism

PHYSIOLOGIC ACTIONS OF VITAMIN D IN CALCIUM HOMEOSTASIS

As a person becomes 25(OH)D deficient, intestinal absorption of calcium and phosphorus decrease, serum ionized calcium levels drop, and a compensatory synthesis and secretion of PTH is stimulated (secondary hyperparathyroidism). Increased plasma PTH levels maintain serum calcium levels by enhancing renal production of 1,25(OH)$_2$D, by increasing bone turnover and bone loss, and by promoting tubular calcium reabsorption and phosphate excretion. Increased 1,25(OH)$_2$D induces intestinal absorption of calcium and phosphorus and stimulates osteoclast activity, which increases the availability of calcium and phosphorus in the blood.

BONE EFFECTS OF VITAMIN D

Rickets/Osteomalacia

Deficiency of vitamin D, calcium, or phosphorus can impair normal mineralization of bone, thereby causing rickets or osteomalacia. In children, inadequate mineralization of the osteoid and cartilage in the growth plates causes rickets, a disease characterized by widening at the end of the long bones, prominent costochondral junctions (rachitic rosary), deformations in the skeleton including frontal bossing, and deformities of the lower limbs causing bowed legs and knocked knees. In adults, failure to mineralize the bone matrix is termed osteomalacia, a disease characterized by generalized bone pain, muscle weakness, waddling gait and pseudofractures, a classical radiologic feature characterized by areas of cortical lucency with surrounding sclerosis in the long bones.

Vitamin D–Dependent Rickets/Osteomalacia

- **Nutritional rickets/osteomalacia.** Vitamin D deficiency is most commonly seen in infants with prolonged breast-feeding who do not receive vitamin D supplementation or adequate exposure to sunlight. All infant formulas in the United States are fortified with at least 400 IU/L of vitamin D. The American Academy of Pediatrics recommends 200 IU/day of vitamin D$_2$ supplementation to all breastfed infants unless they receive at least 500 mL of vitamin D–fortified formula and to all non-breastfed infants who ingest <500 mL of vitamin D–fortified formula. Nutritional rickets/osteomalacia is also seen in elderly people with dark skin and with limited exposure to sunlight. Patients will have low serum calcium and phosphorus and high

PTH levels. In adults, ergocalciferol doses of 50,000 IU weekly for 8 to 10 weeks along with calcium supplementation of 1000 mg/day has been used for rickets treatment. Serum calcium, phosphorus, alkaline phosphatase, and urine calcium/creatinine ratios are measured before and 4 weeks after initiation of therapy, and every 3 months thereafter. Radiographs are obtained to document healing of rachitic changes.

- **Genetic Vitamin D–dependent Rickets**
  - **Vitamin D–dependent rickets type I (VDDR-I)**, also called pseudovitamin D deficiency rickets, usually manifests before 2 years of age. It has an autosomal-recessive inheritance and is linked to chromosome 12q14. It is caused by a defect in renal tubular 1α-hydroxylase enzymes that convert 25(OH)D into the active 1,25(OH)$_2$D. Serum calcium levels are usually low or normal, 25(OH)D levels are normal or high, 1,25(OH)$_2$D levels are low, and PTH is high secondary to hypocalcemia. Serum phosphorus is usually low owing to high PTH and low 1,25(OH)$_2$D levels. Treatment involves replacement with calcitriol (1,25[OH]$_2$D), and the aim of therapy is to maintain serum calcium, phosphorus, alkaline phosphatase, and PTH levels within normal limits.
  - **Vitamin D–dependent rickets type II (VDDR-II)**, also called hereditary vitamin D–resistant rickets (HVDRR), is very rare. It has autosomal-recessive inheritance and is associated with end-organ resistance to calcitriol, resulting from mutations in the gene that encodes the VDR. Affected children are normal at birth, but metabolic bone disease presents early within the first 2 years of life. Serum calcium is low, PTH is high, 25(OH)D is normal to high, and 1,25(OH)$_2$D is normal to high. Treatment involves high doses of calcitriol and calcium. Long-term central venous infusion of calcium is an alternative for severely resistant patients.

Vitamin D–Independent Rickets/Osteomalacia
- **X-linked hypophosphatemic rickets** is an X-linked dominant genetic disorder (Xp22). It is caused by a defect in PHEX (phosphate-regulating endopeptidase), which lyses a circulating factor that causes renal phosphate losses. Patients with this disorder also have defective 1,25(OH)$_2$D synthesis secondary to low levels of plasma phosphorus. Patients have low 1,25(OH)$_2$D, low phosphorus, normal calcium, and normal PTH levels. Treatment includes supplementation with phosphorus and vitamin D.
- **Autosomal-dominant hypophosphatemic rickets**, a mutation in fibroblast growth factor (FGF23) causes increased levels of this phosphatonin leading to large renal losses of phosphate. FGF23 directly inhibits renal 1α-hydroxylase and, therefore, 1,25(OH)$_2$D synthesis. The clinical manifestations and treatment are similar to X-linked hypophosphatemic rickets.
- **Autosomal-recessive hypophosphatemic rickets.** Dentin matrix protein 1 (DMP1) is made in the osteocytes. DMP1 inhibits secretion or production of FGF23. This disease is caused by a homozygous mutation of the *DMP1* gene and results in release of the inhibition of FGF23, thereby causing phosphaturia and osteomalacia. Clinical features are similar to those of autosomal-dominant rickets.
- **Tumor-induced osteomalacia** is characterized by increased production of phosphatonins by sclerosing tumors of mesenchymal origin. Patients have increased renal phosphate losses and a compensatory rise in 1,25(OH)$_2$D synthesis. Treatment includes repletion of phosphorus, tumor resection, and somatostatin analogs.
- **Hypophosphatemia with hypercalciuria.** An autosomal-recessive defect in type 2c Na-PO4 cotransport in the renal proximal tubule. Patients have low phosphorus and a compensatory rise in vitamin D, which causes increased intestinal calcium absorption and hypercalciuria. Treatment includes phosphorous supplementation.

Osteoporosis

Osteoporosis is a systemic disorder characterized by decreased bone mass and microarchitectural deterioration of bone tissue, leading to bone fragility and increased susceptibility to fractures of hip, spine, and wrist. Secondary hyperparathyroidism has been proposed as the principal mechanism connecting vitamin D deficiency, with the pathogenesis of decreased bone mineral density and osteoporosis.

Despite the fact that higher serum 25(OH)D concentrations are associated with higher bone mineral density (BMD) in all population subgroups (NHANES III), the ability of vitamin D supplements to prevent fractures continues to be debated. Vitamin D and calcium supplementation (1000 mg of calcium and 800 IU of vitamin D per day) significantly reduced the risk of hip fractures by 43% and nonvertebral fractures by 32% among 3270 postmenopausal women who were vitamin D–deficient (mean 25[OH]D, 16 ng/mL) and increased 25(OH)D levels to 42 ng/mL after treatment. In a recent meta-analysis, vitamin D supplementation (700–800 IU) reduced hip fractures by 26% and nonvertebral fractures by 23%, compared to subjects without vitamin D supplementation. In contrast, a subgroup analysis of the Women's Health Initiative (WHI) reported that the supplementation of 36,282 postmenopausal women for 7 years with vitamin D_3 (400 IU) and calcium carbonate (1000 mg) failed to prevent hip fractures despite of slight improvement in hip BMD in the treated group when compared to placebo. Several issues have been raised regarding this study that limit its interpretation, including lower rates of adherence to therapy, higher calcium intake at baseline in study participants, and perhaps the selection of a suboptimal vitamin D_3 supplement. In the WHI study, the serum 25(OH)D increased by only ~2.8 ng/mL.

The randomized trial of vitamin D and calcium for the secondary prevention of osteoporosis related fractures in the elderly (RECORD) showed no prevention of a second fracture for patients receiving 1000 mg/day of calcium and 800 IU/day of vitamin D_3. However, multiple questions have been raised altering the interpretation of these results. First, the placebo group was allowed to receive calcium and vitamin D regardless of the intervention. Second, there was poor compliance with the regimen. Reports of compliance in the first year were 60% and 47% in the second year. Third, the achieved mean 25(OH)D concentrations were only 24.8 ng/mL in the vitamin D treatment group. The optimal fracture prevention occurred when 25(OH)D concentrations achieved were at 36 to 40 ng/mL. These concentrations were reached only in trials that gave 700 to 800 IU/day of vitamin D_3 to subjects with mean baseline concentrations between 17 and 31 ng/mL. Therefore, optimal fracture prevention may require intakes of >700–800 IU/day vitamin D_3 in populations with baseline 25(OH)D concentrations <17 ng/mL.

NONCALCEMIC ACTIONS OF VITAMIN D

A growing body of evidence from both rodent models and humans suggests that maintaining optimal vitamin D stores is important for overall health and not just bone health. Although much of the data are correlational at this point, the weight of the evidence suggests that vitamin D deficiency can lead to worsening of known risk factors for cardiovascular disease. The outcomes of prospective randomized controlled clinical trials will be essential.

Type 2 Diabetes Mellitus (DM)

The prevalence of hypovitaminosis D is higher in women with type 2 diabetes. Analysis of NHANES III and Workforce Diabetes Study confirmed that patients with sufficient 25(OH)D levels (>30 ng/mL) have about one-third the risk of developing diabetes or impaired glucose tolerance when compared with those with insufficient vitamin D levels

<24 ng/mL. Studies in rodents have suggested that vitamin D deficiency may lead to impaired insulin secretion and to insulin resistance. In humans, the insulin sensitivity index, as assessed by hyperinsulinemic-hyperglycemic clamps, improves in direct relationship with ambient levels of vitamin D; moreover, interventional studies in vitamin D–deficient subjects have shown improved insulin sensitivity in glucose-intolerant subjects after replacement of vitamin D.

Type 1 Diabetes Mellitus

Type 1 DM is recognized as a T-cell–mediated autoimmune disease. Vitamin D compounds are known to suppress T-cell activation and to alter the antigen-presenting capacity of macrophages and dendritic cells, as well as modulate their cytokine release. These actions may protect beta cells against autoimmune injury. Several epidemiologic studies have described a correlation between geographic latitude and the incidence of type 1 diabetes. A previous study has shown that 25(OH)D levels are lower in patients newly diagnosed with type 1 diabetes compared to healthy controls. The Diabetes Autoimmunity Study in the Young (DAISY) reported that the presence of autoantibodies to islet cells inversely correlated with maternal dietary vitamin D intake during pregnancy. In addition, in patients with rickets, the incidence of childhood diabetes is 3 times higher than the incidence in healthy children. Observational studies have shown that treatment of children with 400 IU or less vitamin D per day did not reduce the risk of developing type 1 DM. However, the only prospective study based on the assessment of vitamin D intake during infancy (of 10,821 children) showed that vitamin D supplementation in infants with doses of 2000 IU/day for a year decreased the risk of developing type 1 DM by 80% by the age of 30 years. Additional studies are needed to determine whether vitamin D should be started during pregnancy and determine the ideal vitamin D doses without side effects.

Vitamin D and Hypertension

Interventional studies suggest that vitamin D replacement decreases blood pressure. In an 8 week treatment study consisting of oral calcium and vitamin D_3 replacement in elderly women with vitamin D deficiency, plasma 25(OH)D levels increased to ≥ 25 ng/mL and systolic blood pressure (SBP) decreased significantly, by 13 mm Hg, compared with the calcium-only treated control group. UVB exposure by skin-tanning sessions increased plasma 25(OH)D levels to 40 ng/mL and decreased blood pressure in mildly hypertensive patients. However, oral administration of 1,25(OH)$_2$D has not shown consistent blood pressure effects, possibly due to discrepancies in the population plasma vitamin D status, as well as different vitamin D doses and duration of the vitamin D replacement.

Vitamin D Suppresses the Renin–Angiotensin System

In animal models, vitamin D downregulates renin gene promoter activity independent of calcium metabolism. Mice lacking the VDR exhibit hypertension and cardiac hypertrophy due to increased renin expression and plasma angiotensin II production. Oral administration of vitamin D in spontaneously hypertensive rats decreased blood pressure as well as improved endothelial cell–dependent vasodilation. In humans, there is an inverse relationship between vitamin D levels and plasma renin levels. Interventional studies with oral synthetic vitamin D replacement lowered plasma renin in nondiabetic vitamin D–deficient patients. This evidence supports the conceptual relationship between vitamin D and the renin–aldosterone system in essential hypertension and the beneficial effect of vitamin D supplementation on blood pressure.

Vitamin D and Cardiovascular Disease

Vitamin D not only alters the hormones involved in the pathophysiology of hypertension and diabetes, but it also has a direct effect on the vasculature. The expression of VDRs and the activation of vitamin D by 1α-hydroxylase enzyme in endothelial (EC) and vascular smooth muscle cells (VSMC) suggest the importance of vitamin D in vascular cell metabolism. Vitamin D deficiency is more prevalent in patients with peripheral vascular disease, and vitamin D levels are inversely correlated with vascular resistance in hypertensive patients. Cardiovascular events are more prevalent during winter months and at increased geographic latitudes where average serum vitamin D levels are the lowest. 25(OH)D levels are significantly lower in patients with stroke, in nondiabetic patients with acute myocardial infarction, and in patients with heart failure. Type 2 diabetic individuals with clinically relevant CVD have lower 25(OH)D concentrations than their vitamin D–sufficient diabetic counterparts without CVD. Also in type 2 diabetic patients, low vitamin D levels are strongly and independently associated with increased carotid artery intima-media thickness (CIMT), a reliable marker of atherosclerosis. Finally, some interventional studies have documented that long-term vitamin D supplementation in nondiabetic, vitamin D–deficient individuals significantly reduced plasma levels of C-reactive protein, tissue matrix-metallo-proteinases (MMP 1 and 9) and its inhibitors (TIMP-1),25 and had beneficial effects on the elastic properties of the common carotid artery in postmenopausal women.

Immunity

The VDR is present in macrophages and T lymphocytes. 1,25(OH)$_2$D acts as an immune system modulator, preventing excessive expression of inflammatory cytokines and increasing the "oxidative burst" potential of macrophages. Most importantly, vitamin D stimulates antimicrobial peptides (cathelicidin and beta-defensin 2) that exist in neutrophils, monocytes, natural killer cells, and in epithelial cells lining the respiratory tract, where they play a major role in protecting against bacteria, viruses, and fungi. African Americans, known to have increased susceptibility to tuberculosis (TB), are reported to have low serum levels of 25-hydroxyvitamin D and inefficient induction of cathelicidin expression. Adding vitamin D to serum from African Americans increased cathelicidin production by macrophages and accelerated rates of TB-microbe killing. Cathelicidin and beta-defensin 2 display broad-spectrum of antimicrobial activity, including antiviral activity, and have been shown to inactivate the influenza virus. Volunteers inoculated with live attenuated influenza virus during winter are more likely to develop fever and serologic evidence of an immune response compared to those inoculated during summer, suggesting a correlation between vitamin D levels and the recurrent seasonality of the influenza epidemics. Vitamin D deficiency predisposes children to respiratory infections. Increased vitamin D levels by UV radiation and cod liver reduces the incidence of respiratory infections in children. This suggests that differences in the ability to produce vitamin D may contribute to susceptibility or resistance to microbial infection.

Antiproliferative Effects

The active vitamin D metabolite, in addition to regulating calcium–phosphate homeostasis and bone mineralization, induces in vitro cell cycle arrest, differentiation, and apoptosis in a variety of cancer cells.

Most observational studies have reported an inverse correlation between vitamin D status, sunlight exposure, and cancer risk and mortality. High 25(OH)D levels at the time of diagnosis or during cancer treatment, may improve prognosis in colon, breast, and prostate cancer. Patients with genetic VDR polymorphism, especially the *Bsm I* genotype bb, have twice the incidence of colon, prostate, and breast cancer. VDR *FokI* polymorphism modifies prostate cancer risk. Men with the less functional *FokI* ff genotype are more susceptible to this cancer in the presence of low 25(OH)D levels.

In colon cancer, the evidence is substantial. Most studies that examined circulating 25(OH)D concentrations and subsequent risk of colorectal cancer or adenoma, found a lower risk associated with higher 25(OH)D concentrations. In the recent analysis in the Nurses' Health Study, colon cancer risk negatively correlates with 25(OH)D concentrations. Patients with 25(OH)D concentrations of 39.9 ng/mL have almost half the relative risk (RR) of developing colon cancer (RR, 0.53; confidence interval [CI], 0.27–1.04) compared to patients with levels <16 ng/mL ($p = 0.02$). Benefit from higher 25(OH)D concentrations was observed for cancers in older women with cancer at the distal colon and rectum, but was not evident for those at the proximal colon.

In a prospective study of 1954 men, vitamin D intake of 233 to 652 IU/day decreased by half the relative risk of developing colon cancer compared to men with a vitamin D intake less than 6–94 IU/day. The WHI, a 7-year prospective study, confirmed that women at enrollment who had low blood vitamin D levels (<15 ng/mL) had a greater than twofold risk of bowel cancer compared to those with vitamin D levels >58.4 nmol/L. However, there was no evidence that treatment with calcium 1000 mg/day and vitamin D (400 IU/day) reduced bowel cancer occurrence. Several issues have been raised regarding this study, mainly the short duration of the study and a dose of 400 IU of vitamin D_3 that was inadequate to raise blood levels of 25(OH)D to a range above 30 ng/mL. Based on these, and previous studies, the estimated optimal serum 25(OH)D concentrations associated with reduced incidence of colonic adenomas is 30 to 35 ng/mL.

In prostate cancer, epidemiologic and laboratory data support the role of vitamin D in the growth and differentiation of human prostatic cells. In a Finnish study, prostate cancer incidence was assessed in 18,966 men, ages 40 to 57 during 14 years. Those men with 25(OH)D levels below 16 ng/mL had a 70% higher incidence rate of prostate cancer than those with levels 16 ng/mL or above. For younger men with 25(OH)D levels below 16 ng/mL, the incidence of prostate cancer was 3.5 times higher than for those with levels of 16 ng/mL or above, and the incidence of invasive cancer was 6.3 times higher. A few small phase II trials showed evidence that 1,25(OH)$_2$D alone or in combination with antimitotic chemotherapy decreases prostate cancer progression, but further studies are needed.

In breast cancer, combined analysis of 1760 women from two trials reporting risk of breast cancer by quintiles of 25(OH)D, showed that a 50% reduction of breast cancer risk was associated with 25(OH)D levels of 50 ng/mL compared to those with levels of 10 ng/mL. In addition, women in the lowest quartile of serum 1,25(OH)$_2$D had a risk of breast cancer 5 times higher than those in the highest quartile. Low 1,25(OH)$_2$D levels were also associated with faster progression of metastatic breast cancer. Animal studies confirmed that 1,25(OH)$_2$D inhibits breast cancer, but interventional studies in humans are still pending.

Myopathy

Muscle weakness is a common clinical feature in patients with vitamin D deficiency. It may affect fracture risk by altering the susceptibility to falls. Combined evidence from five studies including 1237 patients showed that vitamin D intake reduced the risk of falling by 22% (RR, 0.78; 95% CI, 0.64–0.92). In a recent double-blind study, elderly ambulatory subjects taking 700 IU vitamin D plus 500 mg calcium had a 46% decreased risk of falling compared to those taking placebo. Fall reduction was most pronounced in less active women. Poor physical performance and a greater decline in physical performance in 1234 older men and women were found when serum 25(OH)D concentrations were below 20 ng/mL. Hypovitaminosis D myopathy may be present even before biochemical signs of bone disease develop. Full normalization of hypovitaminosis D myopathy demands high-dose vitamin D treatment for 6 months or more. There is also evidence that idiopathic low back pain in patients with vitamin D deficiency markedly improves when levels are restored. Low levels of 25(OH)D are also common in patients with fibromyalgia and chronic refractory nonspecific musculoskeletal pain.

Rheumatoid Arthritis

Rheumatoid arthritis (RA) is one of the most common chronic inflammatory diseases and affects about 1% of the population in the United States. Epidemiologic studies have reported low serum levels of vitamin D and its metabolites in patients with RA. Small interventional studies in RA with high-dose oral alfacalcidol (form of vitamin D) therapy showed a positive effect on disease activity in 89% of the patients, and only 11% of patients showed no improvement. In psoriatic arthritis, oral administration of 1,25-$(OH)_2D_3$ showed an improvement in disease symptoms. In the WHI study, women who received less <200 IU of vitamin D in their diets each day were 33% more likely to develop rheumatoid arthritis than women who received more. These results provide evidence that VDR ligands can be of potential clinical use for the treatment of RA.

Multiple Sclerosis

Epidemiologic data correlate the geographic location and the prevalence of MS. In women, the Nurses' Health Study and Nurses' Health Study II results confirm a protective effect of vitamin D on the risk of multiple sclerosis (MS). The relative risk to develop MS was decreased by 60% when comparing women who had an intake of ≥400 IU/day with women not taking supplemental vitamin. No prospective studies have addressed this hypothesis.

TREATMENT

The vitamin D dose depends on the target concentration of 25(OH)D desired. New clinical research indicates that the vitamin D intake used to prevent rickets is much lower than the requirement for prevention of osteoporosis related bone fractures, cancer, and improvement of the metabolic abnormalities described previously. However, the ideal oral intake of vitamin D that provokes healthy effects without side effects has not been completely elucidated.

Vitamin D is available in two forms for supplementation. Ergocalciferol (vitamin D_2) made from yeast fat exposed to UV light and cholecalciferol (vitamin D_3) obtained from animal fat. Vitamin D_2 is one-third less potent than vitamin D_3 and has a shorter duration of action relative to vitamin D_3 (<14 days). The half-life of 25(OH)D in the circulation is reported to be approximately 1 month in humans. Conventional pharmacology indicates it should take at least four half-lives before a drug's equilibrium is achieved. Increased responsiveness to vitamin D administration is seen more in thin patients with low vitamin D levels at baseline using low vitamin D doses and long duration of vitamin D supplementation. An increased dose of vitamin D does not increase the plasma 25(OH)D levels proportionally. Previous studies indicate that 75% or more of the molecules of vitamin D that enter to the body are catabolized and excreted without becoming 25(OH)D. Generally, 100 IU/day for 8 months increases 25(OH)D levels by 1 ng/mL.

The **current recommendations**, based on the assumption that young and middle-aged adults were more likely than older adults to be exposed to sunlight, are as follows: 200 IU/day for children and adults ≤50 years of age, 400 IU/day for men and women aged 50 to 70 years, and 600 IU/day for those older than 70 years. This recommendation will require revision in the near future. To achieve the current 25(OH)D goal (28–40 ng/mL), a minimum intake of 700–1000 IU/day was determined in groups of younger and older adults exposed to sunshine. Subgroups of the population such as the obese individuals, pregnant women, and patients with nephrotic syndrome and chronic renal failure require 1000 to 2000 IU of vitamin D_3 daily or 50,000 IU of vitamin D_2 every 2 weeks to prevent vitamin D deficiency during the winter months. The Food and Nutrition Board guidelines specify 2000 IU vitamin D_3 as the highest vitamin D intake that healthy adults can consume without risking hypercalcemia. However, some patients may require higher doses; multiple studies have shown that optimal 25(OH)D levels can be achieved safely during winter in all patients at a vitamin D_3 dose of 4000 IU.

In the United States, the only pharmaceutical preparation of vitamin D is vitamin D_2. **The recommended dose of ergocalciferol to treat vitamin D deficiency is 50,000 IU every week for 8 weeks.** If the patient does not achieve 25(OH)D levels >30 ng/mL, then another 8 weeks of therapy is recommended. If the 25(OH)D levels are >30 ng/mL, then follow with maintenance therapy of 50,000 IU every other week or once a month depending on the etiology of the vitamin D deficiency. In patients with obesity, nephrotic syndrome, or malabsorption, or in patients taking anticonvulsants, glucocorticoids, HAART (AIDS treatment), and transplant antirejection medications, ergocalciferol loading doses (50,000 IU/week) should be administered for longer periods (8–12 weeks). If 25(OH)D levels are still <30 ng/mL after a loading dose, repeat for another 8 to 12 weeks of treatment. Maintenance doses in this special subgroup of patients should be 50,000 IU every week or every other week.

Previous reports suggest that IDS RIA or ADVANTAGE CPBA system assays for 25(OH)D might not detect vitamin D_2 levels. These tests will give misleading results and could lead to misdiagnosis and subsequent dangerous consequences for the patient, such as hypervitaminosis D after vitamin D_2 replacement. If you cannot obtain an expected increase in the 25(OH)D level after supplementation, check with the laboratory to determine what type of 25(OH)D assay is used.

Another way to replace vitamin D is to administer it as a single large dose, either orally or through injection. This approach, known as stoss therapy, should be closely monitored by an experienced physician.

The most sensitive clinical index of safety during vitamin D replacement is measurement of urinary calcium. This is measured by **morning calcium-to-creatinine ratio** (normal values are <1 mmol/mmol or <0.35 mg/mg in a well-hydrated patient). An elevated calcium-to-creatinine ratio increases the risk for nephrolithiasis, and increased caution in replacement dosing, hydration, and monitoring should be exercised. However, hypercalciuria cannot be excluded if the urinary creatinine concentration is >40 mg/dL. Given that during vitamin D replacement, serum 25(OH)D is at the plateau concentration by 1 month, we suggest an assessment of serum calcium and urine calcium-to-creatinine ratio 2 to 4 weeks after starting vitamin D replacement therapy. We recommend repeating these studies monthly for 1 or 2 months because the plateau of 25(OH)D concentration may be slightly underestimated in some cases.

Hypersensitivity to vitamin D supplementation can occur in patients with primary hyperparathyroidism, sarcoidosis, TB, or lymphoma. In primary hyperparathyroidism, production of $1,25(OH)_2D$ is persistently upregulated by high PTH concentrations, and $1,25(OH)_2D$ concentrations correlate directly with serum 25(OH)D. However, the current data provide preliminary evidence that vitamin D repletion in patients with mild primary hyperparathyroidism does not promote an increase in serum calcium and has beneficial effects by decreasing PTH levels and bone turnover. Only a small initial increase in urinary calcium excretion was present in 2 of 21 patients in one study. We recommend assessment of plasma calcium and urinary calcium/creatinine ratio in the first 2 weeks of the vitamin D replacement and then monthly during replacement.

Multiple medications can interact with vitamin D. Cholestyramine, Colestipol, mineral oil, Orlistat, and Olestra (a fat substitute) reduce vitamin D absorption. Ketoconazole, following the administration of 300 to 1200 mg daily in healthy men for 7 days, decreased serum $1,25(OH)_2D$ levels. Anticonvulsants, glucocorticoids, HAART (AIDS treatment), and transplant antirejection medications activate the destruction of 25(OH)D and $1,25(OH)_2D$ to inactive compounds.

Sun exposure very efficiently forms vitamin D_3. In summer months, total-body sun exposure for 15 to 30 minutes in Caucasian adults generates about 250 mcg (10,000 IU) of vitamin D_3/day, with no signs of vitamin D–induced intoxication. In a randomized control study in a psychogeriatric nursing home, exposure to UV irradiation with half of the minimal erythematous dose on 1000 cm^2 of the back 3 times per week for 12 weeks increased plasma 25(OH)D to the same levels as those who received oral 400 IU/day of vitamin D_3. Exposure of face, forearms, and hands (total exposed skin area was 426 ± 32 cm^2) to sunlight for 15 minutes and calcium supplementation may be safe and effective in increasing BMD and reducing the risk of fracture in chronically hospitalized elderly women with Alzheimer's disease.

Most tanning beds emit 2% to 6% UVB radiation. In patients with malabsorption, tanning-bed exposure is a potential source of vitamin D supplementation.

TOXICITY

Vitamin D toxicity is extremely rare and generally occurs by accidental or uninformed consumption of very high doses of vitamin D. Toxicity occurred with ingestion of more than 40,000 IU/day, which reflects 4 times the maximum vitamin D (10,000 IU) acquired by sunshine exposure. Concentrations of $1,25(OH)_2D$ are not increased by vitamin D intoxication but free $1,25(OH)_2D$ levels are generally high.

Hypercalcemia (>11 mg/dL) is the main criterion for vitamin D–induced toxicity. The **clinical manifestations** include anorexia, nausea and vomiting, hypotonicity, lethargy, constipation, generalized pain, conjunctivitis, fever, chills, thirst, and weight loss. Hypercalcemia can result in a loss of the urinary concentrating mechanism of the kidney tubule, resulting in polyuria and polydipsia. The prolonged ingestion of excessive amounts of vitamin D and the accompanying hypercalcemia can result in metastatic calcification of soft tissues—including the kidney, blood vessels, heart and lungs—and increased risk for nephrolithiasis.

The only treatment for vitamin D toxicity is to decrease the hypercalcemia by forcing a negative calcium balance. Glucocorticoids, intravenous saline, furosemide, calcitonin, or a bisphosphonate has been used. Because vitamin D is stored in fat, vitamin D intoxication may persist for weeks after vitamin D ingestion is terminated. The elimination half-life of vitamin D is about 3 weeks to one month. Persistent treatment with corticosteroid or an oral bisphosphonate for this period is required.

KEY POINTS TO REMEMBER

- The skin is the main organ responsible for vitamin D production; patients with limited exposure to the sun such as the elderly and those in northern latitudes are at risk for vitamin D deficiency.
- Serum levels of 25(OH)D are the best indicator of vitamin D status.
- The recommended dose of ergocalciferol to treat vitamin D deficiency is 50,000 IU every week for 8 weeks for a target 25(OH)D level >30 ng/mL.
- There is a growing body of evidence that vitamin D is important for overall health and not just bone health. Vitamin D deficiency may be linked to many health problems including hypertension, colorectal cancer, myopathy, diabetes mellitus, cardiovascular disease, rheumatoid arthritis, and multiple sclerosis.

ACKNOWLEDGMENTS

The authors thank Adriana Dusso for her considerate review of this manuscript.

REFERENCES AND SUGGESTED READINGS

Bischoff-Ferrari HA, Giovannucci E, Willett WC, et al. Estimation of optimal serum concentrations of 25-hydroxyvitamin D for multiple health outcomes. *Am J Clin Nutr* 2006;84:18–28.

Bischoff-Ferrari HA, Willett WC, Wong JB, et al. Fracture prevention with vitamin D supplementation: a meta-analysis of randomized controlled trials. *JAMA* 2005;293: 2257–2264.

Dusso AS, Brown AJ, Slatopolsky E. Vitamin D. *Am J Physiol Renal Physiol* 2005;289: F8–F28.

Heaney RP, Davies KM, Chen TC, et al. Human serum 25-hydroxycholecalciferol response to extended oral dosing with cholecalciferol. *Am J Clin Nutr* 2003;77:204–210.

Holick MF. Vitamin D deficiency. *N Engl J Med* 2007;357:266–281.

Hollick MF. Vitamin D: importance in the prevention of cancers, type 1 diabetes, heart disease, and osteoporosis *Am J Clin Nutr* 2004;79:362–371.

Mathieu C, Gysemans C, Giulietti A, et al. Vitamin D and diabetes. *Diabetologia* 2005;48:1247–1257.

Norman PE, Powell JT. Vitamin D, shedding light on the development of disease in peripheral arteries. *Arterioscler Thromb Vasc Biol* 2005;25:39–46.

Schwartz GG, Blot WJ. Vitamin D status and cancer incidence and mortality: something new under the sun. *J Natl Cancer Inst* 2006;98:428–430.

Towler DA, Clemens TL. Vitamin D and cardiovascular medicine. In: Feldman D, Pike JW, Glorieux FH, eds. *Vitamin D,* 2nd ed. San Diego: Academic Press; 2005: 889–910.

Vieth R, Bischoff-Ferrari H, Boucher BJ, et al. The urgent need to recommend an intake of vitamin D that is effective. *Am J Clin Nutr* 2007;85:649–650.

Vieth R. Vitamin D supplementation, 25-hydroxyvitamin D concentrations, and safety. *Am J Clin Nutr* 1999;69:842–856.

Zittermann A, Schleithoff SS, Koerfer R. Putting cardiovascular disease and vitamin D insufficiency into perspective. *Br J Nutr* 2005;94:483–492.

Osteoporosis

Jason S. Goldfeder and Parvin F. Peddi

INTRODUCTION

Osteoporosis, which literally means "porous bone," is a disorder characterized by low bone mass and microarchitectural deterioration of bone that leads to a **decrease in bone mass, enhanced bone fragility**, and a consequent **increase in the risk of fractures**. Osteoporosis is the most common metabolic bone disorder in humans and is generally an asymptomatic condition until complications develop. The prevalence, adverse outcomes, and economic cost associated with osteoporotic fractures, particularly hip fractures, are significant. The association of osteoporosis as an asymptomatic risk factor for fractures is similar to that of hypertension with stroke and hypercholesterolemia with coronary heart disease, with a relative risk (RR) of hip fracture of 2.6 for each 1 standard deviation (SD) decrease in bone mineral density at the hip. Significant advances in diagnostic testing since the early 1990s have made osteoporosis relatively easy to diagnose, and several national societies have developed guidelines endorsing routine screening for osteoporosis. Several pharmacotherapeutic agents that differ in their impact on enhancing bone density, decreasing the rates of fracture at various clinical sites, and side effects are approved for the prevention and treatment of osteoporosis. However, a significant percentage of patients with osteoporosis, including those who have already experienced fractures, are not appropriately diagnosed and treated.

Definition

Before 1994, making a diagnosis of osteoporosis required the presence of a clinical fracture. In 1994, the World Health Organization (WHO) changed the definition of osteoporosis to include criteria based on bone densitometry testing. There are four diagnostic categories based on the comparison of a patient's bone mineral density (BMD) with that of a young adult reference mean (the T score; see Bone Mineral Density Testing in this chapter).

- **Normal:** BMD within 1 SD of the young adult reference mean (T ≥ -1.0)
- **Osteopenia:** BMD between 1 and 2.5 SDs below the young adult reference mean ($-2.5 < T < -1.0$)
- **Osteoporosis:** BMD >2.5 SDs below the young adult reference mean (T ≤ -2.5)
- **Established or severe osteoporosis:** BMD >2.5 SDs below the young adult reference mean (T ≤ -2.5) and the presence of one or more fragility fractures

Classification

Osteoporosis can be classified as primary or secondary. In primary osteoporosis, the deterioration of bone mass is related to aging or decreased gonadal function, typically in postmenopausal women or aging men. Secondary osteoporosis results from chronic conditions or medications that accelerate bone loss (see Risk Factors in this chapter and Table 25-2).

Epidemiology

Approximately 30 million postmenopausal women in the United States have either osteopenia or osteoporosis. The majority of available data on the epidemiology of osteopenia and osteoporosis is in white women. Current estimates of the prevalence of osteoporosis come from the The National Health Nutrition and Examination Survey (NHANES) III epidemiologic study, which was conducted from 1988 to 1994. In this study, which used young white women as the referent for comparison, osteopenia and osteoporosis, respectively, were estimated to be present in 41% and 17% of Caucasian women, 28% and 8% of African American women, and 37% and 12% of Mexican-American women older than 50 years of age. The ratio of the age-adjusted prevalence of osteoporosis in Caucasian versus African American women ranged from 1.5 to 2.8, depending on the site of measurement. The ratio in Caucasian versus Mexican-American women ranged from 0.8 to 1.2. Extrapolating the NHANES data to the current population, the National Osteoporosis Foundation currently estimates that 52% and 20% of postmenopausal white women have osteopenia and osteoporosis, respectively, and that there are currently approximately 22 million and 8 million women of all races in the United States with osteopenia and osteoporosis, respectively.

CAUSES

Pathogenesis

An adult's total bone mineral content is dependent on his or her peak bone mass achieved during early adulthood and his or her level of bone remodeling. Bone remodeling takes place throughout childhood and adulthood and is a result of the balance of concurrent bone resorption and new bone formation. Osteoporosis can result from either poor bone acquisition and the failure to achieve expected peak bone mass or from increased bone remodeling.

Peak bone mass is generally reached at approximately age 25 to 30. Peak bone mass is primarily determined by genetic factors, including race and gender. However, potentially modifiable environmental and metabolic conditions, such as nutritional status, calcium intake, physical activity level, tobacco use, hormonal deficiencies, and other medical comorbidities, can also affect the level of peak bone mass achieved. Black women and men typically achieve higher levels of peak bone mass than white women, which is a key reason why the rates of osteoporosis and fractures are lower in these groups. Adults who do not achieve their predicted peak bone mass are at risk of developing osteoporosis at an earlier age.

When the rate of bone resorption exceeds that of new bone formation, the overall increased rate of bone turnover leads to a net loss of bone mass. Men and women slowly begin to lose peak bone mass at a rate of ~0.5% to 1% per year starting at approximately age 35. The rate of net bone loss is frequently increased after menopause in women, as estrogen deficiency alters cytokine production and enhances osteoclast activity. This accelerated rate of bone loss is most prominent in areas of trabecular bone, such as the spine, and may result in a rate of loss of bone mass of 3% to 5% per year for up to 10 years. The rate of bone loss in areas with more cortical bone, such as the hips, tends to be delayed and less rapid. Because men achieve a higher peak bone mass initially and do not usually go through a rapid period of bone loss, in the absence of secondary disorders, bone loss does not tend to reach levels that increase the risk for fractures until age 65 to 70.

Risk Factors

Several risk factors have been shown to be independently associated with low bone mass (Table 25-1). Some of these risk factors are modifiable and are important to address in a regimen to prevent or treat osteoporosis. There are also multiple chronic medical conditions

TABLE 25-1	RISK FACTORS FOR OSTEOPOROSIS

Female sex
White race
Advanced age
Personal history of a fracture
Family history of osteoporosis/fracture in a first-degree relative
Small body habitus/low body weight (<127 lb)
Sedentary lifestyle/lack of physical activity
Tobacco use
Excessive alcohol intake (>2 drinks/day)
Insufficient intake of calcium or vitamin D
Excessive caffeine intake
Early menopause (age <45 years)
Premature ovarian failure
Medical or surgical menopause

and medications that are risk factors for causing secondary osteoporosis (Table 25-2). Osteoporosis typically results in fractures when adults with low bone density fall. As such, risk factors for falling that are independent of low BMD are important risk factors for experiencing osteoporotic fractures (Table 25-3).

Presentation

Most patients with osteoporosis are asymptomatic until they develop fractures. As such, the history and physical examination are usually not sufficiently sensitive to make a diagnosis of osteoporosis in the absence of diagnostic testing. Once a patient is clinically diagnosed with osteoporosis, the history should focus on assessing for modifiable risk factors (Table 25-1), medical conditions associated with secondary osteoporosis (Table 25-2), and risk factors for falling (Table 25-3).

Screening for Osteoporosis

No randomized, controlled, prospective clinical trial has proven that screening for osteoporosis and subsequent intervention decreases the incidence of osteoporotic fractures or other complications. However, based on the prevalence of the condition, frequency of complications, accessibility of diagnostic testing, and available treatment options, several national societies have issued consensus statements supporting routine screening for osteoporosis (Table 25-4). In general, all groups agree that women who present with fragility fractures in the absence of trauma should be screened, but opinions vary on whether and under what conditions routine screening of asymptomatic adults should be conducted. Of note, although the majority of data on the diagnosis and treatment of osteoporosis is in white women, the recommendations for screening for osteoporosis in women are irrespective of race.

Osteoporotic Fractures

Fragility Fractures

Fragility fractures are the primary cause of morbidity and mortality in adults with osteoporosis. The most common sites for osteoporotic fractures are the **hip**, the **spine**, and the

TABLE 25-2 CAUSES OF SECONDARY OSTEOPOROSIS

Endocrine disorders

Acromegaly

Amenorrhea (primary or secondary amenorrhea of any cause)

Anorexia

Cushing's syndrome/hypercortisolism

Diabetes mellitus, type 1

Hyperparathyroidism

Hyperprolactinemia

Hyperthyroidism

Hypogonadism (primary or secondary)

Porphyria

Genetic/collagen disorders

Ehlers-Danlos

Glycogen storage diseases

Homocystinuria

Hypophosphatasia

Osteogenesis imperfecta

Gastrointestinal/hepatic disorders

Celiac sprue

Chronic cholestatic liver disease

Chronic malabsorptive conditions

Cirrhosis

Gastric bypass/gastrectomy

Hemochromatosis

Inflammatory bowel disease

Hematologic disorders

Amyloidosis

Leukemia/lymphoma

Mastocytosis

Multiple myeloma

Infectious diseases

HIV/AIDS

Metabolic/nutritional disorders

Alcoholism

Hyperhomocystinemia

Hypocalcemia

Vitamin D deficiency

Pulmonary disorders

Chronic obstructive pulmonary disease

Renal disorders

Chronic kidney disease (of any cause)

Renal tubular acidosis

Rheumatologic disorders

Ankylosing spondylitis

Rheumatoid arthritis

Medications

Aluminum

Cyclosporine

Dilantin

Glucocorticoids

Gonadotropin agonists (e.g., Lupron)

Heparin (prolonged use)

Methotrexate

Phenobarbital

Phenothiazines

Protease inhibitors

Thyroxine (excessive replacement)

distal radius (forearm or wrist). Approximately 1.5 million osteoporotic fractures occur each year in the United States, including 700,000 vertebral fractures, 300,000 hip fractures, 200,000 wrist fractures, and 300,000 other fractures. In white women aged 65 to 85, it is estimated that 90% of all vertebral fractures, 90% of all hip fractures, 70% of all forearm fractures, and 50% of all other fractures are attributable to osteoporosis. The corresponding rates in black women are 80% for vertebral fractures, 80% for hip fractures, 60% for forearm fractures, and 40% for all other fractures. In both races, a smaller percentage of fractures can be attributed to osteoporosis in women younger than age 65, but a larger

TABLE 25-3	RISK FACTORS FOR FALLING

History of falls

Dementia

Impaired vision

Poor physical condition/frailty

Foot problems or inappropriate footwear

History of stroke or Parkinson's disease

Environmental hazards

Use of benzodiazepines, anticonvulsants, or anticholinergic medications

percentage can be attributed to osteoporosis in women older than 85. A 50-year-old white woman has an approximate 50% risk of experiencing an osteoporotic fracture during her lifetime, including a 32% risk of a having a vertebral fracture, a 16% risk of having a hip fracture, and a 15% risk of having a wrist fracture. With the anticipated aging of the population, osteoporotic fractures are predicted to increase several-fold worldwide by 2050.

Hip Fractures

Hip fractures are the most devastating cause of morbidity and mortality attributable to osteoporosis. Mortality rates are increased five- to sixfold during the first month after a hip fracture and approximately threefold over the first year, resulting in a 1-year mortality rate

TABLE 25-4	SOCIETAL RECOMMENDATIONS ON ROUTINE SCREENING FOR OSTEOPOROSIS
Group	**Recommendations**
National Osteoporosis Foundation	Screen all women >65 years regardless of risk factors
	Screen younger postmenopausal women with ≥1 risk factor besides sex, race, and menopausal status
U.S. Preventive Services Task Force	Screen all women >65 years regardless of risk factors
	Screen women aged 60–65 years who are at increased risk for fractures primarily based on low body weight (<70 kg) or lack of hormone replacement therapy
NIH	Routine screening is not recommended
American College of Obstetricians and Gynecologists	Screen all women >65 years regardless of risk factors
	Screen postmenopausal women <65 years with additional risk factors
European Foundation for Osteoporosis and Bone Disease	Routine screening is not recommended

from hip fractures in women of 10% to 20%. Fifteen percent to 30% of women require nursing home placement for at least 1 year. Up to one-half of women able to walk before a hip fracture require long-term placement or help with activities of daily living after a hip fracture. Only 30% to 40% of women regain their prefracture level of function. Treatment of hip fractures and their associated complications is responsible for the majority of the cost associated with treating osteoporosis, with cost estimates of $14 billion to treat hip fractures in 1995 and $17 billion in 2001.

Vertebral Fractures

Vertebral fractures are also associated with significant morbidity and mortality. Vertebral fractures tend to be more occult than hip fractures and are often present radiographically, but not clinically. As opposed to hip and wrist fractures, most vertebral fractures are not related to acute trauma and can result from routine everyday activities or minor stresses on the spine such as bending or lifting. Only approximately one-third of radiographically confirmed vertebral compression fractures come to medical attention, and <10% result in hospital admissions. However, asymptomatic vertebral fractures are a major risk factor for subsequent fractures, including hip fractures. Treatment to prevent subsequent hip fractures with antiresorptive therapy is more beneficial in adults with prevalent vertebral fractures. Vertebral fractures are associated with chronic back pain, loss of height, and kyphosis. Having multiple vertebral fractures can result in the development of restrictive lung disease or gastrointestinal complications, such as chronic abdominal pain, constipation, and anorexia. Vertebral fractures have been shown to decrease quality of life across several domains. Most important, long-term prospective studies have shown that the presence of vertebral fractures, whether symptomatic or not, is associated with a 15% to 30% increased rate of overall mortality, including an increased risk of mortality secondary to all cancers, specifically lung cancer, and pulmonary disease.

DIAGNOSIS

Bone Mineral Density Testing

The standard of care for diagnosis and evaluation of adults for osteoporosis is to assess their BMD. Several radiologic tests are available to measure BMD, including central and peripheral dual energy x-ray absorptiometry (DEXA), quantitative computed tomography (CT), and peripheral ultrasonography.

DEXA is the gold standard and is recommended for adults who have had osteoporotic fractures or who are undergoing general screening. DEXA imaging results in a low level of radiation exposure (approximately one-tenth that of a traditional x-ray) and has excellent precision and reproducibility. The most common sites to measure with DEXA are the spine, the hip, and the distal forearm. BMD results are calculated as the bone mineral content divided by the area of bone measured (g/cm^2). In the lumbosacral spine, measurements are generally made at the L1, L2, L3, and L4 vertebrae and then averaged together for a total spine score. At the hip, measurements are made at the femoral neck, greater trochanter, intertrochanteric area, and Ward's triangle, and then averaged. Results of BMD testing are then reported in comparison to reference ranges in SDs as the T score and the Z score.

- The *T score* compares the patient's BMD in SDs with the average peak BMD of young healthy adults of the same gender.
- The *Z score* compares the patient's BMD in SDs with the average BMD of adults of the same age and gender.

The **diagnoses of osteoporosis and osteopenia are made based on the T score.** The Z score can occasionally be helpful if it is very abnormal, as it suggests the possibility of a secondary cause of osteoporosis. Decreased BMD is a strong predictor of subsequent fracture. On average, the risk of fracture approximately doubles for each 1 SD decrease in the T score. Although decreased bone density at one site allows the diagnosis of osteoporosis to be made and increases the risk for fracture at all sites, the best predictor of fracture at a specific site is the bone density at that site. This is most important at the hip, which is the fracture site most associated with morbidity and mortality. For each 1 SD decrease in hip BMD, the risk of hip fractures increases by 2.6-fold, the risk of vertebral fractures increases by 1.8-fold, the risk of wrist fractures increases by 1.4-fold, and the risk of all fractures increases by 1.5-fold. The risk of a subsequent hip fracture associated with decreased BMD at other sites is somewhat lower. This is explained by the fact that different parts of the skeleton are affected differently at different periods and by different medical conditions. In the early postmenopausal period, bone loss occurs most rapidly in the spine. However, in adults older than 65 years, the bone density of the spine may be falsely elevated by osteoarthritis of the spine or vascular calcification. Adults with primary hyperparathyroidism lose bone most rapidly in the distal radius. If insurance coverage allows, bone density testing should be obtained of both the spine and the hip. However, if only one site is covered, bone density testing of the spine is often more helpful in women younger than 65 or within 15 years of menopause, as bone is more apt to be lost more rapidly in the spine, and vertebral fractures are the most common type of fracture in this age group. In women older than age 65, bone density of the hip is often more clinically useful, as hip fractures become more of a clinical concern and the spine bone density has a greater chance of being falsely elevated.

Although results of bone density testing are an important risk factor for subsequent fracture, other factors (particularly age) also play prominent roles. The 10-year risk of experiencing osteoporotic fractures at multiple sites increases significantly with age at the same level of BMD.

Quantitative CT scanning and **central bone densitometry** have a similar ability to predict fractures. Quantitative CT scanning is a measure of volumetric density and reports results in g/cm^3. Quantitative CT can be obtained of the hip or spine and is less affected by superimposed osteoarthritis. However, quantitative CT scanning is more expensive, requires a larger dose of radiation, and is not frequently used clinically.

Peripheral bone density testing can be performed with either DEXA or single x-ray energy absorptiometry. Sites that can be measured include the forearm, finger, and heel. Studies using single x-ray energy absorptiometry that were performed before central DEXA was available found that abnormal results were associated with complications such as hip fractures. Peripheral ultrasonography can be performed on the heel, tibia, and patella. The primary benefits of peripheral DEXA and ultrasonography are the portability of the equipment and the ability of the tests to be performed in a primary care office. However, there are not universally agreed on diagnostic criteria for the different machines available. In addition, the precision of the machines does not allow their use for monitoring response to therapy. Peripheral testing has not been fully endorsed for use in the diagnosis of osteoporosis, but if peripheral testing is performed, abnormal results should be followed up with a central DEXA to establish or confirm the diagnosis.

Plain film x-rays are generally unreliable markers of bone mass, as 20% to 50% of bone must be lost before changes are evident on x-ray. Although not routine, a baseline lumbosacral spine x-ray could be considered in an adult with newly diagnosed osteoporosis to assess for any baseline vertebral fractures, which are a prominent risk factor for subsequent clinical fractures.

Laboratory Evaluation

Multiple laboratory tests are available to evaluate for **secondary causes of osteoporosis** (see Table 25-2). There is not a uniform consensus on how much of a workup, if any, is required in adults with a new diagnosis of osteoporosis. Secondary osteoporosis is more common in premenopausal women and men in whom the threshold for diagnostic testing should be somewhat lower. One study of patients from a tertiary referral center found that most patients would be diagnosed with the combination of a serum calcium, parathyroid hormone (PTH), 24-hour urine for calcium, and thyroid-stimulating hormone (TSH) if the patient was taking levothyroxine (Synthroid). The National Osteoporosis Foundation endorses consideration of limited biochemical testing in some patients with initial tests, possibly including a TSH, PTH, vitamin D level (25OH-VitD), serum protein electrophoresis, and 24-hour urine for calcium and cortisol. Other tests to consider if disorders are suggested by the history and physical examination include assessment of renal and liver function, testosterone screening, and luteinizing hormone (LH) and follicle-stimulating hormone (FSH) levels.

Serum and urinary markers of bone turnover are frequently increased in patients with osteoporosis. Markers of bone formation include serum alkaline phosphatase and osteocalcin. Markers of bone resorption include urinary hydroxyproline, and N- and C-terminal collagen telopeptides. Markers of bone turnover may predict the risk of fracture independent of BMD and allow assessment of the response to treatment, but at this point their role in clinical practice is unclear and testing is generally unnecessary.

TREATMENT

Indications for Treatment

All postmenopausal women should be evaluated for risk factors for osteoporosis. Bone density testing should be performed in all adults with fractures and should be considered in postmenopausal women based on their age and risk factors. The nonpharmacologic and lifestyle recommendations should be suggested to all adults, including those who do not meet the criteria for specific pharmacologic therapy for osteoporosis, to prevent the development of osteoporosis. The following are indications to initiate specific therapy for osteoporosis. (It is important to be aware that the prospective randomized controlled pharmacologic trials for the treatment of osteoporosis have taken place mainly in white women [85%–>95% in most treatment trials], so limited data are available on the therapeutic benefit of pharmacologic agents in minority groups.)

- All adults with osteoporotic fractures of the hip or spine
- Adults with a T score ≤ -2.0 SD who do not have specific risk factors for osteoporosis
- Adults with a T score of ≤ -1.5 SD who have risk factors for osteoporosis

Nonpharmacologic Treatment Options

Adults with osteoporosis should be encouraged to stop smoking and avoid excessive alcohol intake. **Weight-bearing exercise** should be encouraged. Multiple small observational and randomized controlled trials have shown that regular exercise can help maximize peak bone mass in young women, decrease age-related bone loss, actually improve BMD in some circumstances, and help maintain muscle balance and strength. The goal should be to exercise for 30 to 60 minutes at least 3 times per week. High-impact weight-bearing activities, such as brisk walking, jogging, weight lifting, and racket sports, are beneficial forms of exercise. Non–weight-bearing activities, such as swimming, are of more questionable benefit. Exercise has never been proven to prospectively decrease the risk of fracture, but it does improve function and decrease the rate of falls. Patients should be assessed for reversible causes of falls such as overmedication, neurologic or vision problems, and poor footwear. For patients at high risk of falling, hip protectors worn under their clothes have been shown to decrease the rate of hip fractures by 60%. A combined aggressive program of nonpharmacologic treatment has been shown to decrease the rate of hip fractures by up to 25%.

Pharmacologic Treatment Options

Calcium and Vitamin D

Adequate intake of calcium is essential to achieve peak bone mass in early adulthood and to maintain bone mass throughout postmenopausal life. Vitamin D increases calcium absorption in the intestine and calcium reabsorption in the kidney. Vitamin D is supplied both in the diet and in the conversion from skin precursors in the presence of sunlight. Elderly adults, especially those who are chronically ill or institutionalized, frequently have a high prevalence of vitamin D deficiency, as they have limited exposure to sunlight. The majority of clinical trials have found that **supplementation with calcium and vitamin D** has a modest beneficial effect on BMD. Most important, one study of elderly women in nursing homes found that supplementation with calcium and vitamin D decreased the rate of hip and other fractures. In essentially all of the randomized, placebo-controlled clinical trials with antiresorptive and bone-forming agents, patients in both the placebo and treatment groups received supplemental calcium and either received supplemental vitamin D or had serum levels checked with supplementation if vitamin D levels were low.

The recommended daily allowance of calcium varies somewhat in different consensus guidelines, but in general is at least 1000 to 1200 mg/day (Table 25-5).

Foods rich in calcium include milk, yogurt, cheeses, sardines, and fortified juices. The average daily calcium intake in adults from nondairy foods is 250 mg/day. The estimated amount of elemental calcium in common dairy products is as follows:

- 8 oz glass of milk: 300 mg
- 8 oz of yogurt: 400 mg
- 1 oz of cheese: 200 mg
- Fortified juices: varies

Essentially all of the clinical trials in adults with osteoporosis that have included dietary assessments of calcium intake have found that the dietary calcium intake of most adults is significantly below recommended levels. As such, most adults both with and without osteoporosis require calcium supplementation. There are a multitude of calcium supplements available, most as either calcium carbonate or calcium acetate. It is important to realize that

TABLE 25-5	RECOMMENDED DAILY CALCIUM INTAKE	
Organization	**Age (years)**	**Recommended Daily Allowance of Elemental Calcium**
National Osteoporosis Foundation	All ages	1200 mg/day
National Institutes of Health	11–24	1200–1500 mg/day
	25–50	1000 mg/day
	50–65	Men: 1000 mg/day Women on HRT: 1000 mg/day Women not on HRT: 1500 mg/day
	>65	1500 mg/day

HRT, hormone-replacement therapy.

the recommendations for calcium are for elemental calcium and that many over-the-counter calcium supplements are labeled by the amount of calcium carbonate or acetate per pill. Calcium salts are best absorbed when taken between meals. The recommended daily allowance of vitamin D is 400 to 800 IU orally daily, with the higher amount recommended for adults at highest risk of being vitamin D deficient. Foods rich in vitamin D include fortified milk and cereals, egg yolks, and liver. Some calcium supplements include vitamin D (Os-Cal D).

Bisphosphonates: Alendronate (Fosamax), Risedronate (Actonel), Ibandronate (Boniva), and Zoledronic acid (Zometa, Reclast)

The bisphosphonates are the best agents currently available for treating osteoporosis. Bisphosphonates bind to mineralized bone and inhibit osteoclast activity. Bisphosphonates inhibit both bone resorption and bone formation but **inhibit bone resorption** to a greater degree. Alendronate, risedronate, and ibandronate are the three oral bisphosphonates approved by the Food and Drug Administration (FDA) for osteoporosis (Table 25-6). All three agents have been shown to **improve bone density** at various sites in the skeleton and **decrease the rates of total, hip, and symptomatic and asymptomatic vertebral fractures** (only vertebral fractures have been shown to decrease in the published ibandronate trials). Randomized controlled trials showing a benefit in reducing fractures have lasted up to 4 years. Sustained benefit in improving bone density has been shown with as long as 10 years of treatment with alendronate and 7 years of risedronate. Alendronate and risedronate are the only agents to date that have been consistently shown to decrease hip fractures in patients with osteoporosis. However, the significant decrease in hip fractures has primarily been seen only in patients with established osteoporosis (T < -2.5) who have preexisting vertebral fractures. The benefit in absolute terms in reducing fractures of all types with both agents is more prominent in patients with preexisting vertebral fractures.

Bisphosphonates should be taken early in the morning with a glass of water at least **30 minutes before any food or other medications** to prevent retention of the pills in the esophagus. Antacids and calcium limit their absorption. In the randomized, placebo-controlled trials with alendronate, risedronate, and ibandronate, there was no significant difference in the rate of gastrointestinal side effects between the agents and placebo. However, in clinical practice, esophageal and gastric side effects and complications have been reported, reinforcing the need for proper dosing. Once-a-week formulations of alendronate and risedronate are available for both osteoporosis prevention and treatment and may increase compliance. Ibandronate is available in a once-a-month formulation.

Zoledronic acid, also called Zometa and Reclast, is a parenterally administered bisphosphonate. A recent study showed that annually administered Zometa can be at least as efficacious, if not more beneficial, compared to oral bisphosphonates. The HORIZON study (Health Outcomes and Reduced Incidence with Zoledronic Acid Once Yearly) was a multicenter, randomized, double-blind, placebo-controlled trial involving postmenopausal women with osteoporosis who were randomized to placebo versus annual 5 mg intravenous zoledronic acid infusions, and who were followed for 3 years while also receiving calcium and vitamin D in both arms. Treatment with zoledronic acid reduced the risk of vertebral fractures by 70%, hip fractures by 41%, and nonvertebral fractures by 25%. Repetition of this study as well as head-to-head comparison trials of zoledronic acid with oral bisphosphonates will be needed to determine first-line treatment. However, annual infusions of zoledronic acid may provide the answer to current difficulties with regimens of oral bisphosphonates.

Osteonecrosis of the jaw has been recognized as a complication of nitrogen-containing bisphosphonate therapy. Fewer than 50 cases have been reported in the literature in patients on oral bisphosphonates. Most of the reported cases were associated with use of intravenous bisphosphonates in patients with metastatic bone disease. It is unclear whether the lower rate in patients treated for osteoporosis is due to lower doses of bisphosphonates used or to cancer predisposing to higher risk of this condition. In the study of yearly

| TABLE 25-6 | AVAILABLE AGENTS FOR OSTEOPOROSIS: DOSING AND SIDE EFFECTS | | | | |

Agent	FDA Approved for Prevention	Dose for Prevention	FDA Approved for Treatment	Dose for Treatment	Side Effects
Alendronate (Fosamax)	Yes	5 mg p.o./day 35 mg p.o. once/week	Yes	10 mg p.o./day 70 mg p.o. once/week	Abdominal pain, dyspepsia, nausea, esophagitis, musculoskeletal pain
Risedronate (Actonel)	Yes	5 mg p.o./day 35 mg p.o. once/week	Yes	5 mg p.o./day 35 mg p.o. once/week	Abdominal pain, dyspepsia, gastritis, esophagitis
Ibandronate (Boniva)	Yes	2.5 mg p.o./day	Yes	2.5 mg p.o./day or 150 mg p.o./month or 3 mg i.v. every 3 months	Abdominal pain, dyspepsia, back pain, myalgias
Zoledronate (Zometa, Reclast)	No	Not applicable	Yes	5 mg i.v once a year	Myalgias, arthralgias, fever, atrial fibrillation
Raloxifene (Evista)	Yes	60 mg p.o./day	Yes	60 mg p.o./day	Hot flashes, leg cramps, lower extremity edema, increased risk of DVT/PE
Estrogen (alone or with a progesterone); multiple combinations available	Yes	Multiple types Usually 0.625 mg p.o./day conjugated estrogen	No	Not applicable	Vaginal bleeding, breast tenderness increased risk of CHD, stroke, DVT/PE, breast cancer

TABLE 25-6	AVAILABLE AGENTS FOR OSTEOPOROSIS: DOSING AND SIDE EFFECTS *(Continued)*				
Agent	FDA Approved for Prevention	Dose for Prevention	FDA Approved for Treatment	Dose for Treatment	Side Effects
Calcitonin (Miacalcin)	Yes	100 IU intranasally/ day	Yes	200 IU intranasally/ day	Nasal congestion, rhinorrhea
Teriparatide (Forteo)	No	Not applicable	Yes	20 mcg s.c./day	Dizziness, leg cramps, headache, nausea, mild hypercal-cemia
Strontium Ranelate	No	Not applicable	No	2 g p.o./day	Diarrhea, gastritis

CHD, coronary heart disease; DVT, deep vein thrombosis; PE, pulmonary embolism.

zoledronic acid for the treatment of osteoporosis mentioned previously, there were only two cases of potential osteonecrosis of the jaw, one in the placebo group and one in the treatment arm, which were both managed successfully with surgery.

Estrogen-/Hormone-Replacement Therapy

Much has changed in the role of estrogen-replacement therapy (ERT) in prevention and treatment of osteoporosis in recent years. ERT improves bone density by inhibiting osteoclast activity. Little of the clinical data assessing the impact of estrogen have been in women with documented osteoporosis. As a result, most of the data on estrogen are more appropriate to interpret for prevention rather than treatment of osteoporosis. In addition, until the recent publication of the Women's Health Initiative (WHI), most of the fracture data with estrogen was from observational trials.

The WHI answered many important questions about the use of ERT for prevention of chronic conditions. The WHI was the first large-scale prospective randomized, controlled trial that individually found that combination estrogen–progesterone replacement therapy decreased the rate of fractures. Total fractures, vertebral fractures, hip fractures, and other osteoporotic fractures were decreased by 24%, 34%, 34%, and 23%, respectively. Although the rate of colon cancer also decreased by 37%, overall, the rate of adverse events, including a 29% increase in coronary heart disease, a 41% increase in stroke, a 111% increase in deep venous thrombosis/pulmonary embolism, and a 26% increase in breast cancer, exceeded the benefits, including fracture reduction. Similar rates of fracture reductions were found in the estrogen-alone group in women of the WHI who previously had a hysterectomy, with less of the adverse effects seen in the combination estrogen/progesterone group.

Little prospective data actually exist in patients with known osteoporosis; only one published small trial found a decrease in vertebral fractures with transdermal estrogen. Based on the lack of data in treating known osteoporosis and the balance of adverse events shown in the WHI, ERT has fallen out of favor for the prevention or treatment of osteoporosis. ERT is actually not FDA-approved for the treatment of osteoporosis; other forms of therapy are more potent with less toxicity to use in prevention.

Raloxifene (Evista)

Raloxifene is a selective estrogen receptor modulator that exhibits proestrogen effects on certain tissues and antiestrogen effects on other tissues. Raloxifene exhibits beneficial effects on bone by blocking the activity of cytokines that stimulate osteoclast-mediated bone resorption. Raloxifene has been shown in randomized controlled trials lasting up to 3 to 4 years to **improve BMD** at the spine and the hip and to **decrease the rate of new vertebral fractures** (MORE study). Raloxifene has not been found to have a significant impact on hip or total nonvertebral fractures. Therefore, the ideal candidate for raloxifene is a woman who has predominantly decreased BMD at the spine with more preserved levels of bone density at the hip, especially a woman who cannot tolerate a bisphosphonate. Raloxifene decreases total cholesterol and low-density lipoprotein (LDL) cholesterol in a manner similar to estrogen, but does not raise high-density lipoprotein (HDL) cholesterol and triglycerides as estrogen does. Raloxifene does not reduce hot flashes. It does increase the risk of deep venous thrombosis and pulmonary embolism in a fashion similar to estrogen. However, raloxifene does not stimulate the endometrium or breast and does not increase the risk of endometrial hyperplasia or cancer or breast cancer. In fact, a significant decrease in estrogen receptor–positive breast cancer as a secondary end point was found in a large clinical trial with raloxifene.

Considering the adverse cardiovascular events associated with estrogen use, the RUTH study was undertaken to study the cardiovascular impact of raloxifene. In a large prospective randomized controlled trial of 10,101 postmenopausal women with coronary heart disease (CHD) or risk factors for CHD followed for a median of 5.6 years, no significant difference in the risk of primary coronary events was found between the raloxifene and placebo groups. The study showed a similar decrease in the risk of breast cancer found in earlier studies of raloxifene but also found an increased risk of venous thromboembolism and fatal strokes in the treatment arm, although total all-cause mortality was similar between raloxifene and the placebo group. Therefore, these risks need to be weighed against the benefits of reducing vertebral fractures and the risk of breast cancer in women considered for raloxifene therapy.

Calcitonin (Miacalcin)

Calcitonin is an endogenous peptide that enhances BMD by **inhibiting osteoclast activity**. Calcitonin is available in both subcutaneous and intranasal forms, but the intranasal route is the one that has been most studied in osteoporosis. The beneficial effects on BMD of the spine are generally less with calcitonin than with most of the other agents available to treat osteoporosis. Minimal to no impact has been seen on BMD of the hip. In the Prevent Recurrences of Osteoporotic Fracture (PROOF) study, the 200 IU/day dose was found to decrease vertebral fractures after 5 years. There was not a dose-dependent response for vertebral fractures and there was not a significant benefit in decreasing hip or nonvertebral fractures. Calcitonin is typically a **second- or third-line agent** for the treatment of osteoporosis and is primarily reserved for patients with either contraindications to or intolerable side effects from other agents, particularly bisphosphonates. However, intranasal calcitonin has been found to be **beneficial in treating the pain of acute vertebral compression fractures**.

Teriparatide (Forteo)

Teriparatide is a recombinant formulation of the active 34 N-terminal peptide portion of parathyroid hormone. Although continuous exposure to PTH (as in patients with primary hyperparathyroidism) leads to increased bone resorption, intermittent exposure has been shown to stimulate bone formation. Teriparatide is the first pharmacologic agent that primarily increases bone formation by **stimulating osteoblast activity**. As opposed to all of the other agents for osteoporosis that work by decreasing bone turnover more than new bone formation, teriparatide works by stimulating new bone formation more than it stimulates bone resorption.

Teriparatide has been studied in high-risk women with a history of vertebral fractures for up to 2 years when administered by daily subcutaneous injections. The improvement in bone density was greater than that seen with any of the other available agents for osteoporosis (Table 25-7). Spinal fractures and total nonvertebral fractures decreased significantly, but the trial was too small and too short for there to be enough hip fractures to assess that end point. Because of its significant cost, teriparatide should generally be **reserved for patients with severe or established osteoporosis**, particularly those who cannot take or have had unsuccessful results with bisphosphonates. Mild hypercalcemia occasionally develops. Rats that were treated with high doses of teriparatide had an increased rate of developing osteosarcomas. Although this has not been seen in human trials, teriparatide's package insert contains a black-box warning about osteosarcomas. Teriparatide is contraindicated in patients with preexisting hypercalcemia or metastatic bone disease and in those at increased risk for osteosarcoma, such as

TABLE 25-7	AVAILABLE AGENTS FOR OSTEOPOROSIS: IMPACT ON BONE MINERAL DENSITY (BMD) AND FRACTURES				
Agent	Increase in BMD of Spine	Decrease in Rate of Vertebral Fractures	Increase in BMD of Hip	Decrease in Rate of Hip Fractures	Decrease in Rate of Nonvertebral Fractures
Alendronate (Fosamax)	6%–13%	40%–55%	4%–7%	50%–55%	20%–47%
Risedronate (Actonel)	5%–11%	40%–60%	2%–5%	40%–60%	20%–40%
Ibandronate (Boniva)	3%–5%	50%–60%	2%–5%	Studies not powered	Studies not powered
Zoledronate (Zometa, Reclast)	4%–7%	70%	3%–6%	41%	25%
Raloxifene (Evista)	3%	30%–50%	2%	Not significant	Not significant
Estrogen/ hormone replacement therapy[a]	4–7%	34%–40%	2%–4%	34%–36%	24%–27%
Calcitonin (Miacalcin)	1%–2%	33%	No change	Not significant	Not significant
Teriparatide (Forteo)	8%–14%	65%–70%	3%–5%	Studies not powered	53%
Strontium Ranelate	14%	40%	8%	36%	Not studied

[a]Data for estrogen-/hormone-replacement therapy are from studies in postmenopausal women and not in women with known osteoporosis.

patients with Paget's disease, prior radiation therapy to bone, and in children. Treatment is not recommended for >2 years.

Strontium Ranelate

Strontium ranelate is a new agent, recently approved for use in Europe, which increases calcium uptake and bone formation as well as inhibiting bone resorption. It is orally administered, and in a randomized controlled trial, daily dosing reduced the risk of vertebral fractures by 40%. Hip fractures were reduced by 36% in a subgroup of patients (≥74 years and with femoral neck BMD T score ≤−3). It was well tolerated with no significant adverse events reported. Strontium ranelate is not currently approved by the FDA.

Combination Therapy

Several different combination regimens have been studied with variable results. Studies assessing combination regimens have primarily studied the impact on BMD and have not been large enough or long enough to assess fracture risk. Adding alendronate or risedronate to regimens of patients already taking hormone-replacement therapy (HRT) has been shown to improve bone density compared to placebo. Combination therapy with alendronate and HRT was shown to improve bone density more after 3 years than either agent alone. Larger trials are needed to study whether this improvement in bone density with two agents that have a similar mechanism of action translates into better fracture results. In the absence of such data, the possible adverse effects of HRT need to be considered before initiating dual therapy.

Adding teriparatide to HRT has been shown to improve BMD. The most promise was held for combining teriparatide with a bisphosphonate using the most potent agents for bone resorption and bone formation. However, there have been conflicting data in this area. Several studies, including one in men, have found that combination therapy with teriparatide and alendronate is less effective than teriparatide alone at improving BMD and increasing new bone formation, whereas another study found small improvements in BMD in women previously treated with alendronate with daily or cyclic treatment with teriparatide (daily PTH for three months followed by three months off medication). Starting a bisphosphonate after completing 2 years of teriparatide makes theoretical sense, and in a recent study, BMD improvements with one year of teriparatide therapy were maintained or improved with subsequent alendronate but lost if therapy was not followed by a bisphosphonate. Therefore, this sequence is possibly the best type of combination therapy, although more studies are needed to validate this finding.

Impact of Other Medical Therapies on Fractures

Two common forms of medical therapy that have been thought to possibly impact the risk of osteoporotic fractures are **thiazide diuretics** and **hepatic 3-methylglutaryl coenzyme A (HMG-COA) reductase inhibitors**. Thiazide diuretics are thought to be helpful because they decrease urinary calcium excretion. A large population cohort study found that adults taking thiazide diuretics experienced significantly fewer hip fractures, especially if they had been receiving treatment for >1 year. Initial case-control studies with HMG-COA reductase inhibitors suggested an association of the agents with less hip fractures, but more recent studies have not found a significant benefit.

FOLLOW-UP

Follow-up of patients with osteoporosis includes **monitoring for complications, side effects, and response to treatment**. Continued assessment should take place for modifiable risk factors for fall such as gait disorders, visual problems, or sedating medications (see Table 25-3). Height should be followed on a regular basis to screen for asymptomatic vertebral fractures. In general, antiresorptive therapy needs to be continued long term, as the beneficial effect on BMD is lost over time after stopping treatment, especially with HRT. BMD should be reevaluated after 12 to 18 months to assess response to therapy. Repeat measurements made sooner than that can be difficult to interpret, as the expected change in bone density over a shorter period may be similar to the precision of the machine. BMD changes generally need to be at least 3% to be considered significant, as the precision of most bone densitometers is approximately 1% to 1.5%. Repeat measurements need to be made on the same bone density machine to allow results to be accurately compared. Patients who are being screened for osteoporosis but are not on treatment should wait at least 2 years before undergoing repeat bone density testing.

Osteoporosis in Men

Much less is known about osteoporosis in men than women. The prevalence of osteoporosis and osteoporotic fractures is less common in men than women because men achieve a higher peak bone mass, lose bone at a slower rate, and have a shorter life expectancy. Men typically have a BMD that is 8% to 18% greater at different sites than women. Men begin to experience complications from osteoporosis ~15 to 20 years later than women. Complications of osteoporosis are significant in men, as a 50-year-old man has a 13% lifetime risk of an osteoporotic fracture. Approximately 30% of hip fractures occur in men, and men have higher mortality rates after hip fractures than women. Men have a 31%, 1-year mortality after a hip fracture, 79% are in a nursing home or assisted living facility at 1 year, 60% have a permanent disability, and only 41% return to prior level of functioning.

Estimates of the prevalence of osteoporosis in men depend on the bone density cutoff used to make a diagnosis of osteoporosis. There are differences of opinion on whether male or female bone density cutoffs should be used. Two percent to 6% of men older than 50 years of age meet the diagnostic criteria for osteoporosis, with the number varying based on whether female or male cutoffs are used for comparison. BMD testing should be considered in men with nontraumatic fractures, osteopenia on x-rays, use of chronic steroids, hypogonadism, hyperparathyroidism, and other risk factors for secondary osteoporosis. There are no universal consensus guidelines for routine screening in men, although some experts recommend considering screening in men older than age 70 or 75. The most recent Canadian guidelines recommend screening men older than age 65. Men are more likely than women to have secondary osteoporosis. A laboratory evaluation, including testosterone screening, is generally recommended in men, as 30% to 60% have a specific cause of their osteoporosis.

Nonpharmacologic therapy, including weight-bearing exercise, smoking cessation, decreasing alcohol intake, and decreasing fall risks, are recommended to men just as they are to women. **Calcium and vitamin D supplementation** is recommended. **Alendronate** has been shown to improve bone density and decrease the rate of vertebral fractures in men. Alendronate is FDA-approved for osteoporosis, including steroid-induced osteoporosis, and risedronate is approved for steroid-induced osteoporosis. Teriparatide has been shown to improve BMD and is another option for men. Testosterone replacement with intramuscular injections, topical patches, or topical gels should be prescribed for men with documented hypogonadism. Studies have consistently found that a small percentage of men with fragility fractures are diagnosed with and treated for osteoporosis.

KEY POINTS TO REMEMBER

- The clinical consequences of osteoporosis are primarily related to fragility fractures, which most commonly occur at the spine, hip, and wrist.
- The key part of the evaluation in patients with suspected osteoporosis is to evaluate their bone density by DEXA. Osteoporosis and osteopenia are defined as T scores >2.5 and 1 to 2.5 SDs below the young adult reference mean.
- All patients with osteoporotic fractures, a T score < -2.0, or a T score < -1.5 with additional risk factors should be treated for osteoporosis.
- It is vital to ensure that all patients with osteoporosis have an adequate intake of calcium and vitamin D, which usually requires supplementation.
- ERT and HRT can prevent the development of osteoporotic fractures, but this benefit must be weighed against the increased risk of several adverse outcomes.
- Bisphosphonates (alendronate, risedronate, and ibandronate) are generally the first-line agents in the treatment of osteoporosis as they are the only treatment options that have been proven to decrease the development of vertebral and hip fractures.
- New medication regimens including parathyroid hormone monotherapy or in sequence with bisphosphonates and strontium ranelate hold further promise for osteoporosis treatment.

REFERENCES AND SUGGESTED READINGS

Barrett-Connor R, Mosca L, Collins P, et al. Effects of raloxifene on cardiovascular events and breast cancer in postmenopausal women. *N Engl J Med* 2006;355: 125–137.

Black DM, Bilezikian JP, Ensrud KE, et al. One year of alendronate after one year of parathyroid hormone (1-84) for osteoporosis. *N Engl J Med* 2005;353:555–565.

Black DM, Cummings SR, Karpf DB, et al. Randomized trial of effect of alendronate on risk of fracture in women with existing vertebral fractures. *Lancet* 1996;348: 1535–1541.

Black DM, Delmas PD, Eastell R, et al. Once-yearly zoledronic acid for treatment of post-menopausal osteoporosis. *N Engl J Med* 2007;356:1809–1822.

Black DM, Greenspan SL, Ensrud KE, et al. The effects of parathyroid hormone and alendronate alone or in combination in postmenopausal osteoporosis. *N Engl J Med* 2003; 349:1207–1215.

Blake GM, Fogelman I. Applications of bone densitometry for osteoporosis. *Endocrinol Metab Clin North Am* 1998;27:267–288.

Brunader R, Shelton DK. Radiologic bone assessment in the evaluation of osteoporosis. *Am Fam Physician* 2002;65:1357–1364.

Cauley JA, Seeley DG, Ensrud K, et al. Estrogen replacement therapy and fractures in older women. *Ann Intern Med* 1995;122:9–16.

Chapuy MC, Arlot ME, Duboeuf F, et al. Vitamin D3 and calcium to prevent hip fractures in elderly women. *N Engl J Med* 1992;327:1637–1642.

Chestnut CH, Silverman S, Andriano K, et al. A randomized trial of nasal spray salmon calcitonin in postmenopausal women with established osteoporosis: the prevent recurrence of osteoporotic fractures study. *Am J Med* 2000;109:267–276.

Chestnut CH, Skag A, Christiansen C, et al. Effects of oral ibandronate administered daily or intermittently on fracture risk in postmenopausal osteoporosis. *J Bone Miner Res* 2004;19:1241–1249.

Cramer JA, Amonkar MM, Hebborn A, et al. Compliance and persistence with bisphosphonate dosing regimens among women with postmenopausal osteoporosis. *Curr Med Res Opin* 2005;21:1453–1460.

Cummings SR, Black DM, Nevitt MC, et al. Bone density at various sites for prediction of hip fractures. *Lancet* 1993;341:72–75.

Cummings SR, Black DM, Thompson DE. Effect of alendronate on risk of fractures in women with low bone density but without vertebral fractures. *JAMA* 1998;280:2077–2082.

Delmas PD, Bjarnason NH, Mitlak BH, et al. Effects of raloxifene on bone mineral density, serum cholesterol concentrations and uterine endometrium in postmenopausal women. *N Engl J Med* 1997;337:1641–1647.

Ettinger B, Black DM, Mitlak BH, et al. Reduction of vertebral fracture risk in postmenopausal women with osteoporosis treated with raloxifene. *JAMA* 1999;282:637–645.

Ettinger MP. Aging bone and osteoporosis: strategies for preventing fractures. *Arch Intern Med* 2003;163:2237–2246.

Finkelstein JS, Hayes A, Hunzelman JL, et al. The effects of parathyroid hormone, alendronate, or both in men with osteoporosis. *N Engl J Med* 2003;349:1216–1226.

Greenspan SL, Resnick NM, Parker RA. Combination therapy with hormone replacement and alendronate for prevention of bone loss in elderly women. *JAMA* 2003;289: 2525–2533.

Harris ST, Watts NB, Genant HK, et al. Effects of risedronate treatment on vertebral and nonvertebral fractures in women with postmenopausal osteoporosis. *JAMA* 1999;282: 1344–1352.

Hulley S, Furberg C, Barrett-Connor E, et al. Noncardiovascular disease outcomes during 6.8 years of hormone therapy: heart and estrogen/progestin replacement study follow-up (HERS II). *JAMA* 2002;288:58–66.

Kado DM, Browner WS, Palermo L. Vertebral fractures and mortality in older women. *Arch Intern Med* 1999;159:1215–1220.

Kannus P, Parkkari J, Niemi S. Prevention of hip fracture in elderly people with the use of a hip protector. *N Engl J Med* 2000;343:1506–1513.

Looker AC, Orwoll ES, Johnston CC, et al. Prevalence of low femoral bone density in older U.S. adults from NHANES III. *J Bone Miner Res* 1997;12:1761–1768.

Lufkin EG, Wahner HW, O'Fallon WM, et al. Treatment of postmenopausal osteoporosis with transdermal estrogen. *Ann Intern Med* 1992;117:1–9.

Marshall D, Johnell O, Wedel H. Meta-analysis of how well measures of bone mineral density predict occurrence of osteoporotic fractures. *BMJ* 1996;312:1254–1259.

McClung MR, Geusens P, Miller PD, et al. Effect of risedronate on the risk of hip fracture in elderly women. *N Engl J Med* 2001;334:333–340.

Melton LJ, Thamer M, Ray NF, et al. Fractures attributable to osteoporosis: Report from the National Osteoporosis Foundation. *J Bone Miner Res* 1997;12:16–23.

Meunier PJ, Roux C, Seeman E, et al. The effects of strontium ranelate on the risk of vertebral fracture in women with postmenopausal osteoporosis. *N Engl J Med* 2004;350: 459–468.

National Osteoporosis Foundation. *Physician's Guide to the Prevention and Treatment of Osteoporosis.* Washington, DC: National Osteoporosis Foundation; 2003.

Neer RM, Arnaud CD, Zanchetta JR, et al. Effect of parathyroid hormone (I-34) on fractures and bone mineral density in postmenopausal women with osteoporosis. *N Engl J Med* 2001;344:1434–1441.

Nelson HD, Helfand M, Woolf SH, et al. Screening for postmenopausal osteoporosis: a review of the evidence for the U.S. Preventive Services Task Force. *Ann Intern Med* 2002;137:529–541.

NIH Consensus Development Panel on Optimal Calcium Intake. Optimal calcium intake. *JAMA* 1994;272:1942–1948.

NIH Consensus Development Panel on Osteoporosis Prevention, Diagnosis, and Therapy. Osteoporosis prevention, diagnosis, and therapy. *JAMA* 2001;285:785–795.

Orwoll E, Ettinger M, Weiss S, et al. Alendronate for the treatment of osteoporosis in men. *N Engl J Med* 2000;343:604–610.

Reid IR, Brown JP, Burckhardt P, et al. Intravenous zoledronic acid in postmenopausal women with low bone mineral density. *N Engl J Med* 2002;346:653–661.

Rosen CJ. Postmenopausal osteoporosis. *N Engl J Med* 2005;353:595–603.

Schoofs MW, van der Klift M, Hofman A, et al. Thiazide diuretics and the risk for hip fracture. *Ann Intern Med* 2003;169:476–482.

Todd JA, Robinson RJ. Osteoporosis and exercise. *Postgrad Med* 2003;79:320–323.

Torgerson DJ, Bell-Syer SEM. Hormone replacement therapy and prevention of nonvertebral fractures—a meta-analysis of randomized trials. *JAMA* 2001;285:2891–2897.

U.S. Preventive Services Task Force. Screening for osteoporosis in postmenopausal women: recommendations and rationale. *Ann Intern Med* 2002;137:526–528.

Woo SB, Hellstein JW, Kalmar JR. Bisphosphonates and osteonecrosis of the jaws. *Ann Intern Med* 2006;144:753–756.

World Health Organization. WHO technical report series 843. Assessment of fracture risk and its application to screening for postmenopausal osteoporosis. Geneva: World Health Organization; 1994.

Writing group for the PEPI trial. Effects of hormone replacement on bone mineral density. Results from the postmenopausal estrogen/progestin interventions (PEPI) trial. *JAMA* 1996;276:1389–1396.

Writing group for the Women's Health Initiative Investigators. Risks and benefits of estrogen plus progestin in healthy postmenopausal women. Principal results from the Women's Health Initiative randomized controlled trial. *JAMA* 2002;288:321–333.

Paget's Disease

Jason S. Goldfeder and Parvin F. Peddi

INTRODUCTION

Paget's disease is a disorder of focal abnormal bone turnover characterized by **increased skeletal remodeling, hypertrophy, and abnormal bone structure** that lead to mechanically weaker bone. Paget's disease can be localized to one skeletal area (monostotic Paget's disease), or it can simultaneously affect multiple parts of the skeleton (polyostotic Paget's disease). It was first described in 1877 by Sir James Paget and is also referred to as **osteitis deformans**. Pain is the most common symptom of Paget's disease, and multiple complications can occur, but the majority of patients are asymptomatic and are diagnosed incidentally after abnormalities are found on laboratory tests or x-rays done for other reasons. Treatment decisions in patients with Paget's disease are based on symptoms, the areas of the skeleton that are involved, and the degree of bone turnover.

Epidemiology

Paget's disease is the second most common metabolic bone disorder in older adults after osteoporosis. It has a distinctive geographic distribution throughout the world. Paget's disease occurs most commonly in western Europe, especially Great Britain, North America, Australia, and New Zealand. It is uncommon in Asia, Africa, and the Middle East. Paget's disease is a disorder of the elderly and is extremely uncommon in adults younger than age 40 years. The prevalence increases significantly each decade after age 50. Population studies using x-rays and autopsies have found prevalence rates of 1% to 3% in adults older than age 50 in the United States. The prevalence of symptomatic Paget's disease is several-fold lower. Prevalence and incidence rates are higher in men than women. The prevalence of Paget's disease is similar in both white and African American populations. Since the 1980s, the prevalence of Paget's disease has declined in several countries, including the United States, Great Britain, and Australia.

Etiology

The exact etiology of Paget's disease has been debated for several decades and remains somewhat unclear. A **viral infection of osteoclasts** has been postulated since the 1970s. Viruses that have been proposed as possible causative agents include members of the paramyxovirus family, such as respiratory syncytial virus and the measles virus, and canine distemper virus. Indirect evidence supporting a viral etiology has included the description of viral-like inclusion bodies in osteoclasts on electron microscopy and viral-like antigens on immunohistochemical studies. However, no viral pathogen has ever been cultured from bone or detected in polymerase chain reaction (PCR) testing.

Genetic factors also appear to play a role in Paget's disease. Up to 15% to 30% of patients with Paget's disease (40% in one isolated Spanish study) have a positive family history. The mode of transmission appears to be autosomal dominant. The relative risk of developing Paget's disease is increased sevenfold in first-degree relatives of those with

Paget's disease. Familial cases typically are diagnosed in patients at a younger age and have a more aggressive disease course. Possible susceptibility genes have been located on chromosomes 6 and 18. In addition, a homozygous gene deletion on chromosome 8 has recently been discovered that leads to osteoprotegerin deficiency, which can result in juvenile Paget's disease. The leading hypothesis for the development of Paget's disease is that a viral infection of osteoclasts in genetically susceptible hosts acts to trigger the increased osteoclast activity that initiates the enhanced bone turnover.

Pathophysiology

Normal bone remodeling depends on the coupled metabolic response of bone-forming osteoblasts and bone-resorbing osteoclasts. The primary abnormality in Paget's disease is enhanced osteoclast activity. The osteoclasts in patients with Paget's disease are multinucleated and are markedly increased in number and size. Pagetic osteoclasts have up to 100 nuclei compared to the normal 5 to 10 nuclei. The increased osteoclastic activity results in three distinct phases of the disease. Different parts of the skeleton may simultaneously go through different stages:

- The **initial osteolytic phase** is characterized by intense bone resorption by the abnormally large osteoclasts, usually in the long bones or the skull.
- In the **mixed osteolytic/osteoblastic phase**, active bone resorption by osteoclasts is coupled with increased bone formation by reactive osteoblasts.
- The **late sclerotic phase** is characterized primarily by continued new bone formation, resulting in the overproduction of thickened disorganized bone of poor quality.

PRESENTATION

The majority of patients with Paget's disease are **asymptomatic**, and the disease is diagnosed incidentally on x-rays done for other reasons or in the follow-up of an elevated alkaline phosphatase. Recent studies have found that only 5% to 30% of patients with Paget's disease are symptomatic. Paget's disease predominates in the axial skeleton and long bones. There is only one skeletal area involved (monostotic Paget's disease) in 10% to 30% of patients, whereas the remainder have multiple foci of disease (polyostotic Paget's disease) that may be at different stages of disease. Once the initial sites of disease have been detected, it is uncommon for new foci of disease to develop. The rates of skeletal involvement by location are shown in Table 26-1.

TABLE 26-1	FREQUENCY OF SKELETAL SITES INVOLVED IN PAGET'S DISEASE (%)
Skeletal Site	**Frequency of Involvement**
Pelvis	72
Lumbosacral spine (esp. L3–4)	58
Femur	55
Thoracic spine	45
Sacrum	43
Skull	42
Tibia	35
Humerus	31
Scapula	23
Cervical spine	14

TABLE 26-2	POSSIBLE COMPLICATIONS IN PAGET'S DISEASE
Organ System	**Possible Complications**
Long bones	Fractures
Neurologic	Spinal stenosis
	Chronic headaches
	Cranial neuropathies (especially II, V, VII, VIII)
	Noncommunicative hydrocephalus
	Dementia
	Seizure disorder
Dental	Loss of teeth/malocclusion
ENT	Deafness
	Tinnitus
	Vertigo
Rheumatologic	Hyperuricemia/gout
	Increased susceptibility to seronegative spondyloarthropathies, psoriatic arthritis
Cardiovascular	Increased vascular disease
	High-output heart failure
	Valvular heart disease (aortic > mitral)
Metabolic	Hypercalcemia (usually with immobility)
	Primary hyperparathyroidism
Tumors	Benign giant cell tumors
	Malignant sarcoma

ENT, ear, nose, and throat.

Common Symptoms

The two most common symptoms in adults with Paget's disease are **bone pain** and **joint pain**. Bone pain typically is constant and deep-seated and may be worse at night. Pain frequently increases with weight bearing. The severity of pain does not always correlate with the severity of the x-ray findings and tends to be more prominent in advanced lytic lesions. Secondary osteoarthritis and corresponding pain frequently develop, particularly in weight-bearing joints, such as the hip and the knee. Several mechanisms contribute to the development of osteoarthritis, including uneven bony expansion resulting in an uneven base for articular cartilage, limited joint space due to bony overgrowth, and altered joint mechanics secondary to bony deformities. Bony deformities include bowing of the limbs, kyphosis or scoliosis of the spine, and enlargement of the skull (osteoporosis circumscripta). Local skin warmth may also occur secondary to increased bony vascularity.

Complications

Multiple complications can occur in patients with Paget's disease (Table 26-2), although most are infrequent. **Fractures** are one of the most common complications and occur in 6% to 7% of patients. Fractures occur most commonly in the femur, tibia, and humerus and are often associated with poor healing and nonunion. Multiple possible **neurologic complications** can occur because of either direct nerve root compression by expanding bone or diversion of blood flow to bone. Spinal stenosis is the most common of the neurologic complications. Deafness occurs in 10% to 30% of patients with disease affecting the skull. Most of the cardiovascular complications are much less common than previously thought, particularly high-output heart failure. Because Paget's disease is a focal process, bone marrow involvement and the development of anemia or thrombocytopenia do not occur.

Malignant Sarcomatous Degeneration

Malignant sarcomatous degeneration is an uncommon but severe and usually life-threatening complication of Paget's disease. It occurs in <1% of patients and occurs most commonly in those with severe polyostotic disease. Sarcomas occur more commonly in men than women and usually occur in older adults. The majority of tumors are osteosarcomas, whereas much smaller percentages are malignant fibrous histiocytomas, fibrosarcomas, and chondrosarcomas. The most common bones involved, in descending order, are the femur, humerus, pelvis, skull, and facial bones. Malignant transformation may be heralded by a sudden or severe increase in pain, a palpable mass, an increase in the alkaline phosphatase, or a pathologic fracture. The prognosis is poor, with a 50% mortality rate at 6 months and a 5-year survival rate of only 5% to 15%. A small percentage of patients with limb-bone sarcomas without evidence of metastatic disease can be treated with wide surgical excision/amputation and aggressive chemotherapy and/or radiation therapy.

MANAGEMENT

Diagnostic Evaluation

The evaluation of patients with Paget's disease includes plain films, a bone scan, and laboratory assessment of markers of bone turnover. The order in which the tests are obtained typically depends on whether the patient is diagnosed based on symptoms or incidentally. Symptomatic patients are usually diagnosed after x-rays are obtained to evaluate the cause of pain. Characteristic features on plain films include localized bony enlargement, cortical thickening, sclerotic changes, and osteolytic areas. A bone scan should subsequently be obtained to assess what additional parts of the skeleton are involved.

A **bone scan** is the best test for extent of disease and should be performed in all patients with Paget's disease. The bone scan is more sensitive, but less specific than traditional x-rays. It can pick up 15% to 30% of lesions that are not detected by plain films. It is sometimes difficult to differentiate Paget's disease from metastatic bone disease, and bone biopsy in these instances may be warranted. Subsequent plain x-rays can be obtained of painful areas or high-risk areas that are abnormal on the bone scan (spine, skull, and joints) to assess for the degree of abnormalities. Markers of bone turnover should also be obtained (see subsequent text).

The most frequent way Paget's disease presents clinically is in asymptomatic patients who are found to have an **elevated alkaline phosphatase**. Sources of an elevated alkaline phosphatase include the liver and bone. If there are no other evident abnormalities on routine liver function tests (aspartate aminotransferae [AST], alanine aminotransferase [ALT], and bilirubin), a serum gamma-glutamyltransferase (GGT) should be obtained to further rule out occult hepatic disease. If the GGT is normal, a bone scan should be obtained to assess for lesions consistent with Paget's disease. X-rays should be obtained of abnormal areas to confirm the diagnosis of Paget's disease.

Several laboratory tests are available to assess the degree of bone formation and bone resorption. There is not uniform agreement about which tests are necessary, particularly with regard to bone resorption. The alkaline phosphatase is the most useful clinical marker of bone formation to assess the degree of osteoblast activity. The **alkaline phosphatase level correlates well with the extent of disease on bone scan**. Bone-specific alkaline phosphatase is more specific than the total alkaline phosphatase, but it is more difficult to obtain. It can be considered in patients with monostotic Paget's disease who may have a normal total alkaline phosphatase. Serum osteocalcin and procollagen type I C-terminal peptide are additional markers of bone formation that have been studied, but they are less reliable and should not be routinely obtained. Serum calcium and phosphorous concentrations are usually normal, and hypercalcemia in ambulatory patients suggests presence of a second disorder such as primary hyperparathyroidism.

Laboratory markers of bone resorption assess the degree of osteoclastic activity. The majority of available tests are urinary measurements that are obtained from the second voided morning urine after an overnight fast. Several different tests have been evaluated. Two of the most clinically useful are urinary **type I collagen pyridoline crosslinks** and **N-telopeptide**, which have supplanted urine hydroxyproline as the tests of choice for bone resorption. These tests of bone resorption often have to be sent to a referral laboratory.

At the time of initial diagnosis, markers of both bone formation and bone resorption should be obtained. The alkaline phosphatase is sufficient to serve as the sole marker for **monitoring disease activity** in many patients, particularly those with primarily increased osteoblastic activity. However, patients with a normal alkaline phosphatase or high levels of osteoclastic activity should have markers of bone resorption followed. The effectiveness of treatment is typically judged by the degree of decline in markers of bone turnover, percentage of decline, and the time required until the markers normalize.

Additional radiographic testing is generally unnecessary except to evaluate for complications. A computed tomography (CT) or magnetic resonance imaging (MRI) is most commonly used to evaluate for neurologic complications, such as spinal stenosis. A bone biopsy is usually not required to make a diagnosis of Paget's disease and is obtained primarily when concern arises for malignant sarcomatous degeneration.

Treatment

The primary goals of treatment are to decrease pain and decrease the rate of bone turnover to prevent progression of disease and the development of complications.

Pharmacologic Therapy

Therapeutic options have significantly improved since the early 1990s with the development of more potent bisphosphonates. **Bone pain** is the one indication for which there is proven benefit of treatment from randomized controlled clinical trials. Most experts recommend treating asymptomatic patients who are at risk for developing complications based on the skeletal sites involved and the degree of bone turnover. However, there are no randomized, prospective clinical trial data to support this approach. Asymptomatic disease in areas that are at low risk for developing complications, such as the ribs, scapula, distal bones, or the sacrum, generally does not require treatment. The following are generally accepted **indications to initiate treatment:**

- Symptomatic disease: bone pain, deformities, or neurologic symptoms
- Asymptomatic patients with evidence of increased bone turnover at risk for complications based on the areas involved
  - Lytic lesions in long bones with a high risk for developing fractures
  - Disease in proximity of joints with risk of developing secondary osteoarthritis
  - Disease in the spine because of the risk of spinal stenosis
  - Disease in the skull because of the risk of deafness and cranial nerve dysfunction
- Patients preparing for elective orthopedic surgery on involved joints should receive treatment for at least 6 weeks to decrease bony vascularity

TABLE 26-3	TREATMENT OPTIONS IN PATIENTS WITH PAGET'S DISEASE
Agent	**Dose**
First-line agents	
Alendronate (Fosamax)	40 mg p.o. q.d. for 6 months
Risedronate (Actonel)	30 mg p.o. q.d. for 2 months
Pamidronate (Aredia)	30–60 mg i.v. q.d. for 3 days or
	30 mg i.v. q week for 6 weeks or
	30 mg i.v. q month for 6 months
Zoledronate (Zometa, Reclast)	5 mg i.v. × 1 dose
Second-line agents	
Tiludronate (Skelid)	400 mg p.o. q.d. for 3 months
Etidronate (Didronel)	400 mg p.o. q.d. for 6 months
Calcitonin (Miacalcin)	50–100 IU i.m. q.d. for 6–12 months
	200–400 IU intranasally q.d. for 6–12 months
Agents currently being investigated	
Ibandronate (Boniva)	2 mg i.v. × 1 dose

A **second-generation bisphosphonate** is recommended for treatment in patients requiring therapy (Table 26-3). When used to treat Paget's disease, bisphosphonates are given as pulse courses of therapy at higher doses than are traditionally used to treat osteoporosis. Alendronate (Fosamax), risedronate (Actonel), and pamidronate (Aredia) are recommended as first-line agents (Table 25-3). These agents typically decrease bone turnover, as measured by the decline in serum alkaline phosphatase, by 60% to 80%. Bone markers are normalized in approximately 50% to 70% of patients. Etidronate (Didronel) and tiludronate (Skelid) are older bisphosphonates that are less effective on improving symptoms and markers of bone turnover. **Supplemental calcium and vitamin D** are recommended to prevent defective bone mineralization, although this is much less common with the newer bisphosphonates. The oral bisphosphonates should be taken with water only. The patient should remain upright, and food and other medications should be avoided for at least 30 minutes to decrease the likelihood of developing esophageal complications. Newer intravenous bisphosphonates such as zoledronate and neridronate are currently being studied as well and in a recent randomized trial were found superior to pamidronate in achieving response in patients with single intravenous infusions. In another study, a single infusion of zoledronate led to better results than daily oral risedronate. Zoledronate was just approved by the FDA in April 2008 for the treatment of Paget's disease.

Calcitonin (Miacalcin) is another second-line agent that can be considered in patients who are unable to tolerate bisphosphonates. Calcitonin is more effective in Paget's disease when given intramuscularly than when given via inhalation. The rates of bone turnover are decreased by approximately 50% and normalized in approximately 25% of patients. Symptoms and bone turnover usually recur soon after stopping therapy. Plicamycin (Mithracin) and gallium nitrate (Ganite) are experimental agents with potential serious adverse effects that can be considered in patients with severe disease that does not respond to bisphosphonates, but only after referral to an expert in bone metabolism.

Surgery

Surgical therapy is **indicated for complications** of Paget's disease. The most common indication for surgery is a joint replacement, usually of the hip or the knee, for secondary osteoarthritis. Other reasons to consider surgical intervention are for a complicated or non-healing fracture, bowing deformities of long bones, spinal stenosis, and focal nerve root compression syndromes. Bisphosphonate therapy is typically prescribed for at least 6 weeks before elective surgery to decrease bone vascularity and the risk of intraoperative bleeding.

Follow-Up

Follow-up of patients with Paget's disease includes **monitoring their symptoms** and **markers of bone turnover,** occasionally supplemented with plain film x-rays. Symptoms should initially be monitored every 3 months in those on therapy and every 6 to 12 months in those not on treatment. The markers of bone resorption typically improve quickly within days, whereas the markers of bone formation take longer to improve, often up to 1 month. The goal of therapy is to normalize the markers of bone turnover. The **alkaline phosphatase** is the easiest of the markers of bone turnover to follow and is usually the only one needed in follow-up. The alkaline phosphatase should be checked every 3 to 4 months during therapy until it normalizes. The urine type I collagen pyridoline crosslinks or N-telopeptide should be followed in those with highly active lytic disease, especially if the alkaline phosphatase is relatively normal. The alkaline phosphatase should be followed annually in those not on treatment. Repeat x-rays should be obtained after 1 year of treatment in those with high-risk lytic lesions. Other indications for subsequent x-rays are new symptoms or worsening of stable symptoms, trauma, a concern for a fracture, and concern for sarcomatous degeneration.

Patients whose alkaline phosphatase normalizes on therapy should have it serially followed. Retreatment with another course of a bisphosphonate should be considered if the alkaline phosphatase increases by >20% to 25% above the posttreatment nadir.

KEY POINTS TO REMEMBER

- Paget's disease is a disorder of enhanced osteoclast activity that leads to increased bone remodeling, bony hypertrophy, and abnormal bony architecture.
- The primary risk factors for developing Paget's disease are advanced age, a positive family history, and male gender.
- Paget's disease predominates in the axial skeleton, long bones, and skull.
- Most patients with Paget's disease are asymptomatic and are diagnosed after finding an isolated elevated alkaline phosphatase.
- The most common symptoms of Paget's disease are bony pain and joint pain related to secondary osteoarthritis.
- Multiple complications can develop in patients with Paget's disease, but most are uncommon except for fractures, spinal stenosis, and hearing loss.
- The initial diagnostic evaluation should include a bone scan, x-rays of high-risk areas, and measurement of the serum alkaline phosphatase and urinary markers of bone resorption.
- Symptomatic patients and those who are asymptomatic but have evidence of disease in high-risk areas, such as long bones, near joints, the spine, and the skull, should be treated, but asymptomatic patients who do not have disease in high-risk areas can be followed without treatment.

(*continued*)

KEY POINTS TO REMEMBER (Continued)

- Standard therapy for Paget's disease is a several-month course of high doses of a bis-phosphonate.
- The goal of treatment is to normalize markers of bone turnover, particularly the alkaline phosphatase. Retreatment should be considered in patients whose markers of bone turnover increase by >25% over their posttreatment nadir.

REFERENCES AND SUGGESTED READINGS

Altman RD, Bloch DA, Hochberg MC, et al. Prevalence of pelvic Paget's disease of bone in the United States. *J Bone Miner Res* 2000;15:461–465.

Ankrom MA, Shapiro JR. Paget's disease of bone (osteitis deformans). *J Am Geriatr Soc* 1998;46:1025–1033.

Delmas PD, Meunier PJ. The management of Paget's disease of bone. *N Engl J Med* 1997; 336:558–566.

Delmas PD. Biochemical markers of bone turnover in Paget's disease of bone. *J Bone Miner Res* 1999;14(Suppl 2):66–69.

Drake WM, Kendler DL, Brown JP. Consensus statement on the modern therapy of Paget's disease of bone from a western osteoporosis alliance symposium. *Clin Ther* 2001;23:620–626.

Fraser WD. Paget's disease of bone. *Curr Opin Rheumatol* 1997;9:347–354.

Hadjipavlou AG, Gaitanis IN, Kontakis GM. Paget's disease of bone and its management. *J Bone Joint Surg* 2002;84:160–169.

Hamdy RC. Clinical features and pharmacologic treatment of Paget's disease. *Endocrinol Metab Clin North Am* 1995;24:421–435.

Harrington KD. Surgical management of neoplastic complications of Paget's disease. *J Bone Miner Res* 1999;14(Suppl 2):45–48.

Hosking DJ. Prediction and assessment of the response of Paget's disease to bisphosphonate treatment. *Bone* 1999;24(Suppl 5):69S–71S.

Kaplan FS. Surgical management of Paget's disease. *J Bone Miner Res* 1999;14(Suppl 2):34–38.

Klein RM, Norman A. Diagnostic procedures for Paget's disease. Radiologic, pathologic, and laboratory testing. *Endocrinol Metab Clin North Am* 1995;24:437–450.

Leach RJ, Singer FR, Roodman GD. Genetics of endocrine disease. The genetics of Paget's disease of the bone. *J Clin Endocrinol Metab* 2001;86:24–28.

Lombardi A. Treatment of Paget's disease of bone with alendronate. *Bone* 1999;24(Suppl 5):59S–61S.

Lyles KW, Siris ES, Singer FR, et al. A clinical approach to diagnosis and management of Paget's disease of bone. *J Bone Miner Res* 2001;16:1379–1387.

Merlotti D, Luigi G, Martini G, et al. Comparison of different intravenous bisphosphonate regimens for Paget's disease of bone. *J Bone Miner Res* 2007;22(10):1510–1517.

Ooi CG, Fraser WD. Paget's disease of bone. *Postgrad Med J* 1997;73:69–74.

Poncelet A. The neurologic complications of Paget's disease. *J Bone Miner Res* 1999; 14(Suppl 2):88–91.

Reddy SV, Menaa C, Singer FR, et al. Cell biology of Paget's disease. *J Bone Miner Res* 1999;14(Suppl 2):3–7.

Reid, IR, Miller P, Hosking D, et al. Comparison of a single infusion of zoledronic acid with risedronate for Paget's disease. *N Engl J Med* 2005;353:898–908.

Roux C, Dougados M. Treatment of patients with Paget's disease of bone. *Drugs* 1999;58:823–830.

Russell RGG, Rogers MJ, Frith JC, et al. The pharmacology of bisphosphonates and new insights into their mechanisms of action. *J Bone Miner Res* 1999;14(Suppl 2):53–65.

Selby PL, Davie MWJ, Ralston SH, et al. Guidelines on the management of Paget's disease of bone. *Bone* 2002;31:366–373.

Singer FR. Update on the viral etiology of Paget's disease of bone. *J Bone Miner Res* 1999; 14(Suppl 2):29–33.

Siris ES. Goals of treatment for Paget's disease of bone. *J Bone Miner Res* 1999;14(Suppl 2):49–52.

Staa TPV, Selby P, Leufkens HGM, et al. Incidence and natural history of Paget's disease of bone in England and Wales. *J Bone Miner Res* 2002;17:465–471.

Tiegs RD, Lohse CM, Wollan PC, et al. Long-term trends in the incidence of Paget's disease of bone. *Bone* 2000;27:423–427.

Tiegs RD. Paget's disease of bone: indications for treatment and goals of therapy. *Clin Ther* 1997;19:1309–1329.

Whyte MP, Obrecht SE, Finergan PM, et al. Osteoprotegerin deficiency and juvenile Paget's disease. *N Engl J Med* 2002;347:175–184.

Whyte MP. Paget's disease of the bone. *N Engl J Med* 2006;355:593–600.

Standards of Care for Diabetes Mellitus

27

Janet B. McGill

INTRODUCTION

Standards of care for patients with diabetes are developed by consensus committees both in the United States and abroad to facilitate the application of evidence-based medicine to all patients with diabetes. The stated goals of these committees are to provide practical guidelines for health-care providers that will reduce the risk of morbidity and mortality from acute and chronic complications of diabetes. Health-care providers are expected to know the health risks associated with diabetes, and to be able to develop treatment strategies for individual patients to attain the stated targets. Third party payers are beginning to utilize these treatment targets as benchmarks for evaluation of services and for payment. Although individual patients may require modification of treatment targets, providers should strive to achieve the stated goals in the majority of patients with diabetes.

Standards of care for patients with diabetes have been established by the American Diabetes Association (ADA), the American Association of Clinical Endocrinologists (AACE), and the European Association for the Study of Diabetes (EASD) in conjunction with the European Society of Cardiology (ESC). Other groups have addressed specific comorbid conditions, such as the Joint National Committee for the Study of Hypertension (JNC VII) and the Adult Treatment Panel (ATP). Most of the recommendations are similar; however, there are key differences that will be pointed out in this chapter. Original studies and grade of evidence supporting the recommendations discussed in this chapter are referenced in the consensus documents. Diagnostic and treatment strategies have been discussed in Chapter 28, Diabetes Mellitus Type 1, and Chapter 29, Diabetes Mellitus Type 2.

SCREENING FOR DIABETES

Screening for type 1 diabetes mellitus (T1DM) is generally not recommended, even in relatives of persons with T1DM. The ADA recommends that screening for type 2 diabetes mellitus (T2DM) begin at age 45 with a check of fasting glucose, particularly in persons with a body mass index BMI of ≥25. If the fasting glucose is 100 to 125 mg/dL, a 2-hour oral glucose tolerance test (OGTT) using 75 g of glucose is recommended. Persons at higher than usual risk should be screened earlier and followed more closely. High-risk characteristics include a history of gestational diabetes or having delivered a baby weighing more than 9 pounds, obesity, family history of diabetes, history of polycystic ovarian syndrome (PCOS), hypertension, sedentary lifestyle, dyslipidemia characteristic of the metabolic syndrome, a prior test indicating impaired glucose tolerance (IGT) or impaired fasting glucose (IFG), or a history of vascular disease. The EASD and ECS recommend using a risk-assessment tool such as the FINnish Diabetes Risk Score (FINDRISC) to assess the

10-year risk of T2DM, and performing laboratory testing on persons at high risk. The European groups specifically recommend testing post-prandial glucose in persons with vascular disease. Diagnostic criteria for diabetes are covered in Chapter 29, Diabetes Mellitus Type 2, Table 29.2. Although a hemoglobin A1c (HbA1c) is not recommended for screening purposes, a study from the NHANES population suggested that an HbA1c >5.8% provides the best sensitivity and specificity for abnormal glucose regulation and should, therefore, be followed up with a fasting glucose test or even a glucose tolerance test.

Screening for diabetes in pregnancy is important to ensure optimal fetal outcomes. The current ADA recommendation includes doing a risk assessment at the first prenatal visit, and testing for diabetes in women who are obese, have a family history of diabetes, a previous history of gestational diabetes mellitus (GDM), a history of PCOS, or previous large-for–gestational-age infant. A fasting blood sugar >85 mg/dL should be followed with a 75-g OGTT. Women at low risk early in pregnancy should undergo testing for GDM between 24 and 28 weeks of pregnancy. A 1-hour glucose value of ≥140 mg/dL on an initial nonfasting screen using 50-g oral glucose (glucose challenge test) identifies ~80% of women with GDM, and should be followed with a 3-hour, 100-g OGTT. GDM is diagnosed if two of the following glucose values are exceeded: fasting ≥95 mg/dL, 1-hour ≥180 mg/dL, 2-hour ≥155 mg/dL, or 3-hour ≥140 mg/dL. Women with GDM should also be tested at 6 to 12 weeks postpartum to detect persistence of diabetes, and followed more closely in subsequent years.

PREVENTION OF DIABETES

Several studies have shown that diabetes can be prevented with either lifestyle modification or with medication. All three consensus groups recommend counseling in lifestyle management to reduce weight in those who are overweight and to increase physical activity. Studies of lifestyle management that have resulted in weight loss of ≥5% through diet and exercise have demonstrated a 32% to 58% reduction in the progression to diabetes. Medications that have proved effective in preventing diabetes include metformin, acarbose, rosiglitazone, Xenical, and troglitazone. Medication intervention for the prevention of diabetes is not specifically recommended at this time, but increased surveillance of glycemic status is recommended, and clinical judgment is advised.

GLYCEMIC CONTROL

Targets for glycemic control in diabetes reflect evidence from randomized controlled trials that have demonstrated protection from long-term microvascular complications and reduction in macrovascular events as blood glucose is lowered toward normal levels. In pregnancy, glycemic targets are lower than in nonpregnant adults to mimic nondiabetic pregnant women, and to ensure optimal fetal outcomes.

The two primary ways to monitor glycemic control are **self-monitored blood glucose (SMBG)** and **hemoglobin A1c (HbA1c)**. Continuous glucose monitoring using a real-time sensor that measures glucose concentration in the interstitial fluid has become an ancillary method for glucose monitoring and management. SMBG is generally checked before meals and at bedtime, with periodic checks of glucose during the post-prandial period and during sleep. The frequency of SMBG ranges from 1 to 4 or more readings per day, depending on the intensity of therapy and risk of hypoglycemia. The HbA1c reflects blood glucose levels over the previous 2 to 3 months. The HbA1c should be monitored every 3 months until a patient reaches goal, and then every 6 months if the patient is at target and stable. The goals for glycemic control should be set for the individual patient

TABLE 27-1	GLYCEMIC TARGETS FOR ADULTS WITH DIABETES			
Glycemic Parameter	ADA	AACE	EASD	Pregnancy
Hemoglobin A1c	<7.0%*	≤6.5%	≤6.5%	Near normal
Fasting and pre-prandial blood glucose	90–130 mg/dL	<110 mg/dL	≤108 mg/dL	60–90 mg/dL
Post-prandial blood glucose	<180 mg/dL	<140 mg/dL	≤135 mg/dL	≤120 mg/dL

*Using a DCCT-referenced assay.

AACE, American Association of Clinical Endocrinologists; ADA, American Diabetes Association; EASD, European Association for the Study of Diabetes.

based on age, risk of hypoglycemia, and presence of comorbidities. Normalization of HbA1c may be appropriate for many patients. Guidelines for glycemic control established by consensus groups are listed in Table 27-1.

The ADA stipulates that the HbA1c goal for individual patients may be near normal (<6%) if possible to achieve without hypoglycemia, and that less stringent targets may be appropriate for very young patients, very old patients, those with a history of severe hypoglycemia or limited life expectancy. Targets for children are adjusted to permit scrupulous avoidance of serious hypoglycemia.

Note that capillary blood glucose levels are 10% to 15% lower than plasma glucose levels. Newer blood glucose meters are calibrated to report plasma glucose values, so each patient should be informed whether his or her meter reports blood or plasma glucose values. If there is a discrepancy between SMBG values reported by the patient or depicted in meter readings and the A1c, it may be useful to measure SMBG 1 to 2 hours after meals. Persistently high A1c despite lower than expected blood glucose readings, or wide fluctuations in blood glucose, should prompt further investigation, which is often done best by a certified diabetes educator. The correlation between HbA1c and mean plasma glucose is depicted in Table 27-2.

TABLE 27-2	CORRELATION BETWEEN HbA1c AND MEAN PLASMA GLUCOSE	
HbA1c %	Mean Plasma Glucose	
	mg/dL	mmol/L
6	135	7.5
7	170	9.5
8	205	11.5
9	240	11.5
10	275	15.5
11	310	17.5
12	345	19.5

HbA1c, Hemoglobin A1c.

TREATMENT RECOMMENDATIONS

The ADA and EASD have developed a consensus statement on the management of hyperglycemia in diabetes. The basic tenets are early intervention with medical nutrition therapy aimed at achieving and maintaining normal weight, and exercise for both weight control and fitness. Diabetes education by qualified educators is suggested for all patients when the illness is diagnosed, as needed to achieve glycemic goals and when insulin is initiated. Nutrition recommendations need to be individualized with consideration to the patient's level of overweight, ethnicity, diabetes therapy and food choices. Aerobic exercise of at least 150 minutes per week and supplemental repetitive resistance training are recommended for all adults with diabetes in the absence of contraindications. Medication intervention should normally begin with metformin, with other agents added sequentially to achieve glycemic targets. Earlier treatment with insulin is recommended to correct blood glucose level >250 to 300 mg/dL at presentation or any time in the course of treatment. Hypoglycemia is a limiting factor in the glycemic management of diabetes. Glucose values <70 mg/dL should be treated with 15 to 20 g of glucose (preferred) or other carbohydrate, and rechecked. Persons at risk for severe hypoglycemia should have a prescription for glucagon, and instructions for use by a companion.

CARDIOVASCULAR DISEASE

Cardiovascular disease is the leading cause of mortality in patients with diabetes. Diabetes confers an increased risk of acute coronary syndrome, myocardial infarction, heart failure, atrial fibrillation, stroke, peripheral vascular disease and sudden death that is 2 to 5 times the risk in nondiabetic comparator groups. Persons with diabetes also experience greater morbidity after vascular events, and interventions such as coronary angioplasty may not be as effective at reducing morbidity and mortality in diabetic patients compared to nondiabetic comparison groups. Although the increased risk is not entirely explained by usual risk factors, studies have shown that the risk of cardiovascular events can be reduced by aggressive management of hypertension, lipids, and use of antiplatelet agents in patients with diabetes, and that the benefits of treatment of each risk factor in diabetes may exceed the benefits in lower risk cohorts. Consequently, healthcare providers are expected to address cardiovascular risk in a comprehensive manner, and achieve targets that are more stringent for blood pressure, lipids, and healthy lifestyles than in nondiabetic patients.

LIFESTYLE

Smoking cessation is critically important for persons with diabetes, and counseling regarding smoking cessation should be documented in medical records. Studies have shown that high levels of physical activity, either as part of a daily work routine or for pleasure, are associated with reduced cardiovascular risk in both primary and secondary prevention that is equivalent to first-line pharmacologic therapy. Healthcare providers should assess the level of physical activity in patients with diabetes, and provide encouragement to reach the target of 150 minutes of aerobic exercise weekly or 10,000 steps daily. Physical limitations should be addressed and alternative exercise programs developed in selected patients. Nutrition advice specific to cardiovascular risk reduction includes avoidance of trans and saturated fats, increased intake of fiber, and intake of five or more servings of fruits and vegetables daily. Reduction of salt intake is advised in persons who are hypertensive. This advice should be provided to all patients as part of routine healthcare visits, and included in medical nutrition therapy instructions.

HYPERTENSION

Hypertension is present in more than 75% of persons with T2DM, and more than one-half of persons with T1DM. Blood pressure reduction has been shown to reduce the frequency of myocardial infarction, cerebrovascular disease, and diabetes-related deaths. In addition, blood pressure reduction slows the progression of nephropathy, retinopathy, and vision loss. Blood pressure should be checked at every visit in patients with diabetes. Lifestyle modifications and medical treatment should be considered if the blood pressure is >130/80 mm Hg. All of the consensus guidelines suggest using angiotensin-converting enzyme (ACE) inhibitors (ACEIs) or angiotensin receptor blockers (ARBs) as initial therapy because of proven benefit in lowering cardiovascular mortality and progression of both retinopathy and nephropathy. Second- and third-line treatment with diuretics, β-blockers, or calcium channel blockers should be tailored to the individual patient. β-Blockers are indicated in patients who have had a myocardial infarction, heart failure, or for rate control in atrial fibrillation. Vasodilating agents such as carvedilol or nebivolol may be particularly useful in patients with diabetes, since they do not worsen insulin resistance or symptomatic peripheral vascular disease. Although the target blood pressure in diabetes is <130/80 mm Hg, physicians should be aware that risk of cardiovascular events doubles when the blood pressure increases from 115/75 mm Hg to 135/85 mm Hg, quadruples at 155/95 mm Hg, and so on. Consequently, the AACE suggests a lower target blood pressure of 120/75 mm Hg in patients with high-risk conditions such as nephropathy. Use of ACEIs in diabetic patients with blood pressure below the stated target of 130/80 mm Hg and with retinopathy or microalbuminuria may provide protection from progression of these complications. ACEIs and ARBs have been associated with birth defects, so caution is advised in premenopausal women, especially those women who indicate a desire to become pregnant or who are not using adequate birth control.

HYPERLIPIDEMIA

Diabetic patients should have a **fasting lipid profile** (total cholesterol, low-density lipoprotein [LDL] cholesterol, high-density lipoprotein [HDL] cholesterol, and triglycerides) **checked yearly**. Lipid targets for patients with diabetes are listed in Table 27-3.

Therapy is initially directed toward meeting the LDL cholesterol goal. A secondary goal is to raise HDL cholesterol above the gender-specific target. For those with triglycerides ≥200 mg/dL, current National Cholesterol Education Program/Adult Treatment Panel III guidelines have established a non–HDL cholesterol (total – HDL cholesterol) target of <130 mg/dL as the secondary goal. If the triglyceride level is >500 mg/dL, therapy should first be directed at lowering triglycerides to prevent pancreatitis. HMG-CoA reductase inhibitors (statins) have provided the greatest benefit in patients with diabetes, and should be considered first-line therapy. Combination therapy with fibrates, fish oil, or niacin may be needed in selected patients to achieve HDL and triglyceride targets. Additional LDL lowering with ezetimibe or a bile acid sequestrant may be required to reach LDL targets. For specific recommendations on treatment of hyperlipidemia, please refer to Chapter 32, Diagnosis, Standards of Care, and Treatment for Hyperlipidemia.

RETINOPATHY

Patients with diabetes are at risk for retinopathy. Diabetic retinopathy poses a serious threat to vision and is the leading cause of blindness in middle-aged Americans. To monitor for this complication, **yearly dilated ophthalmologic evaluations** are recommended. Newly

TABLE 27-3 LIPID TARGETS FOR PERSONS WITH DIABETES

	ADA, AACE, ATP III	EASD/ESC[a]
Total cholesterol		<4.5 mmol/L (174 mg/dL)
LDL cholesterol	<100 mg/dL	<2.5 mmol/L (97 mg/dL)[b]
• DM + CVD	<70 mg/dL, or ↓ by 30%–40% regardless of baseline	<1.8 mmol/L (70 mg/dL)
• DM older than age 40	↓ by 30%–40% regardless of baseline using a statin	
HDL	>40 mg/dL in men >50 mg/dL in women	>1 mmol/L (39 mg/dL) in men >1.2 mmol/L (46 mg/dL) in women
Triglycerides	<150 mg/dL If >500 mg/dL, lowering TG becomes a priority	>1.7 mmol/L (151 mg/dL) is a marker for increased vascular risk; begin treatment when >2.3 mmol/L (189 mg/dL) and LDL is at target
Non-HDL (TC-HDL)	<130 mg/dL (especially for those with TG >200 mg/dL)	0.8 mmol/L (31 mg/dL) above stated LDL goal

AACE, American Association of Clinical Endocrinologists; ADA, American Diabetes Association; ATP, Adult Treatment Panel; CVD, cardiovascular disease; DM, diabetes mellitus; EASD, European Association for the Study of Diabetes; ESC, European Society of Cardiology; HDL, high-density lipoprotein; LDL, low-density lipoprotein; TC, total cholesterol; TG, triglycerides.

[a]With the Third Joint European Societies Task Force on Cardiovascular Disease Prevention in Clinical Practice.

[b]Includes patients with type 1 diabetes.

diagnosed T1DM patients should have an initial dilated eye examination within 3 to 5 years after onset of their disease. Persons with T2DM should have a comprehensive eye examination at the time of diagnosis and yearly thereafter. Women who are planning a pregnancy, or who present early in pregnancy, should have a comprehensive eye examination due to the risk of development or progression of retinopathy during pregnancy. Laser photocoagulation therapy has been the mainstay treatment for preservation of vision in diabetic retinopathy, but it does not restore lost vision. Close ophthalmologic follow-up is recommended to determine the timing and extent of laser or other therapies.

NEPHROPATHY

Diabetic nephropathy accounts for nearly 50% of end-stage renal disease in the United States and is a leading cause of diabetes-related morbidity and mortality. Typically, the earliest sign of diabetic nephropathy is microalbuminuria. The most common screening test for kidney damage due to diabetes is measurement of the microalbumin-to-creatinine ratio in a spot urine sample. **Microalbuminuria** is defined as a microalbumin:creatinine ratio of

30 to 300 mcg/mg, and **macroalbuminuria** is defined as microalbumin:creatinine ratio of ≥300 mcg/mg. Macroalbuminuria carries a worse prognosis with regard to progression of kidney disease and need for renal replacement therapy. Testing for albuminuria should be performed in patients with T1DM within 5 years of diagnosis and in patients with T2DM at the time of diagnosis and repeated annually. For an accurate initial diagnosis, microalbuminuria should be confirmed in two of three tests within 3 to 6 months to eliminate positive tests due to transient conditions such as exercise, urinary tract infections, hematuria, viral illness, and hyperglycemia. Once microalbuminuria is diagnosed, treatment should begin with either an **ACEI or an ARB** (even if normotensive), hypertension should be treated to goal, and glycemia should be normalized. These treatments can slow the progression of diabetic nephropathy. If the patient develops clinical macroalbuminuria (>300 mcg/mg or 300 mg/24 hours) modest dietary protein restriction to 0.8 g/kg/day may help slow progression of this renal complication.

Similarly, serum creatinine should be measured annually in patients with both T1DM and T2DM. Calculation of estimated glomerular filtration rate (eGFR) should be done using the Cockroft-Gault formula if the creatinine appears to be normal (<1.0 mg/dL), the Modification of Diet in Renal Disease (MDRD) equation if the reduced clearance is suspected. The MDRD eGFR formula can be found at: www.kidney.org/professionals/ kkdoqi/gfr_calculator.cfm. Recent studies have shown that kidney function can decline in the absence of albuminuria and retain pathologic features of diabetic nephropathy. Careful attention to blood pressure and glycemic control, and the use of ACEIs or ARBs can slow the progression of kidney disease. When the eGFR is <60 mL/minute/1.73 m^2 by the modified MDRD formula, testing for anemia, vitamin D, and parathyroid hormone should be undertaken and abnormal values treated. A referral to a nephrologist is recommended in all patients with eGFR <60 mL/minute/ 1.73 m^2, regardless of etiology.

NEUROPATHY

Neuropathy is considered a microvascular complication of diabetes, which can present in several forms. The most common are distal symmetric sensorimotor diabetic polyneuropathy (DPN) and autonomic neuropathy involving gastrointestinal, genitourinary, and cardiovascular systems, as well as contributing to hypoglycemic unawareness. Focal neuropathy is less common, and typically presents acutely. Evaluation of possible neuropathy should begin with a history of symptoms such as pain, numbness, and paresthesias in the feet or hands, or with early satiety. A **neurologic examination should be performed annually** and should evaluate deep tendon reflexes and various sensory modalities (pain/temperature, vibration, light touch, and joint position sense). Sensory testing with a 10-g monofilament detects the presence or absence of "protective sensation." Defects in more than one testing modality suggest DPN in the absence of other causes, and loss of monofilament sensation and vibration predicts foot ulcers. Although there is no specific therapy that alters the course of DPN, strict control of blood glucose, with attention to reducing glucose fluctuations, may prevent progression. Symptomatic pain relief can be attained through the use of some anticonvulsant medications and some antidepressants. Foot care is particularly important in patients with DPN.

LOWER EXTREMITY COMPLICATIONS

Patients with diabetes develop foot problems owing to a combination of vascular and neurologic compromise and poor wound healing. DM is the leading cause of nontraumatic lower extremity amputation in the United States. **Annual foot examinations** should include evaluation of touch and vibration sense (Semmes-Weinstein 10-g monofilament and 128 mHz tuning fork), deep tendon reflexes, and pedal pulses. At every visit, the feet should be visually inspected for skin breakdown, callus, discoloration, or signs of vascular or neurologic disease. Patients should be educated on the importance of well-fitting shoes and frequent inspection of their feet. Those with bony deformities may require custom-molded shoes. Foot ulcerations, should they occur, require treatment by a multidisciplinary team to ensure healing and prevent recurrence.

ANTIPLATELET THERAPY

Treatment with low-dose aspirin has been shown to reduce recurrence of cardiovascular events, including myocardial infarction (~30%) and stroke (~20%) in persons with diabetes. It is, therefore, strongly recommended for persons with both T1DM and T2DM who are older than age 40, and may be used in patients older than 30 years of age who have additional risk factors. The suggested dose of aspirin is 75 to 162 mg/day, which may be used in combination with other antiplatelet agents such as clopidogrel for prevention of recurrence of vascular problems in patients who are at high risk.

SCREENING FOR CARDIOVASCULAR DISEASE

The ADA recommends that patients with diabetes who complain of angina, with or without a history of coronary heart disease, undergo noninvasive stress testing for coronary heart disease. The ADA suggests screening exercise stress testing in patients with any of the following: typical or atypical cardiac symptoms, abnormal resting electrocardiogram (ECG), peripheral or carotid occlusive arterial disease, and age >35 years with sedentary lifestyle planning to begin a vigorous exercise program. A consultation with a cardiologist is recommended regarding further workup of patients with an abnormal exercise ECG.

IMMUNIZATIONS

Influenza vaccine should be administered annually to patients with diabetes, beginning each October. The pneumococcal vaccine should be administered once the diagnosis of diabetes is established. Other specific vaccines are left to clinical judgment.

IN-PATIENT MANAGEMENT

Hyperglycemia in hospitalized patients is recognized as an important modifiable contributor to increased morbidity and mortality. Persons with diabetes (whether previously diagnosed or not) are admitted to the hospital more often than individuals without diabetes, and the stress of acute illness and surgery can cause hyperglycemia in previously nondiabetic individuals. Therefore, more than half of patients in some intensive care units (ICUs) and 25% of ward patients will require management of hyperglycemia. In a joint consensus statement, the ADA and AACE made the following recommendations:

- Identify all patients with a known diagnosis of diabetes clearly in the medical record.
- Measure blood glucose on admission, and institute point-of-care glucose testing in all patients with a prior diagnosis of diabetes, in those with hyperglycemia identified in the hospital, and in those with high-risk medical or surgical illnesses or procedures.

- Target blood glucose for non–intensive care unit (ICU), nonpregnant patients is 80 to 110 mg/dL pre-meal and ≤180 mg/dL post-meal.
- Target blood glucose for ICU patients is 80 to 110 mg/dL.
- Use of continuous insulin infusion is generally required in ICU settings, to treat diabetes hyperglycemic emergencies, and in labor and delivery.
- Scheduled subcutaneous insulin for medical and surgical ward patients should include the following components:
  - Basal insulin using an intermediate (NPH) or long-acting (glargine or detemir) insulin preparation, which should be marked "Do not hold."
  - Prandial insulin using a rapid-acting preparation (lispro, aspart, glulisine), with orders to give immediately with the meal, and held if the meal is missed or not eaten.
  - Correction factor using a rapid-acting preparation (lispro, aspart, glulisine), to be given at prespecified times, and at intervals at least 4 hours apart to avoid stacking doses.
- Orders for treatment of hypoglycemia with oral carbohydrate source if mild and the patient is able to take oral nutrients (intravenous if unable to handle oral intake), should be prespecified, along with re-test intervals and physician notification.
- Safety is of paramount importance in the management of inpatient hyperglycemia, so a systems approach with appropriate training, boundaries, and monitoring is needed to ensure success.
- Follow-up of patients who were hyperglycemic during their hospital stay is appropriate, either to adjust newly instituted therapy or to perform diagnostic testing for diabetes.

Optimum care of patients with diabetes prevents acute complications and reduces the risk of development of long-term complications of this disease. This can be accomplished through patient education, regular health screening, medical care, laboratory evaluation, and timely referral to specialists.

KEY POINTS TO REMEMBER

- Tight glycemic control reduces the microvascular complications of diabetes.
- Glycemic targets for most patients with diabetes are near normal, but can be modified for safety in individual patients.
- The most important facet of diabetes care may be to identify and treat cardiac risk factors, such as hypertension, hyperlipidemia, sedentary lifestyle, and cigarette smoking, with antiplatelet therapy, lifestyle modification, and smoking cessation.
- Screen for albuminuria and serum creatinine annually and start an ACEI or ARB if evidence of kidney damage.
- Provide/refer patients for annual dilated retinal examinations.
- Inspect the feet at each visit and provide a yearly comprehensive foot examination.
- Develop expertise in the treatment of hyperglycemia in hospitalized patients to reduce morbidity and mortality.

REFERENCES AND SUGGESTED READINGS

AACE Diabetes Mellitus Clinical Practice Guidelines Task Force. American Association of Clinical Endocrinologists medical guidelines for clinical practice for the management of diabetes mellitus. *Endocr Pract* 2007;13:4–68.

AACE Hypertension Task Force. American Association of Clinical Endocrinologists medical guidelines for clinical practice for the diagnosis and treatment of hypertension. *Endocr Pract* 2006;12:196–222.

American Diabetes Association. Standards of medical care in diabetes–2007 (position statement). *Diabetes Care* 2007;27:S4–S41.

Chobanian AV, et al. The seventh report of the Joint National Committee on prevention, detection, evaluation, and treatment of high blood pressure (the JNC 7 report). *JAMA* 2003;289:2560–2572.

Executive summary of the third report of the National Cholesterol Education Program (NCEP) expert panel on detection, evaluation, and treatment of high blood cholesterol in adults (Adult Treatment Panel III). *JAMA* 2001;285:2486–2497.

Grundy SM, Cleeman JI, Merz NB, Brewer HB, Clark LT, Hunninghake DB, Pasternak RC, Smith SC, Stone NJ, for the Coordinating Committee of the National Cholesterol Education Program. Implications of recent clinical trials for the national cholesterol education program adult treatment panel III guidelines. *Circulation* 2004; 110:227–239.

Harris MI, Klein R, Welborn TA, et al. Onset of NIDDM occurs at least 4–7 years before clinical diagnosis. *Diabetes Care* 1992;15:815–819.

Klein R, Klein BE. Vision disorders in diabetes. In: Harris MI, et al., eds. *Diabetes in America*, DHHS publication number 85-1468. Washington, DC: United States Government Printing Office; 1985.

The ACE/ADA Task Force on Inpatient Diabetes. American College of Endocrinology and American Diabetes Association consensus statement on inpatient diabetes and glycemic control. *Diabetes Care* 2006;29:1955–1962.

The Task Force on Diabetes and Cardiovascular Diseases of the European Society of Cardiology (ESC) and of the European Association for the Study of Diabetes (EASD). Guidelines on diabetes, pre-diabetes, and cardiovascular diseases: executive summary. *Eur Heart J* 2007;28:88–136.

Diabetes Mellitus Type 1

28

Janet B. McGill

INTRODUCTION

Type 1 diabetes mellitus (T1DM) is an illness in which autoimmune destruction of pancreatic beta cells causes **insulin deficiency** and **hyperglycemia**. The overall prevalence of the disease is 0.25% to 0.5% of the population, or 1 of 400 children and 1 of 200 adults in the United States. The incidence of T1DM is increasing in developed countries, and it is appearing at younger ages. The peak onset occurs at age 10 to 12 years; however, it can be diagnosed from a few months of age into the ninth decade of life. Males and females are equally affected. T1DM accounts for 5% to 10% of all cases of diabetes and needs to be accurately diagnosed so that insulin therapy is not delayed or withheld inappropriately. Insulin deficiency can lead to acute metabolic decompensation known as **diabetic ketoacidosis (DKA)**; however, insulin excess can produce life-threatening hypoglycemia. Chronic hyperglycemia is the root cause of disabling microvascular complications and contributes to macrovascular disease. The treatment goal of T1DM is normalization of blood glucose (BG) by physiologically based insulin replacement therapy.

Etiology and Pathogenesis

The autoimmune process that **selectively destroys pancreatic beta cells** is T-cell mediated with an unknown antigenic stimulus. Environmental factors, including coxsackie and rubella viruses, and dietary factors, such as early exposure to cow's milk, have been implicated. Insulitis (lymphocytic infiltration of pancreatic islets) is an early finding, followed by apoptosis of beta cells, which leads to their virtual absence later in the disease course. Antibodies to beta-cell antigens can be found in the majority of patients before diagnosis, and for some time after the onset of clinical diabetes. These disease markers are antibodies to glutamic acid decarboxylase (GAD65), to tyrosine phosphatases IA-2 and IA-2 beta, and to insulin (IAA). Of these markers, GAD65 is positive in 80% of children and adults near the time of diagnosis, whereas IA-2 and IAA are positive in ~50% of children and are less likely to be present in adults. The presence of two antibodies has high sensitivity and specificity for rapid progression to insulin dependency and may help clarify the diagnosis in some patients. In cases of T1DM in which no evidence of autoimmunity can be detected, the classification used is idiopathic T1DM.

Several organ-specific **autoimmune diseases occur with increased frequency in patients with T1DM**, including autoimmune thyroiditis (Hashimoto's and Graves' diseases), Addison's disease, pernicious anemia, celiac sprue, vitiligo, alopecia, and chronic active hepatitis. In a study of 265 adults with T1DM, the risk of thyroid disease was 32% for the proband, 25% for siblings, and 42% for parents, with females more commonly affected than males. The risk of developing autoimmune thyroid disease increases with age, so periodic screening should continue throughout adulthood in patients with T1DM and their family members.

The **genetic susceptibility** to T1DM is manifested by linkage with several gene loci and association with HLA-DR and DQ. The *IDDM1* gene located in the HLA region of chromosome 6p21.3, and the *IDDM2* gene in the region 5′ upstream of the insulin gene on chromosome 11p15.5 contribute 42% and 10%, respectively, to the observed familial clustering. In the family of a patient with T1DM, the risk of an identical twin developing T1DM is 30%, an offspring is 6%, and a sibling is 5%. The striking familial discordance supports the importance of environmental factors.

Pathogenesis of Complications

Patients with both T1DM and T2DM are susceptible to organ dysfunction that is caused by long-term exposure to hyperglycemia and which leads to devastating morbidity and mortality. The **microvascular complications** of diabetes are retinopathy, nephropathy, and neuropathy. Although they share some pathogenic features, they may not appear at the same time or with the same severity in all individuals with diabetes. The pathogenesis of each of these complications includes increased oxidative stress or the generation of reactive oxygen species with inadequate scavenger activity. **Advanced glycation end-products** are formed by processes of glycation and/or oxidation of proteins, nucleotides, and lipids, and have intrinsic cellular toxicity. High glucose and reactive oxygen species levels have been shown to increase diacylglycerol and stimulate protein kinase C activity, causing alterations in intracellular signal transduction and production of cytokines and growth factors. Glucose enters peripheral nerves by mass action, is converted first to sorbitol by aldose reductase, and then to fructose by sorbitol dehydrogenase. These saccharides produce osmotic stress, increase glycation, and cause alterations in the NADH/NAD ratio, which collectively contribute to nerve fiber damage and loss. Diabetic retinopathy is associated with the adverse effects of hyperglycemia on the vascular endothelium and upregulation of cytokines such as vascular endothelial growth factor. In renal mesangial cells, hyperglycemia induces transforming growth factor β, which stimulates matrix synthesis and inhibits matrix degradation. Investigational agents that target these processes are currently in clinical development.

PRESENTATION

History

T1DM develops most commonly in childhood but can present at any age. Because 80% of cases occur without a positive family history, symptoms may be overlooked until hyperglycemia reaches critical levels. The **prodromal symptoms are related to hyperglycemia** and include weight loss, polyuria, polydipsia, polyphagia, and blurred vision. If ketoacidosis is present, the patient might complain of abdominal pain, nausea, vomiting, myalgias, and shortness of breath and exhibit changes in mental and hemodynamic status.

In previously diagnosed patients, the **history of present illness** should document the duration of the illness, frequency of hyper- and hypoglycemia, results of self-monitored BG (SMBG) testing, dietary habits, and the status of any microvascular or macrovascular complications. The history of present illness or medication history should **record the insulin regimen in detail** and should provide an assessment of adequacy of or problems with the regimen. In female adolescents and adult women, menstrual, sexual, and gestational histories should be elicited, and the method of birth control should be documented. Smoking behavior, alcohol and drug use, and socioeconomic status and social support are all important factors in the care of a patient with T1DM.

Physical Examination

If the patient presents in **DKA**, signs of dehydration and acidosis, such as tachycardia, orthostatic hypotension, and dry mucus membranes, might be evident. Fruity odor to the breath reflects the presence of ketones. Routine follow-up physical examinations should document height, weight, and Tanner staging in children to determine that growth and development are advancing normally. Blood pressure and heart rate are important measures for all patients with T1DM. At least annually, the physical examination should include skin, funduscopic, oral, thyroid, and cardiovascular examinations, as well as sensory testing and foot screening. Dilated eye examination by an ophthalmologist is recommended at 3 to 5 years of T1DM duration, with scheduling of repeat examinations based on clinical findings.

Diagnostic and Laboratory Evaluation

The diagnosis of T1DM is typically made when a **random plasma glucose ≥200 mg/dL** is accompanied by signs and symptoms of diabetes (e.g., DKA). If the diagnosis of T1DM versus T2DM is unclear and the patient has not had DKA, testing for antibodies to GAD65, IA-2B (also known as *ICA*), or IAA or C-peptide level can be useful. C-Peptide levels are typically low or undetectable in patients with T1DM. **Hemoglobin (Hb)A1c** should be measured 2–4 times per year, and a lipid profile, serum creatinine and electrolytes, and urine microalbumin-to-creatinine ratio should be checked at least annually in adolescents and adults. Screening for thyroid antibodies is recommended, and thyroid-stimulating hormone (TSH) should be checked annually if the patient is antibody positive or has a goiter.

MANAGEMENT

Treatment Goals

The goal of diabetes treatment is to **maintain the BG as close to normal as possible** and to **avoid hypoglycemia**. All patients with T1DM require insulin therapy, and early achievement of a near-normal HbA1c has been shown to preserve residual beta-cell function and to reduce long-term complications. The Diabetes Control and Complications Trial (DCCT) and its follow-up study have shown that every 1% reduction in HbA1c reduces retinopathy by 33%, microalbuminuria by 22%, and neuropathy by 38%. Tight control for the first 5 to 10 years of diabetes confers long-term risk reduction, supporting the hypothesis that hyperglycemia induces organ toxicity that can be self-perpetuating (glycemic memory). In children, the therapeutic goals include ensuring normal growth and development and the scrupulous avoidance of severe hypoglycemia at young ages. In the postpubertal adolescent and adult patient, maintenance of normal blood pressure, achievement of target lipid levels, smoking cessation, aspirin use in patients older than age 40, and preconception counseling are important treatment parameters. (Please refer to Chapter 27, Standards of Care for Diabetes Mellitus, for detailed recommendations.)

Glucose Monitoring

Patients with T1DM should be encouraged to do **SMBG** at least 4 times daily so that appropriate insulin adjustments can be made based on ambient glucose levels. These recommendations may be modified for children with school considerations. Increased monitoring is required during acute illnesses, for intense exercise, and before and during pregnancy. Alternate site testing; rapid readings; and meters with averaging, graphing, and download functions have helped patients with the challenging task of SMBG. Periodic monitoring during the nighttime is recommended for all patients to check for nocturnal hypoglycemia. Continuous glucose monitoring is now available from more than one manufacturer. It tests interstitial fluid glucose, which correlates with plasma glucose and provides real-time readings.

Dietary Therapy

Dietary therapy involves **individualized assessment and instruction** and is most effectively provided by a registered dietitian. The caloric requirement for people with moderate physical activity is approximately 35 kcal/kg/day, with significant variation. The usual diet for patients with diabetes provides 50% of calories derived from carbohydrates and fiber. Protein should make up 10% to 20% of calories and <30% should come from fat, keeping saturated fat to a minimum. Individualized instruction should consider the patient's caloric needs, ethnicity, habits, constraints, and the prescribed insulin regimen. Most patients are instructed in either an exchange system or carbohydrate-counting techniques and use meal planning as an integral part of their diabetes treatment. Review of dietary principles is a cost-effective way to help the patient achieve treatment targets.

Insulin Therapy

Insulin therapy must be individualized, and numerous regimens have been used. The DCCT and other studies have clearly demonstrated that patients are more likely to achieve glycemic targets using **intensified insulin therapy with basal and bolus components** than with conventional therapy with one or two injections. Intensive insulin therapy is provided by either multiple daily injections (MDIs) or continuous subcutaneous insulin infusion (CSII) using an insulin pump. Insulin pharmacokinetic properties are highlighted in Table 28-1.

Decisions about the appropriate insulin regimen should be made with the patient's abilities and scheduling constraints in mind. In general, patients need an **intermediate- or**

TABLE 28-1	INSULIN TYPES AND PHARMACOKINETICS[a]		
Insulin	**Onset**	**Peak**	**Duration**
Rapid acting[b]			
Insulin aspart (NovoLog)	10–20 minutes	1–3 hours	3–5 hours
Insulin lispro (Humalog)	10–15 minutes	1–2 hours	3–4 hours
Insulin glulisine (Apidra)	10–20 minutes	1 hour	3–4 hours
Short acting			
Regular ("R")	0.5–1.0 hour	2–4 hours	4–8 hours
Intermediate acting			
NPH ("N")[c]	1.5–3 hours	4–10 hours	10–18 hours
Long acting			
Insulin detemir (Levemir)	1–2 hours	None	Up to 24 hours
Insulin glargine (Lantus)[d]	2–3 hours	None	24 hours

[a]Insulin pharmacokinetics show significant inter- and intrasubject variation. The onset, peak, and duration may be influenced by the dose administered, the injection site, skin temperature, and other less well-defined factors.

[b]Rapid-acting insulin should be administered immediately before or after meals. Also suitable for insulin pump use.

[c]Cloudy, suspended formulations require resuspension by rolling and tipping (but not shaking) the vial before administration. Resuspension is a potential source of erratic pharmacokinetics.

[d]Do not mix with any other type of insulin in the same syringe due to incompatible pH. Clear preparation, no resuspension needed.

TABLE 28-2	INSULIN DOSING REGIMEN	
Time	Dose	Regimen
Before breakfast	0.4 × TDD	NPH
	0.2 × TDD	Humalog, NovoLog, or Regular
Before dinner	0.2 × TDD	Humalog, NovoLog, or Regular
	0.2 × TDD	NPH (this dose is some times given at bedtime)

long-acting insulin to cover basal needs and a rapid- or short-acting insulin to provide meal coverage. When initiating or changing an insulin regimen, an estimation of total daily insulin dose (TDD) should be made. Individual requirements vary, but usually range from 0.5 to 1 U/kg/day, with the majority of patients requiring approximately 0.7 U/kg/day.

Historically, the most widely prescribed regimen was "split-mixed," which used NPH as the basal insulin and a short- or rapid-acting analog before breakfast and dinner (Table 28-2).

Use of this regimen presumed that the patient would eat lunch at a standard time, because the morning NPH is likely to peak at about midday. Patient scheduling problems and the erratic pharmacokinetics of NPH have made this regimen less popular.

The most commonly prescribed regimens for patients with T1DM by endocrinologists are MDI or CSII. These regimens use the concepts of basal and bolus (pre-meal) dosing. The basal dose is generally 45% to 55% of the TDD, ~0.4 U/kg/day, and is often given in one injection of insulin glargine or detemir at bedtime. If NPH is used, the dose will be about 0.2 U/kg, twice a day. The basal insulin dose is adjusted so that the fasting BG is routinely within the target of 80 to 120 mg/dL, and there is <30 mg/dL variation between evening and morning values. Changes in weight, exercise, persistent hyperglycemia, or frequent hypoglycemia should prompt reconsideration of the basal insulin dose.

Bolus doses are administered to cover caloric intake and to correct high BG readings. Pre-meal bolus doses are determined by one or more of the following methods:

- Fixed amount before each meal, ~0.13 U/kg or one-sixth of the TDD
- Fixed dose before each meal as above plus a sliding scale "correction factor" (see subsequent text) based on the pre-meal SMBG
- Carbohydrate counting plus "correction factor" uses variable amounts depending on anticipated carbohydrate intake and the pre-meal SMBG

Both the patient and the physician need to learn important concepts to succeed in the use of MDI regimens. If fixed amounts of pre-meal insulin are to be used, the patient should have a clear idea of the prescribed meal plan and be able to follow it precisely. Alternatively, the patient can adjust the pre-meal dose based on the anticipated carbohydrate content, which allows greater flexibility. To do this, the physician or diabetes educator must determine the "insulin-to-carbohydrate" ratio, which can be calculated by dividing 500 by the TDD. A patient who takes 50 U of insulin daily needs 1 U of insulin for every 10 g of carbohydrate intake. The patient needs to learn which foods contain carbohydrate, how to estimate the grams of carbohydrate in the serving provided, and how to calculate the pre-meal dose. Additional adjustments are sometimes made for high-fat meals or for meals that have high fiber content. Occasional postprandial SMBG is needed to test whether the "insulin-to-carbohydrate" ratio is correct or whether the patient has been able to estimate the carbohydrate content of the meal appropriately.

In addition to covering calories, the patient must be able to compensate for high or low BG readings. An individualized sliding scale, known as the **correction factor** is determined, which provides the number of units to be added (or subtracted) to each pre-meal dose. The correction factor is estimated by dividing 1800 by the TDD.

Sample Calculations

Example 1: An overweight patient takes 60 U of insulin daily. His current BG is 178 mg/dL, and he is about to eat a meal with 90 g of carbohydrate. His physician has told him that his target SMBG is 120 mg/dL. What dose of rapid-acting insulin should he take?

Insulin-to-carbohydrate ratio = 500/60 = 1 U insulin/8.33 g
Correction factor = 1800/60 = 30 (predicts that 1 U insulin drops the BG 30 mg/dL)
90 g carbohydrates/8.33 g/U insulin = ~10 U insulin to cover carbohydrates.
SMBG – target BG = 178 mg/dL – 120 = 58 mg/dL. He will take 2 U insulin as correction.

Thus, the patient should take 12 U of rapid-acting insulin.

Example 2: A thin, insulin-sensitive patient takes 30 U of insulin per day. If this patient has a current BG of 178 mg/dL and is about to eat the same meal as the patient in Example 1, how much insulin should she use?

Insulin to carbohydrate ratio = 500/30 = 1 U insulin/16.66 g
Correction factor = 1800/30 = 60 (predicts that 1 U insulin will drop the BG 60 mg/dL)
90 g carbohydrates/16.66 g/U insulin = ~5 U insulin to cover carbohydrates.
SMBG – target BG = 178 – 120 = 58 mg/dL. She will take 1 U insulin as correction.

Thus, this patient should take 6 U of rapid-acting insulin.

Continuous Subcutaneous Insulin Infusion

Insulin pump therapy has become an accepted alternative to MDI and has both advantages and disadvantages. Technologic advances have contributed to smaller pumps with features such as multiple basal rates, dose calculators, and alternate dosing modalities. CSII systems now include continuous glucose monitoring, which assist with dosing adjustments. CSII offers the patient with T1DM the greatest flexibility, and is more socially acceptable than needles and syringes for frequent dosing. Insulin pumps are the size of a pager and contain 180 to 300 U of insulin in a specialized syringe that is connected to a subcutaneous (SC) catheter by thin tubing. The SC catheter should be changed and repositioned every 3 days. The pump is pre-programmed to infuse the basal rate of insulin, but the patient must activate the pump to deliver bolus doses at the time of the meal or when a correction is needed. Only rapid-acting insulin is used. Diabetes education from an educator experienced in CSII is necessary to teach the patient how to use the pump, which requires several hours of instruction.

Insulin dose prescribing is conceptually similar to MDI; however, the TDD is reduced 10% to 20%, and the basal rate (equal to one-half of the new TDD) is divided by 24 and programmed as an hourly rate. For example, a patient taking 48 U/day with MDI will need approximately 20 U for basal requirements, or ~0.8 U/hour to start. The basal rate can be adjusted to accommodate nighttime low BG, morning rise, and increased or decreased activity during the day. The basal rate can be temporarily reduced for exercise or the pump can be put in suspended mode for hypoglycemia. Bolus dosing is handled similarly to MDI, with a key exception. Today's insulin pumps can administer doses in very small quantities, so the correction factor can be prescribed as a fraction. The opportunity to give smaller doses is helpful for children and insulin-sensitive patients.

The **major disadvantage** of CSII is the high cost of an insulin pump and supplies. Because only rapid-acting insulin is used, if there is a pump or catheter failure, the BG can rise quickly and DKA can ensue within 12 hours of the interruption of insulin delivery. Another potential disadvantage is the risk of catheter-site infection, which is minimized by instruction in semi-sterile techniques.

Adjusting Insulin Doses

Insulin dose adjustments or changes to the insulin regimen are made after evaluating SMBG values and looking for patterns. The efficacy of a specific rapid-acting insulin dose is monitored by the SMBG that follows the dose in question (e.g., postprandial or noon SMBG reflects the breakfast dose of rapid-acting insulin). Intermediate and long-acting insulin doses are evaluated by scrutinizing the SMBG after the injection (e.g., morning SMBG to determine adequacy of evening dose), and review of overall frequency of hyper- and hypoglycemia. Diabetes educators are often skilled at insulin dose adjustments and provide a valuable resource for patients who are experiencing problems keeping their glucose values near the target range. Diabetes education is cost-effective and necessary to achieve tight glycemic control while avoiding hypoglycemic episodes.

Pramlintide (Symlin), a synthetic analog of the beta-cell secretory product amylin, is approved for use as adjunctive therapy to insulin in patients with T1DM. It is given as a separate injection of 15 to 45 mcg before meals, and helps to reduce post-prandial glucose excursions by suppressing glucagon and enhancing satiety. It has a modest effect on HbA1c of about 0.5%, and may contribute to modest weight loss. Side effects are nausea, vomiting, and increased risk of hypoglycemia. Insulin adjustments are needed when pramlintide is prescribed.

DIABETIC KETOACIDOSIS

DKA is the direct result of insulin deficiency; however, dehydration and excess counter-regulatory hormones (glucagon, epinephrine, and cortisol) are accelerating factors. Typically, an **exacerbating factor** can be identified: new diagnosis of diabetes, omission of insulin doses, infections, pregnancy, trauma, emotional stress, excessive alcohol ingestion, myocardial infarction, stroke, intercurrent illness, hyperthyroidism, Cushing's disease, or, rarely, pheochromocytoma. The major clinical features of DKA are hyperglycemia, dehydration, acidosis, abdominal pain, nausea, vomiting, change in hemodynamic status, and altered mental status.

Pathophysiology

The pathophysiology of DKA begins with insulin levels that are insufficient to support peripheral glucose uptake and to suppress hepatic gluconeogenesis. Hyperglycemia is further driven by increases in the counterregulatory hormones glucagon, catecholamines, cortisol, and growth hormone. Activation of catabolic pathways in muscle and fat produce amino acids and free fatty acids, which fuel hepatic gluconeogenesis and ketone production. The osmotic diuresis imposed by hyperglycemia causes marked fluid and electrolyte losses, further stimulating catecholamine release. Catecholamines are antagonistic to insulin action and contribute to increased lipolysis, which pumps free fatty acids into the circulation that then undergo fatty acid oxidation to ketone bodies. Volume depletion decreases renal blood flow, which contributes to reduced excretion of glucose and ketones

TABLE 28-3	DIFFERENTIAL DIAGNOSIS OF ANION-GAP ACIDOSIS (THE MUDPILES MNEMONIC)
Condition	**Clinical Associations**
M: methanol ingestion	Visual impairment/blindness; osmol gap between the calculated and measured osmolality (seen with any alcohol ingestion)
U: uremia	History of renal failure; increased serum urea and creatinine
D: diabetic ketoacidosis	History of diabetes, hyperglycemia
P: paraldehyde	Formaldehyde-like breath odor; increased paraldehyde level
I: iron; isoniazid	Increased serum iron level; patient may have elevated hepatic transaminases with isoniazid toxicity
L: lactic acidosis	May be due to hypovolemia/sepsis, infarction, metformin, cyanide, hydrogen sulfide, CO, methemoglobin; lactate levels are elevated
E: EtOH; ethylene glycol	Osmol gap between the calculated and measured osmolality (seen with any alcohol ingestion); increased EtOH level seen with EtOH intoxication; calcium oxalate crystals seen in the urine with ethylene glycol
S: salicylates	Tinnitus, increased salicylate level, may have a concurrent respiratory alkalosis

EtOH, ethanol.

and increased serum levels of creatinine and potassium. Acidosis ensues when the levels of acetone, acetoacetate, and β-hydroxybutyrate exceed the buffering capacity of bicarbonate and the respiratory response. Low $PaCO_2$ reflects the respiratory effort and the severity of the metabolic acidosis. The presence of an anion gap and low bicarbonate in the setting of high BG and an ill-appearing patient should prompt immediate treatment for DKA while confirmatory laboratory evaluation is under way. The differential diagnosis for anion-gap acidosis is outlined in Table 28-3.

Symptoms

The symptoms of DKA are nonspecific and include anorexia, nausea, vomiting (coffee ground emesis in 25%), abdominal pain, and myalgias or weakness. Polyuria and polydipsia are characteristic of high BG, but may become blunted due to vomiting, reduced renal clearance, and altered mental status as the severity of DKA worsens. Hyperpnea is noted with mild acidosis, and the patient may complain of shortness of breath. Kussmaul breathing is a sign of a critically ill patient. The physical examination reveals tachycardia, hypotension, or orthostatic hypotension, dry mucous membranes, poor skin turgor, abdominal tenderness, and other signs of clinical events that may have prompted the DKA episode. Mental status can be normal or severely compromised. Signs of a concurrent illness or event that precipitated the DKA may be present.

Laboratory Findings

Laboratory findings of DKA include the following: glucose >250 mg/dL, glycosuria, an elevated anion gap (normal gap is ≤12), and the presence of serum or urine ketones. The anion gap is calculated as follows: (Anion gap = $Na^+ - [Cl + HCO_3]$). The serum bicarbonate is typically <15 mEq/L, the P_{CO_2} <40 mm Hg, and the arterial pH <7.3. Creatinine and K^+ are generally increased above baseline. If hypokalemia is present at the time of diagnosis, the patient has severe K^+ depletion and requires careful monitoring. Often the initial potassium level is high, and the ECG should be checked for signs of hyperkalemia, which include peaked T waves, shortened QT intervals, widened QRS complexes, and flattened or absent P waves. Later in the course of treatment, if hypokalemia occurs, a repeat ECG might show ST-segment depression, flattened or inverted T waves, a prolonged QT interval, and appearance of U waves. Hyponatremia may be present, but the measured serum sodium should be corrected for the high glucose (add 1.6 to the reported sodium for every 100 mg/dL that the glucose is >100 mg/dL), and may be further depressed by high triglycerides. Amylase and lipase may be elevated via unclear mechanisms, do not necessarily indicate pancreatitis, and resolve with treatment of the DKA.

Treatment

Clinical Evaluation and Triage

Intensive care admission is required for patients with hemodynamic instability or mental status changes, for pediatric patients, or if frequent monitoring is not possible on a medical ward. Hemodynamic monitoring may be required for patients in shock, with possible sepsis, with DKA complicated by myocardial infarction, or in patients with end-stage renal disease or chronic heart failure. Nasogastric tube placement may be needed for patients with hematemesis or for comatose patients.

Fluids and Electrolytes

Fluid resuscitation in adults should begin with normal saline at 1 L/hour unless there is a contraindication (chronic heart failure, end-stage renal disease). The typical total body water deficit is 4 to 6 L, sodium deficit is 7 to 10 mEq/kg, K^+ deficit is 3 to 5 mEq/kg, and PO_4 deficit is 5 to 7 mmol/kg. If the corrected sodium is normal or high on repeat testing, change the intravenous fluids to 0.45% NaCl; continue 0.9% saline if it is low. When the K^+ drops to <5.0 mEq/L and the patient has adequate urine output, add 20 to 30 mEq K^+ to each liter of intravenous fluid. Plan to correct the water and salt deficits over 24 hours, slower in children. The starting fluid administration rate for children should be 10 to 20 mL/kg/hour and should not exceed 50 mL/kg over the first 4 hours of therapy.

Patients presenting with DKA have a total body PO_4 depletion due to osmotic diuresis, although this may not be apparent on presentation because insulin deficiency and acidosis cause PO_4 to shift out of cells. Serum PO_4 levels decrease with insulin therapy. Except in very severe cases of hypophosphatemia (serum PO_4 <1.0 mg/dL) or concomitant cardiorespiratory compromise, routine administration of PO_4 has not been shown to be beneficial and may, in fact, be harmful because excess replacement can cause hypocalcemia.

Bicarbonate should not be routinely administered to patients in DKA unless the serum pH is <7.0 or the patient has life-threatening hyperkalemia.

Insulin and Glucose

Initial intravenous loading bolus 0.1 to 0.15 U/kg of regular (R) insulin followed by continuous infusion 0.1 U/kg/hour (100 units R insulin/100 mL normal saline solution). Children should not receive intravenous bolus doses of insulin; begin with the infusion.

Monitor serum glucose every hour and expect the BG to decline by 50 to 75 mg/dL/hour. A slower response could indicate insulin resistance, inadequate fluid resuscitation, or improper insulin delivery. As the acidosis clears, the glucose is likely to fall more rapidly. When the serum glucose is <250 mg/dL, add 5% dextrose to the intravenous fluids, and decrease the insulin infusion rate by up to one-half. If the glucose infusion rate is kept stable, the insulin infusion requirements will be more predictable. Continue intensive insulin therapy and monitoring until the patient is tolerating oral intake and the anion-gap acidosis has resolved. As the acidosis resolves, the anion gap closes, arterial and venous pH rise, and serum bicarbonate rises. The American Diabetes Association position paper regarding the treatment of DKA states that criteria for the resolution of DKA include a glucose <200 mg/dL, a serum bicarbonate ≥18 mEq/L, and a venous pH >7.3.

Patients recovering from DKA may develop a transient non–anion gap hyperchloremic metabolic acidosis that occurs because of urinary loss of "potential bicarbonate" in the form of ketoanions and their replacement by chloride ions from intravenous fluids. This non–anion-gap acidosis is transient and has not been shown to be clinically significant, except in renal failure.

Common error: The hyperglycemia will respond to treatment faster than the acidosis will resolve. **Do not decrease or discontinue the insulin infusion when glucose levels approach the normal range.** This can lead to worsening of the ketoacidosis. Instead, continue the intravenous insulin infusion, but adjust the dose and/or add 5% dextrose. If 5% dextrose is infused at excessively rapid rates, the BG will increase, and the transition to SC insulin will be delayed.

Monitoring

- Fingerstick BG every hour during insulin infusion.
- Electrolytes, blood urea nitrogen (BUN), and creatinine levels every 2 to 4 hours until the K^+ has stabilized and the anion gap acidosis is resolved.
- Serum ketones or β-hydroxybutyrate level by fingerstick on admission only. Use of the fingerstick β-hydroxybutyrate test to follow DKA treatment is under review.
- Intake and output, weight.

Transition to Subcutaneous Insulin. Continue the intravenous insulin infusion and intravenous fluids until the acidosis has cleared, the glucose is <250 mg/dL, and the patient is able to eat. **Note:** It is possible for the patient to attempt a small or clear liquid meal while on an insulin drip, but the drip rate may need to be increased for the meal hour and then returned to the usual rate. Make the transition to subcutaneous insulin before a meal or at bedtime, but not during the middle of the night or between meals. If the patient has been previously diagnosed, give the usual pre-meal insulin dose plus any correction factor, and cover basal needs with intermediate- or long-acting insulin. For example, if the drip can be stopped at noon, give a pre-meal dose of short-acting insulin according to the patient's usual schedule and add a partial dose of NPH to cover until dinner or bedtime. Start basal insulin (NPH, detemir [Levemir], or glargine [Lantus]) and short-acting insulin 1 to 2 hours before stopping the insulin drip. Reduce the rate of intravenous dextrose to ≤100 mL/hour or discontinue it if the patient is able to eat. Note that intravenous fluids may need to be continued until the serum creatinine has returned to baseline.

Problem Solving. Recurring DKA should prompt additional history to search for precipitating causes. Insulin pump malfunction, noncompliance with insulin doses, social distress, medication problems, or concomitant illness should warrant attention of an experienced diabetes care provider. Newly diagnosed patients require additional time in the hospital for the institution of an insulin regimen and diabetes education.

CHRONIC COMPLICATIONS

Care of the patient with T1DM includes screening for microvascular and macrovascular complications, and the application of proven therapies to reduce morbidity and mortality. The best-studied intervention in T1DM is the use of angiotensin-converting enzyme (ACE) inhibitors (ACEIs) to prevent progression of microalbuminuria to macroalbuminuria and slow the progression of diabetic nephropathy. ACEIs may also slow the progression of retinopathy. ACEIs should be started if blood pressure increases above the normal range for the patient's age or when microalbuminuria is identified. ACEIs should be avoided in premenopausal women who are not using effective birth control, are planning a pregnancy, or who are pregnant, due to the risk of birth defects. Blood pressure control, lipid parameters, and other prevention measures are covered in Chapter 27, Standards of Care for Diabetes Mellitus, and Chapter 29, Diabetes Mellitus Type 2.

KEY POINTS TO REMEMBER

- Several organ-specific autoimmune diseases occur with increased frequency in patients with T1DM, including autoimmune thyroiditis (Hashimoto's and Graves' diseases), Addison's disease, pernicious anemia, celiac sprue, vitiligo, alopecia, and chronic active hepatitis.
- Dietary therapy is a crucial component of therapy for patients with T1DM.
- Insulin therapy for T1DM is commonly given as either MDI or CSII, both of which use the concepts of basal/bolus dosing with pre-meal dose adjustments.
- In DKA, remember that even though initial serum levels of K^+ may be elevated, patients are actually total body K^+ depleted. Add K^+ to intravenous fluids when serum K^+ is <5 and the patient has adequate urine output.
- During treatment of DKA, hyperglycemia will respond faster than acidosis to treatment with insulin and intravenous fluids. Make sure the anion gap acidosis has resolved before transitioning to subcutaneous insulin.
- Once DKA has resolved, start basal subcutaneous insulin and short-acting subcutaneous insulin 1 to 2 hours before turning off the insulin drip.

REFERENCES AND SUGGESTED READINGS

American Diabetes Association. Standards of medical care in diabetes. *Diabetes Care* 2004;27:S15–S46.

Atkinson MA. Maclaren NK. The pathogenesis of insulin-dependent diabetes mellitus. *N Engl J Med* 1994;331:1428–1436.

Bode BW, ed. *Medical Management of Type 1 Diabetes*, 4th ed. Alexandria, VA: American Diabetes Association; 2004.

Brownlee M. Biochemistry and molecular cell biology of diabetic complications. *Nature* 2001;414:813–820.

Chen Q, Kukreja A, Maclaren NK. Classification of the autoimmune polyglandular syndromes. In: Gill RG, Harmon JT, Maclaren NK, eds. *Immunologically Mediated Endocrine Diseases*. Philadelphia: Lippincott Williams & Wilkins; 2002:167–187.

Cook A. Etiology/pathogenesis of type 1 diabetes. In: Gill RG, Harmon JT, Maclaren NK, eds. *Immunologically Mediated Endocrine Diseases*. Philadelphia: Lippincott Williams & Wilkins; 2002:287–301.

DeWitt DE, Hirsch IB. Outpatient insulin therapy in type 1 and type 2 diabetes mellitus. Scientific Review. *JAMA* 2003;289:2254–2264.

Eisenbarth GS. Update in type 1 diabetes. *J Clin Endocrinol Metab* 2007;92:2403–2407.

Imagawa A, Hanafusa T, Miyagawa J, et al. for the Osaka IDDM Study Group. A novel subtype of type 1 diabetes mellitus characterized by a rapid onset and an absence of diabetes-related antibodies. *N Engl J Med* 2000;342:301–307.

Kitabchi AE, Umpierrez GE, Murphy MB, et al. for the American Diabetes Association. Hyperglycemic crises in diabetes. *Diabetes Care* 2004;27(Suppl 1):S94–S102.

Kitabchi AE, Umpierrez GE, Murphy MB, et al. Management of hyperglycemic crises in patients with diabetes. *Diabetes Care* 2001;24:131–153.

Lewis EJ, Hunsicker LG, Bain RP, et al. For the Collaborative Study Group. The effect of angiotensin-converting enzyme inhibition on diabetic nephropathy. *N Engl J Med* 1993; 329:1456–1462.

Ratner RE, Hirsch IB, Neifing JL, et al. Less hypoglycemia with insulin glargine in intensive insulin therapy for type 1 diabetes. U.S. study group of insulin glargine in type 1 diabetes. *Diabetes Care* 2000;23:639–643.

The Diabetes Control and Complications Trial Research Group. The effect of intensive treatment of diabetes on the development and progression of long-term complications in insulin-dependent diabetes mellitus. *N Engl J Med* 1993;329:977–986.

The Writing Team for the Diabetes Control and Complications Trial/Epidemiology of Diabetes Interventions and Complications Research Group. Sustained effect of intensive treatment of type 1 diabetes mellitus on development and progression of diabetic nephropathy. The epidemiology of diabetes interventions and complications (EDIC) study. *JAMA* 2003;290:2159–2166.

Diabetes Mellitus Type 2

Janet B. McGill

INTRODUCTION

Type 2 diabetes mellitus (T2DM) is a metabolic disorder with carbohydrate intolerance as the cardinal feature. T2DM accounts for about 95% of all cases of diabetes in the United States and Canada and is a growing public health concern, with an estimated total prevalence of 18 million among people ≥20 years of age, or 8.7% of the adult population. Diabetes is the sixth leading cause of death in the United States and a leading cause of morbidity and mortality in other countries. Diabetes is the leading cause of end-stage renal disease, blindness in individuals age 20 to 74 years, and nontraumatic limb amputation. The major cause of mortality in diabetes is cardiovascular, and the diagnosis of diabetes confers a two- to fourfold increase in cardiovascular risk.

CAUSES

Etiology and Pathophysiology

The etiology of T2DM is multifactorial. **Insulin resistance** can be identified in most individuals with T2DM, and hyperglycemia develops when insulin secretion by pancreatic beta cells is inadequate to meet the metabolic demand. Insulin resistance is thought to remain relatively stable in adulthood in the absence of weight gain. **Insulin deficiency**, on the other hand, typically follows a period of hyperinsulinemia, which compensates for insulin resistance. Declining insulin response to a carbohydrate stimulus can be identified in persons with impaired glucose tolerance (IGT) or impaired fasting glucose (IFG), but becomes more pronounced when diabetes develops. Progressive beta-cell failure occurs during the lifespan of most individuals with T2DM, giving the appearance of disease progression and the need for additional therapy over time that may include insulin replacement.

Genetic factors are implicated in insulin resistance, but probably account for only 50% of the disordered metabolism. Obesity, especially visceral adiposity, increasing age, and physical inactivity contribute significantly to insulin resistance and, in epidemiologic studies, are the factors associated with increasing incidence of T2DM. Lifestyle modification that includes weight loss and exercise improves insulin resistance and prevents diabetes in high-risk cohorts. Insulin resistance can be induced or aggravated by pregnancy, endocrine disorders such as Cushing's disease, exogenous steroids, protease inhibitors, serious medical or surgical illness, and a number of commonly used drugs. The definitive tests for insulin resistance measure insulin-mediated glucose uptake or hepatic glucose output and are available in research settings. In the clinical setting, insulin resistance is often inferred when features of the metabolic syndrome are present, with or without a diagnosis of diabetes. There are no definitive histopathologic findings of insulin resistance; however, studies have demonstrated a correlation between increased fat in the liver and level of insulin resistance. Fatty acids and triglyceride levels in muscle are also increased in obesity and diabetes.

Before the onset of diabetes, persons with insulin resistance often have elevated insulin and C-peptide levels to meet the increased metabolic demand. **Insulin deficiency relative to the demand required to accommodate insulin resistance leads to hyperglycemia and the diagnosis of T2DM.** The initial defects in insulin secretion are loss of first-phase insulin release and loss of the oscillatory secretion pattern. The clinical correlate of this early defect is postprandial hyperglycemia. Further decline in insulin secretion leads to inadequate suppression of hepatic glucose output and presents clinically as fasting hyperglycemia. Hyperglycemia contributes to impaired beta-cell function and worsening insulin deficiency, a phenomenon known as **glucose toxicity.** Chronic elevation of free fatty acids, another characteristic of T2DM, may contribute to reduced insulin secretion and islet cell apoptosis. Histopathologic changes in the islets of Langerhans in long-standing T2DM include amyloid accumulation and a reduction in the number of insulin-producing beta cells. Longitudinal data from the UK Prospective Diabetes Study (UKPDS) suggest that loss of insulin secretory capacity over time is common in T2DM. Early in the course of diabetes, improvement in insulin secretion can be achieved by reducing insulin resistance and improving hyperglycemia, thereby reducing the functional defects imposed by hyperglycemia and elevated free fatty acids.

The American Diabetes Association (ADA) classifies a heterogeneous group of hyperglycemic disorders as **"Other specific types of diabetes."** The most common of this group of disorders are the *drug- or chemical-induced forms of diabetes.* Typical offending agents include glucocorticoids, nicotinic acid, thiazides, β-adrenergic agonists, the newer atypical antipsychotic agents, and some antiretroviral agents. Hyperglycemia can be relatively mild or quite severe with the institution of these therapies. *Pancreatic disease* can result in partial or complete insulin deficiency. Patients with hemochromatosis or advanced cystic fibrosis may present with nonketotic hyperglycemia. Pancreatitis, pancreatectomy, pancreatic neoplasia, or fibrocalculous pancreatopathy may cause insulin deficiency, and insulin therapy may be needed early in the course of the illness. Diabetes can occur with *other endocrine diseases* such as Cushing's syndrome and acromegaly. Resolution of the diabetes often occurs when the hormone excess is corrected.

Diabetes is a feature of a number of **genetic disorders.** Patients with Down's syndrome, Prader-Willi syndrome, and others may develop diabetes as a consequence of obesity. Mild to moderate nonketotic hyperglycemia that presents in young adults with a family history that suggests a dominantly inherited trait may represent a monogenetic form of diabetes. These cases are referred to as *maturity-onset diabetes in the young* (MODY), and genetic testing may reveal which of the six defects are present. Obesity and insulin resistance are not characteristic features of MODY. Most of the T2DM that is diagnosed in children and teenagers is not MODY, but is rather early onset classic T2DM. Other rare forms of diabetes that present in adulthood include mitochondrial gene defects and defects in the insulin molecule or insulin receptor (type A insulin resistance).

A common clinical problem is the patient who does not have features of insulin resistance and who may not respond to oral hypoglycemic agents as expected. These patients should be tested for autoimmune markers such as anti-GAD65 and ICA antibodies (see Chapter 28, Diabetes Mellitus Type 1). **Latent autoimmune diabetes in adults (LADA)** is an insulin-deficient form of diabetes that develops more slowly than classic type 1 diabetes and is associated with other autoimmune diseases. The majority of patients with LADA require exogenous insulin within 5 years of diagnosis. Later in the course of the illness, patients with LADA may become C-peptide negative and are at risk for ketoacidosis. The prevalence of autoimmune markers in T2DM varies by the population studied from 4% in U.S. populations to 10% in northern European populations such as the UKPDS study cohort. When LADA is suspected, testing for anti-GAD antibodies and C-peptide may help rule in or rule out the diagnosis.

PRESENTATION

Individuals at high risk for the development of T2DM can often be identified before the onset of clinical diabetes. **Risk factors** for the development of T2DM include older age, obesity (body mass index [BMI] ≥ 27 kg/m^2), sedentary lifestyle, history of glucose intolerance (i.e., gestational DM, impaired glucose tolerance, stress hyperglycemia), history of intrauterine growth retardation, family history, and ethnicity. T2DM is 2 to 6 times more prevalent in African Americans, Asians, Hispanic Americans, Native Americans, and Pima Indians than in non-Hispanic whites.

The **metabolic syndrome**, defined as three or more of the characteristics listed in Table 29-1, may precede the diagnosis of T2DM and may confer increased risk of cardiovascular disease.

The **diagnosis of T2DM** is made when the fasting plasma glucose (FPG) is ≥ 126 mg/dL, confirmed on a second sample; or when a random blood glucose (BG) of ≥ 200 mg/dL is accompanied by symptoms; or by finding that the 2-hour BG on a 75-g oral glucose tolerance test is ≥ 200 mg/dL. Patients with impaired fasting glucose or impaired glucose tolerance are at higher risk for the development of T2DM and may be at higher risk for cardiovascular events even in the absence of T2DM. The diagnostic criteria for diabetes and prediabetic conditions are listed in Table 29-2.

Because mild hyperglycemia is asymptomatic, patients presenting with symptoms of polyuria, nocturia, polydipsia, polyphagia, fatigue, weight changes, or blurred vision are likely to have significant BG elevation and may have been undiagnosed for some time. Patients who present with complaints of extremity pain, sexual dysfunction, or visual changes from diabetic retinopathy are likely to have been hyperglycemic for years before being diagnosed with diabetes.

The **medical history** of a patient with diabetes should include documentation of the onset and progression of diabetes, with information about episodes of diabetic ketoacidosis (DKA), prior response to medications, and level of glycemic control. Health behaviors, such as frequency of self-monitoring of BG, use of medical nutrition therapy, and exercise frequency and intensity, should be recorded. Usual BG values and problems with both hyperglycemia and hypoglycemia require assessment to plan changes in therapy. Symptoms of hyperglycemia and hypoglycemia should be elicited to augment a careful review of glucose records or meter readings.

The past medical history (PMH) should record cardiovascular risk factors and cardiovascular event history. Notation should be made of the level of retinopathy, including eye procedures, evidence of nephropathy, history of neuropathy, and history of foot ulceration or joint problems. The most recent eye examination and vaccine status should be recorded. Menstrual history, pregnancy history, and use of contraception need to be addressed in the PMH of adolescent and adult women.

TABLE 29-1	METABOLIC SYNDROME	
Metabolic Syndromecharacteristic	Men	Women
Waist circumference	>40 inches	>35 inches
	>102 cm	>88 cm
Triglycerides	≥ 150 mg/dL	≥ 150 mg/dL
High-density lipoprotein	<40 mg/dL	<50 mg/dL
Blood pressure	$\geq 130/85$ mm Hg	$\geq 130/85$ mm Hg
Fasting glucose	≥ 100 mg/dL	≥ 100 mg/dL

TABLE 29-2	DIAGNOSIS OF DIABETES		
Stage	**Fasting Plasma Glucose (FPG)**	**Oral Glucose Tolerance Test**	**Random Blood Glucose**
Normal	<100 mg/dL	2-hour PG <140 mg/dL	—
Pre-diabetes			
Impaired fasting glucose	≥100 mg/dL and <126 mg/dL	—	—
Impaired glucose tolerance	—	2-hour PG ≥140 mg/dL and <200 mg/dL	—
Diabetes	FPG ≥126 mg/dL, confirmed	2-hour PG ≥200 mg/dL	≥200 mg/dL with symptoms

FPG, fasting plasma glucose; PG, plasma glucose.

The **physical examination** may be completely normal or may include hypertension, obesity, or acanthosis nigricans. Funduscopic examination may be normal or abnormal (dot hemorrhages, exudates, neovascularization, or laser scars). The cardiovascular examination for patients with diabetes should include carotid and peripheral pulses. Examination of the feet, including skin, nails, joints, and sensation with a 10-g Semmes-Weinstein monofilament, should be done at regular intervals. The diagnosis of neuropathy is based on a combination of symptoms and physical findings, with documented decrease in more than one sensory modality (e.g., absent reflexes plus loss of vibratory sensation).

Laboratory Evaluation

Routine laboratory testing of a patient with T2DM should include a fasting lipid profile, hemoglobin A1c (HbA1c), serum creatinine, urine microalbumin (usually done as microalbumin-to-creatinine ratio on a random spot urine sample), and a baseline electrocardiogram (ECG). HbA1c should be done at diagnosis and at least semiannually. If the HbA1c is significantly above the target of 7% and therapy is being changed, it should be checked every 1–3 months. Liver function testing is required for monitoring of statin and thiazolidinedione (TZD) therapies, and should be considered for all patients with insulin resistance due to the increased risk of nonalcoholic fatty liver disease (NAFLD). Patients with T2DM and proteinuria or renal insufficiency require increased surveillance of renal parameters.

MANAGEMENT

T2DM is best managed with a multidisciplinary team, including doctors, diabetes educators, pharmacists, dietitians, and support groups. Diabetes therapy should be individually designed to achieve glycemic, blood pressure, lipid, and prevention targets while accommodating the patient's age, socioeconomic and cultural status. The glycemic target is a HbA1c value of <7%; however, the ADA recommendations state that there is no lower limit, even into the normal range of <6% (see Chapter 27, Standards of Care for Diabetes Mellitus). Treatment options include (Tables 29-3, 29-4, and 29-5):

- Diet and exercise alone
- Noninsulin antidiabetic agents

TABLE 29-3 NON-INSULIN ANTIDIABETIC DRUGS

Drug	Daily Dose	Mode of Action	Efficacy	Advantages	Disadvantages
Biguanide					
Metformin (Glucophage, Glucophage XR, Glumetza) (Riomet, liquid formulation)	500–2000 mg daily, divided doses	Reduces hepatic glucose output	↓ A1c by 1%–2%	No weight gain, may ↓ triglycerides; inexpensive	GI side effects (nausea, diarrhea); risk of lactic acidosis. Avoid if creatinine is >1.4 in women; >1.5 in men; chronic heart failure, age >80 years, liver impairment.
Sulfonylureas (SFUs, second generation)					
Glyburide (DiaBeta, Micronase)	2.5–20 mg divided doses	Stimulate insulin release by receptor mediated, glucose independent mechanism	↓ A1c by 1%–2%	Well tolerated, inexpensive	Hypoglycemia, weight gain, allergy. Use with caution in the elderly or in patients with liver or renal insufficiency.
Glipizide (Glucotrol)	2.5–20 mg, divided doses				
Glimepiride (Amaryl)	2–8 mg q.d.				
Meglitinides					
Repaglinide (Prandin)	0.5–2 mg t.i.d. a.c.	Short-acting insulin secretagogue	↓ A1c by 1%–1.5%	Well tolerated, may have less risk of hypoglycemia compared to sulfonylureas	Hypoglycemia, t.i.d. dosing, more expensive than sulfonylureas
Nateglinide (Starlix)	60–120 mg t.i.d. a.c.				

Thiazolidinediones (TZDs)

Pioglitazone (Actos)	15, 30, 45 mg q.d.;	Insulin sensitizer; reduces insulin resistance peripherally	↓ A1c by 0.8%–1.8%	Pioglitazone: neutral to positive effect on CV outcomes, carotid IMT	Both agents: Weight gain, fluid retention, congestive heart failure, anemia; variable lipid effects, expensive; rare liver toxicity
Rosiglitazone (Avandia)	2, 4, 8 mg q.d. or 2–4 mg b.i.d.				Rosiglitazone: increased risk of MI

Alpha-glucosidase inhibitors (AGIs)

Acarbose (Precose), Miglitol (Glyset)	Both agents: 50–100 mg t.i.d. before meals, start with lower doses	Inhibit gut enzymes that break down carbohydrates	↓ A1c by 0.6%–1.2%	No weight gain	GI side effects, including flatulence, diarrhea, and cramping; rare liver toxicity.

Dipeptidyl peptidase IV inhibitor (DPP IVi)

Sitagliptin (Januvia)	100 mg q.d., 50 mg q.d. in stage 3 CKD, 25 mg q.d. in stage 4 CKD	Increases endogenous GLP-1 by inhibiting the enzyme that breaks down GIP and GLP-1	↓ A1c by 0.6%–1.8%	Weight neutral, well tolerated	Dose adjustment in CKD; risk of hypersensitivity; expensive

(continued)

TABLE 29-3 NON-INSULIN ANTIDIABETIC DRUGS *(Continued)*

Drug	Daily Dose	Mode of Action	Efficacy	Advantages	Disadvantages
Bile acid sequestrant (BAS)					
Colesevelam (WelChol)	3.75 g/day (6 tablets)	Reduction or delay in glucose absorption, or modulation of FXR mediated pathways	↓ A1c by 0.6%–1.0%	Weight neutral, lowers LDL cholesterol	Constipation, increased pill count, possible interaction with absorption of other drugs
GLP-1 Mimetic					
Exenatide (Byetta)	5–10 mcg b.i.d. a.c. by subcutaneous injection	Stimulates insulin secretion, decreases appetite	↓ A1c by 0.5%–1.9%	Satiety effect, promotes weight loss	GI: Nausea, vomiting, diarrhea in one-third. Must be given by injection; risk of pancreatitis; expensive
Amylin Analog					
Pramlintide (Symlin)	30–120 mcg t.i.d. a.c. by subcutaneous injection	Decreases postprandial BG by slowing gastric emptying, inducing satiety, enhancing GLP	↓ A1c by 0.5%	Satiety effect, flattens post-prandial BG	GI: nausea and vomiting. Indicated for use with MDI. Can contribute to hypoglycemia

TABLE 29-4	ORAL COMBINATION PILLS
Trade Name	**Generic Names and Doses**
Glucovance	Glyburide/metformin: 1.25 mg/250 mg; 2.5 mg/500 mg; 5 mg/500 mg
Metaglip	Glipizide/metformin: 2.5 mg/250 mg; 2.5 mg/500 mg; 5 mg/500 mg
Avandamet	Rosiglitazone/metformin: 1 mg/500 mg; 2 mg/500 mg; 4 mg/500 mg, 2 mg/1000 mg, 4 mg/1000 mg
Avandaryl	Rosiglitazone/glimepiride: 2 mg/2 mg;
Actoplus Met	Pioglitazone/metformin: 15 mg/500 mg and 15 mg/850 mg
Duetact	Pioglitazone/glimepiride: 2 mg/30 mg and 4 mg/30 mg
Janumet	Sitagliptin/metformin: 50 mg/500 mg and 50 mg/1000 mg

- Oral or injectable antidiabetic agents plus basal insulin
- Pre-mixed insulin therapy with or without oral agents
- Basal-bolus insulin regimen using intermediate- or long-acting insulin plus a rapid- or short-acting insulin for pre-meal doses and dose adjustments
- Continuous subcutaneous (SC) insulin infusion (via SC insulin pump)

Frequency of SMBG (self-monitored blood glucose) is tailored to the type of therapy and risk of hypoglycemia.

Lifestyle modification, incorporating both diet and exercise, is the first-line therapy for the prevention of diabetes and treatment of new-onset T2DM. Lifestyle modification that includes modest weight loss and adherence to 150 minutes (2.5 hours) of exercise per week is effective in reducing the progression from prediabetes to diabetes. Use of the Dietary Approaches to Stop Hypertension (DASH) diet that is enriched in fruits and vegetables and low in fat and salt has been shown to reduce some indicators of insulin resistance. Individualized medical nutrition therapy is recommended for all patients with diabetes, and generally requires several encounters with a registered dietitian or group education program. The UKPDS study showed that only 3% of patients treated with dietary therapy alone were able to achieve and maintain glycemic control over a 6-year period. Institution of insulin therapy should prompt additional dietary counseling to help the patient maintain consistent caloric intake or to instruct the patient in carbohydrate-counting techniques.

Pharmacologic Treatment

Oral Hypoglycemic Agents

Oral hypoglycemic agents (see Tables 29-3 and 29-4) are classed by mechanism of action: biguanide sensitizers, insulin secretagogues, TZDs, glucosidase inhibitors, and dipeptidyl pepdidase IV inhibitors (DPP IVi). The DPP IVi, sitagliptin (Januvia), acts by inhibiting the enzyme that breaks down endogenous glucagon-like peptide-1 (GLP1) and glucose-dependent insulinotropic polypeptide (GIP). GLP1 stimulates insulin biosynthesis and secretion in a glucose-dependent manner, and reduces the secretion of glucagon and inhibition of gastric emptying. Sitagliptin is weight neutral and does not cause hypoglycemia when used alone or in combination with other nonsecretagogue therapies. Recently, a bile acid sequestrant, colesevelam hydrochloride (WelChol), was shown to lower HbA1c in patients with T2DM, and is under consideration for approval as a diabetes treatment.

Of the oral antidiabetic agents, the insulin secretagogues have the highest risk of hypoglycemia. Metformin cannot be used in patients with reduced creatinine clearance or heart failure due to the risk of lactic acidosis from poor clearance of the drug and its metabolites.

TABLE 29-5 INSULIN REGIMENS FOR DIABETES MELLITUS TYPE 2

Regimen	Oral Agents	Insulin Types	Glucose Monitoring	Starting Doses
Oral agents + basal insulin—*Usual starting regimen*	Continue all types of oral agents. Use submaximal doses of TZDs.	Intermediate (NPH) or long-acting (glargine, detemir).	Fasting and as needed during the day	0.1–0.2 U/kg given at bedtime; increase until fasting plasma glucose is at target.
Pre-mixed insulin, generally bid.—*OK for patients with regular meal schedules*	Continue insulin sensitizers. TZDs: use up to 30 mg pioglitazone, 4 mg rosiglitazone.	70/30 NPH/regular; Humalog mix 75/25; NovoLog mix 70/30.	2–4× daily and as needed to avoid hypoglycemia	0.1 U/kg a.m. and p.m.; increase doses equally until blood glucose near the target range; evaluate with q.i.d. self-monitored blood glucose.
MDI regimens—*Helpful for patients with irregular meal schedules; may be necessary to achieve tight control*	Continue sensitizers at doses above if the patient is insulin resistant and there are no contraindications. Discontinue secretagogues.	Basal insulin: insulin glargine given at bedtime or detemir/NPH/Lente given q.d. or b.i.d.; pre-meal insulin: lispro (Humalog), aspart (NovoLog), glulisine (Apidra) or regular.	4× daily is required: before meals and at bedtime	In general, a total dose of 0.5–2 U/kg will be required. Give 50% as basal; divide the remaining 50% into pre-meal doses. Use adjustable scales ± carbohydrate counting for pre-meal dosing.
Continuous SC insulin infusion—*Many attractive features for patients*	Sensitizers may still be useful for insulin-resistant patients.	Lispro (Humalog) Aspart (NovoLog) and glulisine (Apidra)	4× daily and as needed	Conceptually similar to MDI regimens. Intensive diabetes education is needed.

MDI, multiple daily injection; TZD, thiazolidinedione.

TZDs should not be used in patients who have congestive heart failure due to the risk of edema and worsening clinical status. Rosiglitazone carries a black-box warning about a possible increase in the risk of myocardial ischemic events that was noted when rosiglitazone was compared with placebo. Because the agents have different mechanisms of action, most have been tested for use in combination with the other classes. Appropriate patient-specific prescribing can often provide excellent glycemic control with low risk of hypoglycemia, weight gain, and adverse effects.

Non-insulin Injectable Hypoglycemic Agents

Exenatide (Byetta), a GLP-1 mimetic, is a non-insulin injectable agent for T2DM. Its mode of action is to stimulate insulin biosynthesis and secretion in a glucose-dependent manner and to suppress glucagon. It is administered subcutaneously twice daily in one of two doses, 5 or 10 mcg, depending on patient tolerance. A once weekly formulation of exenatide is in phase 3 clinical development, as are other GLP analogs. Exenatide has a high incidence of gastrointestinal side effects, but has an ancillary benefit of contributing to weight loss while lowering blood glucose. Acute pancreatitis has been reported in patients taking exenatide, although the actual incidence is not known.

Another injectable therapy, pramlintide (Symlin) is approved for use in patients with T2DM who are also taking insulin. It is given in doses of 30 to 120 mcg subcutaneously before each meal. Pramlintide slows stomach emptying and improves satiety, which is reflected in reduced post-prandial glucose and modest weight loss. It is approved for use in patients on multiple daily injection (MDI) insulin regimens, and is most often used in overweight patients.

Insulin

Insulin may be required to achieve glycemic targets in patients with T2DM. In most cases, the oral antidiabetic agents should be continued and a basal insulin dose started at bedtime. If the response to one or more oral agents has been poor, or a contraindication develops, a more complex insulin regimen might be required to achieve glucose targets. **Diabetes education** is highly recommended when insulin is started or when the regimen is changed. The regimen should be tailored to the patient's needs and abilities and doses advanced to avoid prolonged hyperglycemia. Instruction in signs and symptoms of hypoglycemia and in methods of treatment is required. Instruction in the use of **glucagon** should be provided to the patient's household members. The long-acting insulins glargine (Lantus) and detemir (Levemir) have been shown to cause less nighttime hypoglycemia when used with oral agents in an evening dosing regimen. Multiple daily dosing regimens have been used to achieve tight glucose control and reduce the risk of hypoglycemia by carefully adjusting the pre-meal doses according to ambient BG, anticipated carbohydrate intake, and activity level. **Insulin requirements** vary with changes in weight, diet, activity, concomitant medication use, acute illnesses, and infections. Use of oral antidiabetic drugs in combination with insulin may help to reduce the insulin requirement and the complexity of the regimen; however, TZD doses should be submaximal (up to 30 mg pioglitazone [Actos]) to minimize the risk of edema and congestive heart failure (see Table 29-4). Refer to Table 28-1 in Chapter 28, Diabetes Mellitus Type 1, for an overview of insulin types and pharmacokinetics.

Concentrated insulin, as U500 (500 U/mL) is available only as Humulin R, or regular, and is an option for patients who require exceptionally large doses of insulin. An endocrinology consultation should be sought if U500 insulin use is contemplated.

Nonketotic Hyperosmolar Coma

Nonketotic hyperosmolar coma (NKHC) evolves over a period of time but presents emergently when **neurologic deterioration** occurs in the setting of **high glucose levels** and dehydration. Elderly or disabled patients with significant hyperglycemia who are unable to compensate for the free water loss with oral intake are predisposed to develop this syndrome. Patients with NKHC present with a plasma glucose that is generally >600 mg/dL, increased BUN and creatinine, increased serum osmolality, and a free water deficit of 2 to 6 L. Typically, the anion gap is normal or only slightly elevated, and the bicarbonate is >15 mEq/L. The effective serum osmolality is >320 mOsm/kg, calculated ([2 × measured Na (mEq/L)] + [glucose (mg/dL)/18] + [BUN (mg/dL)/3]).

The initial goal of therapy is to **replace volume** and **correct the free water** deficit with the infusion of appropriate intravenous fluids. The nature of the fluids (isotonic vs. hypotonic) administered and the rate of infusion are determined by the clinical circumstances. In general, most patients benefit from intravenous infusion of 1 L normal saline over the first hour. Subsequent fluid management is determined by the patient's hemodynamic status, corrected serum sodium (measured Na + 1.6 mEq/L for every 100 mg/dL over 100 mg/dL glucose), and free water deficit. Careful monitoring of volume status and electrolytes is required to avoid fluid overload or overly rapid correction of hypernatremia. As in DKA, patients in NKHC present with total body K^+ deficit, so K^+ should be added to intravenous fluids as soon as adequate urine output is restored and serum K^+ is <5 mEq/L.

Intravenous insulin can be given as repeated intravenous bolus doses (0.1 U/kg/1–2 hours) or via insulin drip (see Chapter 28, Diabetes Mellitus Type 1, for further details). The glucose may decline more rapidly in NKHC than in DKA, so hourly monitoring of glucose is required. Electrolytes and the clinical status of the patient should be checked every 2 to 4 hours and intravenous fluids adjusted accordingly. Subcutaneous insulin should be instituted after the patient's hydration status is normalized, the patient is able to eat, and the BG is ≤250 mg/dL. The mainstay of treatment is fluid resuscitation; however, care must be exercised in the process of treating elderly patients with tenuous cardiac and renal status. Neurologic changes should be evaluated to rule out stroke or other central nervous system (CNS) conditions. Mortality is high in patients who present with NKHC due to age and underlying conditions.

Goals of Therapy

The goal of diabetes therapy for control of hyperglycemia is essentially to **normalize BG values.** The ADA recommends that every patient achieve an HbA1c of <7%, but adds that there is no lower limit at which benefit is not observed. Other groups recommend that the A1c target be set at ≤6.5%. The overriding message is that treatment should target near normal BG values, with appropriate measures taken to avoid hypoglycemia. These measures might include careful prescribing of oral and injectable antidiabetic therapies, diabetes education, more frequent BG monitoring, occasional nighttime glucose checks, and use of more complex insulin regimens that more closely mimic normal physiology. The BG levels that are needed to achieve these glycemic targets are fasting and pre-meal glucoses, 90 to 130 mg/dL; postprandial, ≤180 mg/dL; and bedtime, 100 to 140 mg/dL.

Blood pressure control is important for prevention of nephropathy and retinopathy and for the preservation of renal function. The blood pressure goal for all patients is <130/80 mm Hg, and lower pressures may be helpful for patients with proteinuria. Angiotensin-converting enzyme inhibitors (ACEIs) are considered first-line therapy for patients with prediabetes and diabetes. Both ACEIs and angiotensin receptor blockers (ARBs) have been shown to slow the loss of renal function in patients with nephropathy. Patients with persistent proteinuria may benefit from the use of ACEI and ARB drugs in combination.

Management of **hyperlipidemia** is considered critical to reduce the risk of cardiovascular morbidity and mortality associated with diabetes. The reader is referred to Chapter 32, Diagnosis, Standards of Care, and Treatment for Hyperlipidemia, for further details about specific treatment goals and modalities. Low-dose aspirin (81–162 mg daily) is recommended for patients age >40 years and can be initiated at younger ages. Smoking cessation should be encouraged for all patients. Although **cardiovascular disease** is the leading cause of morbidity and mortality in patients with diabetes, recommendations for screening with provocative testing have not been elucidated for this high-risk group. In general, any complaints of angina or possible anginal equivalent symptoms warrant evaluation.

Screening and treatment for microvascular complications of diabetes including **retinopathy, neuropathy, and nephropathy** are crucial. Specific recommendations for the management of these entities are covered in detail in Chapter 27, Standards of Care for Diabetes Mellitus.

The incidence and prevalence of T2DM is increasing rapidly, and will severely tax future medical resources. Clinicians in every specialty will be called on to participate in the care of these patients to reduce the morbidity and mortality now observed. Increased awareness and communication of risk to individuals and populations will be critical to prevent or effectively manage this multifaceted illness.

KEY POINTS TO REMEMBER

- At the time of presentation, screen for signs and symptoms of end-organ damage such as retinopathy, nephropathy, and neuropathy.
- When evaluating patients with hyperglycemia, consider secondary causes of diabetes such as medications, genetic disorders, and other endocrinopathies.
- Dietary modification and exercise are crucial components of every treatment regimen.
- Meeting glycemic control targets reduces the rate of diabetic complications.
- Physicians and patients should modify treatment and lifestyle regimens aggressively to achieve glycemic targets unless limited by patient safety (hypoglycemia, comorbid conditions) or circumstances.
- Treatment of hyperlipidemia, hypertension, and tobacco dependence is essential to address the leading cause of mortality in diabetic patients.
- Treatment plans must be tailored to the individual patient's needs and capabilities.

REFERENCES AND SUGGESTED READINGS

American Diabetes Association. Standards of medical care in diabetes. *Diabetes Care* 2007;30(Suppl 1):S4–S41. http://care.diabetesjournals.org/content/vol30/suppl_1/.

Beckman JA, Creager MA, Libby P. Diabetes and atherosclerosis: epidemiology, pathophysiology and management. *JAMA* 2002;287:2570–2581.

Diabetes Prevention Program Research Group. Reduction in the incidence of type 2 diabetes with lifestyle intervention or metformin. *N Engl J Med* 2002;346:393–403.

Diabetes Prevention Program Research Group. Role of insulin secretion and sensitivity in the evolution of type 2 diabetes in the Diabetes Prevention Program. Effects of lifestyle intervention and metformin. *Diabetes* 2005:54;2404–2414.

Ennis ED, Stahl EJVB, Kreisberg RA. The hyperosmolar hyperglycemic syndrome. *Diabetes Rev* 1994;2:115–126.

Executive Summary of the Third Report of the National Cholesterol Education Program (NCEP) expert panel on detection, evaluation, and treatment of high blood cholesterol in adults (adult treatment panel III). *JAMA* 2001;285:2486–2497.

Hunter SJ, Garvey WT. Insulin action and insulin resistance: diseases involving defects in insulin receptor signal transduction, and the glucose transport effector system. *Am J Med* 1998;105:331–345.

Kitabchi AE, Umpierrez GE, Murphy MB, et al. Hyperglycemic crises in patient with diabetes mellitus. *Diabetes Care* 2003;26(Suppl 1):S109–S117.

Narayan KMV, Boyle JP, Thompson TJ, et al. Effect of BMI on lifetime risk for diabetes in the U.S. *Diabetes Care* 2007;30:1562–1566.

Park Y, Zhu S, Palaniappan L, et al. The metabolic syndrome: prevalence and associated risk factor findings in the U.S. population from the third national health and nutrition exam survey, 1988–1994. *Arch Intern Med* 2003;163:427–436.

The Diabetes Control and Complications Trial Research Group. The effect of intensive treatment of diabetes on the development and progression of long-term complications in insulin-dependent diabetes mellitus. *N Engl J Med* 1993;329:977.

Turner R et al. UKPDS 25: autoantibodies to islet-cell cytoplasm and glutamic acid decarboxylase for prediction of insulin requirement in type 2 diabetes. *Lancet* 1997;350:1288–1293.

U.S. 2000 Census Data. http://www.cdc.gov/diabetes.

UKPDS publications. http://www.dtu.ox.ac.uk/index.html?maindoc=/ukpds.

Weyer C, Bogardus C, Mott DM, et al. The natural history of insulin secretory dysfunction and insulin resistance in the pathogenesis of type 2 diabetes mellitus. *J Clin Invest* 1999;104:787–794.

Zimmerman BR, ed. *Medical Management of Type 2 Diabetes*, 4th ed. Alexandria, VA: American Diabetes Association; 1998.

Zimmet P, et al. Global and societal implications of the diabetes epidemic. *Nature* 2001;414:782–787.

Obesity

Richard I. Stein, Joan M. Heins, and
James N. Heins

INTRODUCTION

Obesity is the serious medical condition of having excessive body fat. Because body weight is more easily measured, and correlates fairly well with body fat, excessive body weight is often used as a proxy in classifying obesity. Obesity is associated with numerous major health problems, including type 2 diabetes, hypertension, orthopedic problems, and coronary heart disease, as well as psychosocial problems such as stigmatization, employment discrimination, and poor body image. Among children, obesity is a significant risk factor for being obese in adulthood. Given these health risks, as well as a major rise in the prevalence of obesity in the United States over the last two decades, obesity has recently been declared a global epidemic. Federal health officials have also called obesity the fastest-growing cause of death and disease, and the second leading cause of preventable deaths in the United States.

Definition and Classification

Obesity is usually defined and classified in terms of **body mass index** (BMI), a measure of weight adjusted for height (see Table 30-1 for calculation methods). In adults, an individual with a BMI of 25.0–29.9 kg/m^2 is considered overweight, and one with a BMI $\geq$30.0 kg/m^2 is considered obese. In children and adolescents, because the expected BMI changes during development, obesity is defined based on BMI percentile for sex and age (based on the Centers for Disease Control and Prevention's [CDC's] BMI-for-age growth charts available on-line at http://www.cdc.gov/nchs/about/major/nhanes/growthcharts/datafiles.htm), with the recent recommendation that BMI between 85th and 95th percentile be classified as "overweight" and BMI at or above 95th percentile be classified as "obese." This is a change from previous terminology that avoided the word "obese" in children because of the potential stigmatization. In adults, obesity is further broken down into subclasses according to BMI (Table 30-2).

Epidemiology

Results from national epidemiologic studies from 2003 to 2004 indicate that ~32% of U.S. adults are obese, and an additional 34% are overweight. This represents more than a doubling of the prevalence (15%) of obesity found in similar estimates from 1976 to 1980. For children and adolescents ages 2 to 19, the most recent prevalence estimates indicate 17% of youth are obese (approximately triple the prevalence from 1980), and an additional 17% are overweight. Some postulated reasons for the rising obesity prevalence include increased time spent in sedentary activities such as watching television, decreased time spent in physical activity, and increased food portions (see Causes section later in this chapter).

TABLE 30-1	FORMULAS FOR CALCULATING BODY MASS INDEX (BMI)

BMI = weight (kg) / height squared (m^2)

or

BMI = weight (lb) × 703/height squared (in^2)

Obesity is overrepresented in Hispanics and African Americans among female children, adolescents, and adults, and in Hispanics among male children and adolescents. Less epidemiologic information is available regarding obesity in Native Americans and Alaska Natives, but existing evidence indicates that obesity among these groups is overrepresented in all age groups. In the overall population, recent epidemiologic studies have found no sex differences for obesity in any age group.

Natural History

Weight gain can occur at any age but is more common at certain ages and under certain conditions. Birth weight is a poor predictor of obesity except in children of diabetic mothers, who have a higher risk of becoming overweight during their lifespan. Infants triple their body weight and double in body fat during the first year of life. Those weighing above the 85th percentile have a fourfold increase in risk of obesity compared to non-overweight infants if one or both parents is overweight. An increasing versus decreasing BMI between ages 5 and 7 is associated with a greater risk of adult obesity. Children weighing above the 95th percentile have a 3- to 10-fold higher risk of adult obesity. In adolescence, weight becomes a better predictor of adult weight, with those above the 95th percentile having a 5- to 20-fold greater chance of being overweight as adults. The presence of an overweight parent at any age has been found to greatly increase the risk of obesity for lean as well as obese children. During adulthood, pregnancy, oral contraceptive use, and menopause are

| TABLE 30-2 | CLASSIFICATION OF OVERWEIGHT AND OBESITY BY BMI, WAIST CIRCUMFERENCE AND ASSOCIATED DISEASE RISK |

Classes	BMI	Disease Risk for Type 2 Diabetes, Hypertension, and CVD	
		Waist Circumference Men ≤40 in (≤102 cm) Women ≤35 in (≤88 cm)	Waist Circumference Men >40 in (>102 cm) Women >35 in (>88 cm)
Underweight	<18.5	—	—
Normal	18.5–24.9	—	—
Overweight	25–29.9	Increased	High
Obesity: Class I	30–34.9	High	Very high
Obesity: Class II	35–39.9	Very high	Very high
Obesity: Class III	≥40	Extremely high	Extremely high

BMI, body mass index; CVD, cardiovascular disease.

conditions associated with weight gain for women, whereas transition to a more sedentary lifestyle in later years is associated with weight gain in men.

CAUSES

Obesity is a chronic disease caused by an imbalance between energy intake and energy expenditure that can be attributed to both genetic and environmental factors.

Fat Cells

Obesity is a disease that usually involves an increased number and size of fat cells. A lean adult has approximately 40 billion fat cells, each containing about 0.5 mcg of triglyceride. An obese adult usually has more (up to 120 billion) and larger (each containing up to 1.2 mcg of triglyceride) fat cells. The number of fat cells increases most rapidly in early childhood and late puberty and can increase as much as three to fivefold when obesity occurs at these ages. An increased number of fat cells (hypercellular obesity) is common when obesity develops in childhood.

Energy Intake

Food intake is essential for life, and the senses of taste and smell are fundamental components of the brain's reward mechanism. Determinants of food intake are environmental, cultural, and physiologic (i.e., appetite). Appetite regulation involves physiologic and psychological systems working toward energy homeostasis and hedonic satisfaction. Our understanding of the interactions of these systems is limited. A small imbalance in energy metabolism can, over time, result in obesity. For example, an intake of only 10 kcal/day more than expended (e.g., one stick of gum or one breath mint) could result in a gain of 1 pound in a year.

Appetite control relies upon highly complex cortical processing largely based in the orbital frontal cortex. Pharmacotherapies (see Management section later in this chapter) directed at the reduction of food consumption and appetite are being studied to modulate or influence the activity at these and other centers of the brain.

Energy Expenditure

Total energy expenditure (TEE) comprises resting energy expenditure (REE) for normal cellular and organ function (~70%), thermic cost of digestion (~10%), and physical activity (~20%). The REE of specific tissues varies widely and is not proportionate to their weight (see Table 30-3). Researchers have evaluated the possibility that human obesity is associated with deficits in energy metabolism. REE has been found to be higher in obese subjects than in lean subjects of the same height because of increased lean and adipose tissue cell masses. A small (~75 kcal/day) but potentially significant reduction in the thermic effect of food has been observed in obese subjects and may be related to

TABLE 30-3	WEIGHT AND RESTING ENERGY EXPENDITURE (REE) OF SPECIFIC TISSUES IN A LEAN ADULT	
Tissue	Percent of Body Weight	Percentage Contribution to REE
Organ	10%	75%
Adipose	20%	5%
Skeletal muscle	40%	20%

insulin resistance and decreased sympathetic nervous system activity. Obese individuals expend the same energy as lean individuals (matched for fat-free mass) when their weight is supported (e.g., sitting), but expend more energy during weight-bearing activities owing to the increased effort of carrying more weight. Studies of energy expenditure have not documented major differences in energy metabolism as a cause of obesity, but such studies are limited by being conducted at a single time point in a chronic condition and by being insensitive to small differences that may be additive over time. Therefore, the contribution of variations in energy metabolism to the pathogenesis of obesity remains uncertain.

Genetic and environmental factors influence obesity, both independently and interactively. Our understanding of the relative contribution of each comes from studies of twins, family registries, population-based clinical databases, and epidemiologic research.

Genes

It is estimated that 40% of variation in body mass in humans is a result of genetic factors. This component of human obesity is complex and involves both single genes and interactions among multiple genes. Monogenetic causes of human obesity are rare but have been identified from mutations in genes for leptin, leptin receptor, prohormone convertase 1, pro-opiomelanocortin, melanocortin-4 receptor, and SIM1. The Human Obesity Gene Map Database annually reviews all markers, genes, and mutations associated with obesity phenotypes. In 2005, 176 human obesity cases resulting from single gene mutations in 11 different genes were reported. A number of genetic syndromes are associated with obesity, including Prader-Willi, Bardet-Biedl, and Alström's syndromes. In these syndromes, obesity is accompanied by a constellation of other features, such as mental retardation, renal disease, or short stature. Most of the genetic contribution to human obesity is polygenic, and the specific genes involved are being actively sought.

Environment

A variety of factors in the environment impact eating and activity behaviors, thereby contributing to obesity. The wide availability of food, a trend toward consumption of pre-prepared foods, and an increase in portion sizes all contribute to high caloric intakes. Food also is an important part of social and cultural traditions that promote eating more, more often, and more calorie-dense foods. Physical activity is influenced by diverse environmental factors including mechanization, daily lifestyle routines, and the physical environment. Factors such as remote controls for electronic equipment to suburban living that requires cars to commute, shop, and socialize have systematically reduced opportunities for energy expenditure in routine activities of daily life. The effect of the "built" environment (e.g., food industry, housing, community design, transportation infrastructure) on obesity in the United States is a matter of public health concern, and initiatives are emerging to impact public policy.

DIAGNOSIS

The National Heart, Lung, and Blood Institute's classification of obesity by BMI provides a guide to assess the relative risk of obesity to a patient's health and to determine therapeutic interventions (see Table 30-2). This classification system is based on epidemiologic data demonstrating a relationship between increasing BMI and disease risk. Other factors, such as waist circumference, weight gain since young adulthood, fitness level, and ethnic or racial background, also influence the relation between BMI and overall disease risk. Bouchard classifies obesity into four phenotypes based upon fat distribution (see Table 30-4) with type II (truncal) and type III (visceral) being associated with the greatest metabolic risks, especially hypertension and type 2 diabetes.

TABLE 30-4	CLASSIFICATION OF OBESITY BY FAT DISTRIBUTION
Type I	Overall excess of body mass or percent body fat
Type II	Excess fat in the truncal-abdominal area: android obesity
Type III	Excess fat in the visceral compartment: visceral obesity
Type IV	Excess lower body fat in the gluteofemoral region: gynoid obesity

Adapted from Bray GA. Classification and evaluation of the overweight patient. In: Bray GA, Bouchard C, eds. *Handbook of Obesity: Clinical Applications*, 2nd ed. New York: Marcel Dekker Inc.; 2004:1–32.

Presentation and Evaluation

Obese individuals (BMI ≥30) rarely present to the physician because of their weight. They describe medical problems, often ones related to obesity, but do not identify their obesity as the primary complaint. Obesity is associated with an array of diseases. The relative risk of increasing BMI is presented in Table 30-2. The presence of coronary heart disease and other atherosclerotic diseases (peripheral arterial disease, abdominal aortic aneurysm, symptomatic carotid disease), type 2 diabetes, and sleep apnea place patients in a high-risk category for subsequent complications and mortality. These patients will require aggressive modification of risk factors in addition to the clinical management of the disease. Therefore, the obese patient should be evaluated carefully for short- and long-term morbidities. Discussion of risk associated with obesity includes both identification of factors that contribute to the risk of becoming obese and consideration of the risk that obesity contributes to morbidity and mortality.

Complications

Obesity has been linked with numerous serious and costly medical conditions. **Neurologic complications** include idiopathic intracranial hypertension and stroke. **Pulmonary complications** include obstructive sleep apnea, hypoventilation syndrome, asthma, and dyspnea. **Cardiovascular complications** include coronary artery disease, hypertension, pulmonary hypertension, and venous thromboembolic events. **Gastrointestinal complications** include gastroesophageal reflux disease, nonalcoholic fatty liver disease and steatosis, cholelithiasis, and pancreatitis. **Endocrine complications** include dyslipidemia (defined as elevated triglycerides and low high-density lipoprotein [HDL] level), type 2 diabetes, and polycystic ovary syndrome with hyperandrogenism and menstrual irregularities. **Musculoskeletal complications** include osteoarthritis (particularly of the knees and hips), low back pain, and gout. **Skin manifestations** include varicose veins, lymphedema, cellulitis, acanthosis nigrans, striae, and stasis dermatitis. **Neoplasms** associated with obesity include cancers of the breast, uterus, cervix, esophagus, pancreas, liver, colon, and kidney.

Medical Evaluation

The history should include inquiries into a family history of obesity, medications (e.g., exogenous glucocorticoids), age of onset of weight gain, diet and physical activity history, identification of potential triggers for excessive food intake, life stressors, previous attempts at weight loss, smoking history, and evaluation of socioeconomic status.

Evaluation of the degree of obesity should be an integral part of every patient's physical examination. Several assessment methods can be used, including anthropometric measurements and body composition analyses (e.g., dual energy x-ray absorptiometry

[DEXA], bioelectrical impedance, computed tomography [CT] scans, and magnetic resonance imaging [MRI]), although these studies are more commonly used in the research setting. For clinical practice, calculation of BMI and measurement of waist circumference provide an indication of health risk. For accurate measurements, height and weight should be measured without shoes, and waist circumference measured standing, after a relaxed exhalation, with the measuring tape placed around the abdomen at the iliac crest and parallel to the floor. Many standard scales have a maximum weight capacity that may be inadequate for measuring obese patients. Being unable to take a patient's weight because it is beyond the scale's maximum is humiliating for the patient. Even in less severely obese patients, embarrassment about weight and/or fear of being weighed may cause patients to delay or avoid seeking routine medical care. Therefore, it is essential for clinic staff to have a pre-determined protocol for sensitively handling patients who may be too heavy for the available scale and/or may be uncomfortable being weighed.

The BMI has its limitations. BMI may overestimate body fat in well-muscled individuals and in patients with edema, and BMI may underestimate body fat in elderly patients. Lower cutpoints (reduced by ~6 kg/m^2) are recommended to define obesity for some ethnic groups (e.g., South Asians, Chinese, and Aboriginals) and slightly higher cutpoints for overweight are recommended for African Americans (BMI of 27 kg/m^2). An increased waist circumference is associated with increased risk for type 2 diabetes, hypertension, and cardiovascular disease.

Diagnostic Testing and Laboratory Analysis

Laboratory evaluation is necessary to identify secondary etiologies and to assess for comorbid conditions that may already be present. Unfortunately, too often medical attention is directed to the comorbidity, and the obesity is under-treated. A successful reduction in weight (~10% of body weight) in these situations can be as beneficial as aggressive disease-directed therapy. Testing should include:

- Blood pressure (making sure that the cuff is large enough)
- Routine laboratory tests: fasting blood glucose, fasting lipid panel, thyroid-stimulating hormone (TSH), serum creatinine, and liver function tests
- Additional laboratory tests as indicated to rule out suspected secondary causes of obesity (e.g., 24-hour urine free cortisol to rule out Cushing's syndrome)

Test results will determine: (a) if the obesity is aggravated by or secondary to a disease state (hypothyroidism, etc.), and (b) the absolute risk associated with comorbid conditions (see Table 30-5).

MANAGEMENT

The primary treatments for obesity are therapeutic lifestyle changes, pharmacotherapy, and surgical therapy. Programs for therapeutic lifestyle changes may be conducted by a single interventionist or a multidisciplinary team of professionals with backgrounds in behavior-change, nutrition and/or exercise physiology, among others. Most obese patients derive significant benefit from losing weight, but weight-loss therapy of any kind is contraindicated in some cases, such as those with negative nitrogen balance, and for pregnant or lactating women, although care can be taken to avoid excessive weight gain during pregnancy. For patients with binge eating disorder or bulimia nervosa, or a strong emotional component to their overeating, a referral for specialized care will likely be warranted. Age alone is not a contraindication for treating obesity. Weight loss therapy that minimizes muscle and bone losses is recommended for older persons who are obese and have functional impairments or metabolic complications that can benefit from weight loss. Therapeutic lifestyle

TABLE 30-5 PARAMETERS FOR ASSESSING ABSOLUTE RISK STATUS

Cardiovascular risk factors (3 or more impart a high absolute risk)

Hypertension:	SBP $\geq$140 mm Hg or DBP $\geq$90 mm Hg or current use of antihypertensive agents
Fasting lipids:	LDL cholesterol $\geq$160 mg/dL or
	LDL cholesterol 130–159 mg/dL + 2 or more other risk factors
	HDL cholesterol <35 mg Hg
Glucose:	Impaired fasting glucose (110 and 125 mg/dL) (presence of type 2 diabetes is an independent risk factor for CVD)
Age:	$\geq$ 45 years for men
	$\geq$ 55 years for women (or postmenopausal)

Family history of premature CHD myocardial infarction or sudden death:

—male first-degree relative at $\leq$55 years of age

—female first-degree relative $\leq$65 years of age

Other: Cigarette smoking

CHD, coronary heart disease; CVD, cardiovascular disease; DBP, diastolic blood pressure; HDL, high-density lipoprotein; LDL, low-density lipoprotein; SBP, systolic blood pressure.

change should be considered the primary approach for all patients and will be essential even for those who also receive pharmacotherapy or surgical therapy. Obesity is a chronic disease, and a continuous-care model of treatment will, therefore, be needed for most patients. Behavior changes should be promoted as a permanent lifestyle change, rather than a short-term diet. Patients will need ongoing support for new behaviors, including check-in visits at least monthly during physician-initiated lifestyle-change therapy. Repeated formal weight-loss programs often will be needed over time. Such ongoing care needs should be considered a normal part of the program, so that patients do not feel that they have failed. In addition, given recidivism with behaviors and weight, at least annual follow-up is recommended for obese patients.

Lifestyle-Change Programs

Lifestyle-change programs involve helping a patient modify diet and physical activity behaviors to promote weight loss (or prevent further weight gain). Behavior-modification techniques are typically used as part of the process. Available data indicate that changes in dietary behaviors are most important for achieving initial weight loss, and that increasing exercise is important for maintaining weight loss in the long-term. Behavior changes in dietary intake and physical activity that result in weight loss may be promoted through brief meetings between the physician and patient, but more realistically, the physician may want to refer a patient to another professional (e.g., a dietitian), to a comprehensive medical weight management program, or to a commercial weight-loss program. Whichever of these options is chosen, patients should be educated that for most people a realistic weight loss goal (typically 10% reduction in body weight) is achievable and has clinical health benefits, although this goal may be much less than they are expecting. Discussing realistic goals of therapy upfront may help patients avoid frustration and disappointment down the road.

For physicians prescribing lifestyle change during office visits, the initial suggestion to begin weight-loss therapy should be approached with consideration that most patients will have initiated the visit for a regular check-up or for a comorbid problem and may not have expected a discussion regarding weight. It is essential that the physician tie the need for weight loss to medical issues and not to express or imply disapproval of or blame for the patient's obesity. To do so places at risk the therapeutic alliance that is necessary for successful outcome. *The Practical Guide: Identification, Evaluation, and Treatment of Overweight and Obesity in Adults* is a set of obesity treatment guidelines published by the National Institutes of Health and the North American Association for the Study of Obesity (now called the Obesity Society) in 2000. It includes an algorithm for lifestyle-change therapy that can be conducted during physician office visits. Basic steps include assessing the patient's desire and willingness to make lifestyle changes that would promote weight loss, briefly assessing current eating and physical activity behaviors, and setting concrete goals for making realistic gradual, modest changes to these behaviors, particularly dietary behaviors, to promote an energy deficit (i.e., taking in less calories than expending) that will lead to weight loss. The reader is referred to Brownell & Stunkard's handbook (see References and Suggested Readings) for more details on assessing readiness and setting goals.

An energy deficit of ~3500 calories is associated with 1 lb of weight loss; therefore, an energy deficit of 500 calories per day would be required to lose 1 lb per week. Some patients may not be ready to attempt weight loss but may be willing to modify dietary behaviors to prevent further weight gain. Finally, the physician should do periodic (at least monthly) checks on the patient's progress, praise even modest healthy behavior changes, and set ongoing goals for behavior change to promote further weight loss or maintenance of weight already lost.

When assessing dietary behavior, it is essential for the clinician to be nonjudgmental so that the patient feels more comfortable describing what he or she really eats. Questions should be asked in an open-ended format, most simply by asking patients to describe what they eat in a typical day, from the time they wake up to the time they go to bed. It may also be helpful to ask if eating is different on weekdays (or days they work) than weekends (or days they do not work), as weekends may involve less-structured eating, more snacking, and/or more eating out. Physicians may also choose to have the patient fill out the *Eating Pattern Questionnaire*, a quick tool developed by the AMA (available at http://www.ama-assn.org/ama1/pub/upload/mm/433/weight.pdf) that provides useful information that can be used to initiate the discussion about dietary habits.

One of the most essential behavior-modification tools for helping patients make changes in their dietary behaviors is a **food diary**. This tool can be used to assist with initial assessment of eating behaviors; the patient should be asked to record all foods and drinks for at least 3 days, typically including a weekend day. In addition, patients should be advised to keep a food diary to keep track of changes to eating behaviors over time. The AMA has an excellent formal written food diary on their website. Some on-line sites have free, web-based programs where an individual can enter the foods and drinks he or she has consumed and receive immediate feedback about the calories (and typically some information about the nutrients) contained in those foods and drinks. Web-based food recording may be a good option for some patients (e.g., those who like interactive on-line programs), but can be time-consuming and tedious to complete, particularly at first. Table 30-6 lists the essential features of a food diary, and Table 30-7 has some specific recommendations for reducing caloric intake.

Assessing a patient's current **physical activity level** should be done in a manner similar to the assessment of dietary behaviors by taking a nonjudgmental stance and using open-ended questions and/or structured tools such as the AMA's *Physical Activity Questionnaire* or *Physical Activity Calendar* (these and other helpful, related materials are available at http://www.ama-assn.org/ama1/pub/upload/mm/433/phactivity.pdf). Physical activity can be routinely tracked in a designated section of the food diary. Depending on the patient's risk factors (see Table 30-8), a stress test should be performed before recommending increases in physical activity. Exercise programs should be individualized to avoid exacerbation of medical conditions such as orthopedic problems. In some cases, a referral

TABLE 30-6 BASIC FEATURES OF A FOOD DIARY

Feature	Purpose/Explanation
Overall thoroughness and accuracy	Record all foods and drinks consumed; Reassure of no need to feel self-conscious
Time of each meal/snack/drink	To ensure the patient is not going too long, during waking hours, without eating
Amount of food/drink consumed	Patient should be encouraged to measure when possible, especially during the first 2–3 weeks
Calories	Can be determined from inexpensive nutrition books, nutrition websites, and/or from food labels

to a physical therapist may be warranted to ensure physical activity is done safely, especially for severely obese patients, those with severe orthopedic problems, and those with limited mobility. Table 30-9 provides examples of possible recommendations that can be made for moderate-intensity physical activity; these include hobbies/lifestyle activities (e.g., gardening) and programmatic activities/sports (e.g., running). More modest forms of lifestyle activity can also be recommended, such as taking stairs instead of the elevator.

The Practical Guide has more detailed information about simple ways patients can modify their eating and physical activity, which can easily be discussed during physician office visits. Whatever changes are made, monthly physician visits should be used to monitor progress with goals, set new goals as needed, discuss barriers to reaching goals, and assess weight change. If and when a 10% weight loss goal is reached, the physician and patient can decide if further weight loss or maintaining the weight loss already achieved is the most appropriate next step.

Comprehensive **medical weight management programs**, often affiliated with medical universities, typically involve a multidisciplinary staff of medical, behavioral, nutrition, and exercise professionals. Programs are usually conducted in a group setting, with weekly sessions for the first several months, gradually decreasing to less frequent meetings. Along

TABLE 30-7 SPECIFIC DIETARY CHANGE RECOMMENDATIONS

Example Types of Goals for Reducing Caloric Intake

Reducing portion sizes (specify which foods/drinks)

Reducing or eliminating intake of high-calorie foods, or switching to lower-calorie versions

Reducing fast food or switching to healthier fast food options such as sub sandwiches or salads (with low-calorie dressing)

Eating out less frequently (as restaurants tend to serve very large portions, and the consumer has less control over or knowledge of how the food is prepared)

Reducing or eliminating caloric drinks such as soda, sports drinks, or high-sugar juices

Using meal-replacement products (e.g., nutrition bars and shakes) for 1–2 meals and/or frozen meals for calorically and nutritionally controlled meals.

TABLE 30-8	CRITERIA FOR PERFORMING A STRESS TEST PRIOR TO RECOMMENDING INCREASED PHYSICAL ACTIVITY

Moderate-intensity Physical Activity

Known cardiovascular disease

Known heart murmur

Known pulmonary disease

Known metabolic disease

One or more signs or symptoms of cardiovascular or pulmonary disease

Vigorous-intensity Physical Activity

Any of the criteria above under moderate-intensity physical activity

Age 40 or older

Family history of myocardial infarction or sudden cardiac death

Hypertension

Hypercholesterolemia

Diabetes mellitus

Sedentary lifestyle

Note: In recommending physical activity, care should also be taken to avoid exacerbating or re-injuring orthopedic problems; refer to a physical therapist when appropriate. Adapted from Gill TM, DiPietro L, Krumholz HM. Role of exercise stress testing and safety monitoring for older persons starting an exercise program. *JAMA* 2000;284:342–349.

TABLE 30-9	EXAMPLES OF MODERATE PHYSICAL ACTIVITY

Hobbies and Lifestyle Activities

Raking leaves for 30 minutes

Walking 2 miles in 30 minutes

Pushing a stroller 1.5 miles in 30 minutes

Gardening for 30–45 minutes

Washing windows or floors for 45–60 minutes

Washing a car for 45–60 minutes

Structured Physical Activity and Sports

Running 1.5 miles in 15 minutes

Swimming laps for 20 minutes

Water aerobics for 30 minutes

Dancing fast for 30 minutes

Bicycling 5 miles in 30 minutes

Playing basketball for 15–20 minutes or volleyball for 45–60 minutes

Adapted from *The Practical Guide: Identification, Evaluation, and Treatment of Overweight and Obesity in Adults*, NIH Publication No. 00-4084; 2000.

with nutrition and physical activity information, programs usually focus on behavior modification and cognitive-behavioral topics such as goal-setting, outside factors that cue eating when physically not hungry, problem-solving, changing negative thought patterns that interfere with behavioral change, social support, and relapse prevention.

Nonmedical **commercial programs** are available that cover many of the same topics, although led by individuals of varying qualifications, often including former clients and/or peer counselors trained by the program. Weight Watchers is the only nonmedical commercial U.S. weight loss program that has randomized trial data with long-term follow-up indicating its success. In addition, some commercial programs offer at-home and on-line versions of their programs that may be more convenient for some patients, although no outcome data exist to establish their efficacy. Some commercial programs offer groups located at worksites for added convenience, and some employers offer free or nominal-cost weight-control programs as part of employee wellness initiatives.

Modifying Lifestyle-Change Treatments for Youths

Physician-initiated lifestyle-change, medical weight management programs, and commercial programs may be used to help children and adolescents lose weight as well. Typically, programs for preschool children will involve working primarily with the parents, programs for school-age children will involve parents and children, and programs for adolescents work directly with the youth and have varying degrees of parental involvement. The most important differences in working with children and adolescents are that they may not be motivated to make behavior changes or lose weight even though their parents want them to (indeed, the youths are frequently not the ones seeking out care), and they have far less, if any, control over household food shopping and preparation. Therefore, for school-age children or adolescents, their own motivation should be carefully assessed and parental involvement (or, for adolescents, at least practical support from the parent) will be essential.

Pharmacotherapy

Pharmacotherapy is appropriate for patients with a BMI ≥30 (or BMI ≥27 with obesity-related comorbidities) who have been unable to achieve weight loss goals after actively trying a lifestyle-change program. Weight loss medications should only be used as an adjunct to therapeutic lifestyle-change programs, not as a substitution for such programs, because pharmacotherapy is less effective alone than when used in combination with a comprehensive weight management program. Several medications (e.g., phentermine) are only approved for the short-term treatment of obesity. Only two medications, orlistat and sibutramine, are currently approved for long-term use. Pharmacotherapy for weight loss is only effective as long as the medication is being taken, so we recommend that only medications approved for chronic therapy be used in routine practice.

All of the approved medications act as anorexiants, with the exception of orlistat, which acts by blocking the absorption of dietary fat. Anorexiants act on satiety centers in the brain to decrease the amount of food eaten, the frequency of eating, or both. Methamphetamine is approved by the Food and Drug Administration (FDA) for short-term treatment of obesity, but it is a Drug Enforcement Agency (DEA) schedule II drug and should be avoided because of its addiction and abuse potential. Three anorexiant medications have been taken off the market because of increased risks of either valvular heart disease (fenfluramine and dexfenfluramine) or hemorrhagic stroke (phenylpropanolamine) associated with their use.

Orlistat (Xenical) binds to lipases in the gut lumen and blocks the digestion of dietary fat. Inhibition of fat digestion decreases mixed micelle formation and absorption of long-chain fatty acids, cholesterol, and certain fat-soluble vitamins. Orlistat does not affect the action of systemic lipases or lipases located in other organ systems, because it is minimally (<1%) absorbed from the gastrointestinal tract. The recommended dose is one 120-mg capsule with each meal (up to three times daily) in conjunction with a reduced-calorie diet that contains no more than 30% calories from fat overall and per meal. The most common side effects of orlistat therapy are gastrointestinal events (e.g., fatty/oily stool, increased defecation, fecal urgency). These typically occur early in treatment (within the first 4 weeks), and resolve spontaneously with continued use. In addition, because orlistat blocks the absorption of fat-soluble vitamins and beta-carotene, all patients who are treated with orlistat should take a multivitamin daily, at least two hours before or after ingestion of orlistat. Finally, patients should be forewarned of the possibility of gastrointestinal events during the early period of orlistat use, so they can plan to avoid situations where they do not have easy access to a restroom. Recently, orlistat has become available in 60-mg capsules (Alli) for over-the-counter use.

Sibutramine (Meridia) is a derivative of the amphetamine precursor β-phenylethylamine, which has been chemically modified to eliminate its abuse potential. Sibutramine enhances satiation by blocking the reuptake of monoamine neurotransmitters (serotonin, norepinephrine, and to a lesser extent, dopamine) in the hypothalamus. The most common side effects of sibutramine use are dry mouth, constipation, and insomnia, which are usually mild and transient. Because of its noradrenergic action, sibutramine treatment is associated with a dose-related increase in blood pressure and heart rate (e.g., 10–15 mg/day of sibutramine is associated with increases of 2–4 mm Hg in systolic and diastolic blood pressure, and increases of 4–6 beats/minute in heart rate). Some patients experience much larger increases in blood pressure or heart rate and require dose reduction or discontinuation of therapy. Contraindications for sibutramine include poorly controlled hypertension, coronary heart disease, congestive heart failure, arrhythmias, stroke, severe renal or liver dysfunction, or concomitant monoamine oxidase inhibitor therapy. Recommended starting dose for sibutramine is 10 mg once daily, taken in the morning to avoid sleep disturbance. To promote its mode of action, patients should be advised to pay close attention to when they feel full as a cue for when to end meals. Because of the potential side effects, blood pressure and heart rate should be closely monitored.

If there is no weight loss with either orlistat or sibutramine after 1 to 2 months of use (combined with lifestyle modification), the medication should be discontinued. If weight loss is achieved during the first few months of use, the drug should be continued as long as the patient maintains weight loss and does not experience adverse side effects. As mentioned previously, patients typically regain weight if successful pharmacotherapy is discontinued. Data from randomized controlled trials of orlistat or sibutramine in adolescents are very limited, but appear promising. Finally, when initiating pharmacotherapy for obese patients, prescribing physicians should be aware of the potential financial burden, as these medications are often not covered by insurance plans.

Surgical Therapy
Bariatric surgery may be an appropriate option for patients with a BMI ≥40 (or BMI ≥35 with obesity-related comorbidities). Bariatric surgery is the most effective available treatment for obesity. However, because of its invasiveness, it should be reserved for those who have not achieved adequate weight loss after attempting other, less intensive, treatment options. Contraindications include a history of noncompliance with medical care, certain psychiatric illnesses that may interfere with postoperative regimen compliance (e.g., uncontrolled depression, substance abuse, or personality disorder), or medical comorbidities that increase surgical risk unacceptably. Like pharmacotherapy, surgical treatment should only be used in conjunction with lifestyle change that promotes healthy diet and physical activity. Bariatric surgery is increasingly being considered for the treatment of obese adolescents, but bariatric surgery in adolescents still represents ≤1% of the bariatric surgeries performed in the United States, and systematic outcome data are lacking.

Bariatric surgeries fall into two general categories—those that primarily restrict gastric volume and those (e.g., biliopancreatic diversion) that primarily cause malabsorption. By far the most common surgeries—the Roux-en-Y gastric bypass and laparoscopic adjustable gastric banding—are in the former category.

Patients should be carefully evaluated to determine appropriateness for bariatric surgery. There are no uniformly accepted standards for such evaluations; however, they are best performed by a team approach involving the surgeon, a nurse practitioner or nurse, dietitian, and other specialists/consultants as needed (e.g., psychiatrist/psychologist, cardiologist, pulmonologist). In addition, patients should be advised well in advance about financial aspects of the surgery, especially to verify whether the surgery is a covered benefit with their insurance plan, and if so, to check the specific requirements for approval by their insurance plan, which vary widely. Following surgery, aside from monitoring for complications, patients should be checked for possible changes in their medication regimen if their comorbidities improve with weight loss. For example, weight loss following surgery may be associated with significantly reduced need for diabetes medications.

Roux-en-Y Gastric Bypass

The gastric bypass procedure is the most commonly performed bariatric operation, accounting for more than 70% of the bariatric surgery procedures currently performed in the United States. In this procedure, a small (10–30 mL) proximal gastric pouch is created by either stapling or transecting the stomach. The outlet of the pouch is anastomosed to a segment of jejunum that is brought up to the pouch as a Roux-en-Y limb. Digestive enzymes secreted by the pancreas and bile released from the gallbladder enter the second portion of the duodenum and do not come in contact with ingested foods until they reach the distal anastomoses with the Roux limb. Increasing the length of the Roux limb increases malabsorption and weight loss, and this length can be selected to promote a desired weight loss (e.g., based on the patient's BMI). Specific early complications of this procedure include hemorrhage, gastrointestinal leak with peritonitis, and splenic injury; specific late complications include stomal stenosis, marginal ulcers, staple line disruption, dilation of the bypassed stomach, internal hernias, specific nutrient deficiencies, and dumping syndrome. Depending on the patient's profile, the gastric bypass procedure can be performed laparoscopically by those with specialized surgical skills, and this method has advantages including less wound complications and faster recovery (although operating time may be longer for the laparoscopic procedure).

Laparoscopic Adjustable Gastric Banding

This surgery involves placing a silicone band around the upper stomach, just distal to the gastroesophageal junction. The band is connected to a subcutaneously implanted port that can be accessed percutaneously to change the size of the band circumference by injecting or withdrawing saline. Therefore, band and pouch outlet size can be adjusted over time, as desired, based on rate of weight loss. The incidence and severity of complications for this procedure are lower than after gastric bypass surgery. Specific complications from laparoscopic adjustable gastric banding include band slippage, esophageal dilation, erosion of the band into the stomach, band or port infections, and balloon or system leaks that can diminish weight loss.

Prognosis

Patients in comprehensive behavioral lifestyle-change programs reduce their body weight by an average of approximately 9% after about 5–6 months, but within one year following treatment cessation they regain about 30% to 35% of the weight they have lost. Average weight loss after one year is about 5% of initial body weight, which is still medically significant. There is some evidence that programs for school-age children may have better long-term effects compared to adult programs. Researchers are examining strategies for improving long-term maintenance of behavioral weight loss treatment in adults and children, including lengthening treatment duration, adding specific weight-maintenance education following weight loss, and providing various forms of continuing care (e.g., periodic group meetings, brief individual check-in meetings, mail and phone contact).

For pharmacotherapy, randomized controlled trials indicate that patients taking orlistat lose approximately 4% more of their body weight in the first year than do those taking placebo, and by four years the difference is about 3%. For sibutramine, a dose-ranging study found that patients taking sibutramine lose approximately 3% to 6% more weight, on average, than those on placebo after 6 months, depending on the sibutramine dose. For surgical therapy, data indicate that a gastric bypass results in an average of ~70% reduction of excess weight (i.e., reduction in the difference between current and ideal body weight) by 2 years postsurgery. In the long-term, patients lose approximately 25% of their overall body weight or about 50% of their excess body weight. Meta-analyses indicate that laparoscopic adjustable gastric banding results in somewhat less weight loss (~10% lower reduction in excess body weight), but that this difference becomes less extreme over time. Again, it is important to remember that for a positive prognosis with pharmacotherapy or surgical therapy, adjunctive lifestyle-change therapy will be needed. In addition, for all these treatment modalities, patients' comorbidities such as hypertension, orthopedic problems, and symptoms related to type 2 diabetes, often show notable improvement with weight loss.

Special Topics

Clinics and hospitals will need special equipment and furniture to accommodate obese patients. As two basic examples, extra-large blood pressure cuffs and hospital gowns should be available. The medical office should have wider chairs, including some with (for extra support when moving from supine to standing position) and without (for extra width) arms. Hospitals should have extra-wide wheelchairs, as well as some bariatric hospital beds that can support severely obese patients. A checklist of equipment and tools for office-based obesity care is available on-line from the AMA at http://www.ama-assn.org/ama1/pub/upload/mm/433/officeenvironment.pdf.

KEY POINTS TO REMEMBER

- Obesity is a chronic condition that requires ongoing care, including regular follow-up.
- Obesity is associated with many medical and psychosocial problems, and is steadily rising in prevalence.
- Lifestyle-change therapy is the core treatment approach. Surgical therapy or pharmacotherapy may be warranted, in conjunction with lifestyle-change therapy, if a patient is not successful with a lifestyle-change program alone. Pharmacotherapy only works as long as a drug is taken.
- Lifestyle change to initiate and maintain weight loss is difficult. The physician needs to be supportive and recognize the significant hurdles involved for most patients. Referral to a comprehensive weight management program or experienced professional can help patients achieve successful weight loss.

ACKNOWLEDGMENTS

The authors are indebted to Dr. Samuel Klein, Professor of Medicine and Nutritional Science, Washington University School of Medicine, for his considerate review of this chapter and to Ms. Jamie Manwaring for her feedback on an earlier draft.

REFERENCES AND SUGGESTED READINGS

Berkowitz RI, Fujioka K, Daniels SR, et al. Effects of sibutramine treatment in obese adolescents—a randomized trial. *Ann Intern Med* 2006;145:81–90.

Bray GA. Classification and evaluation of the overweight patient. In: Bray GA, Bouchard C, eds. *Handbook of Obesity: Clinical Applications*, 2nd ed. New York: Marcel Dekker Inc.; 2004:1–32.

Brownell KD, Stunkard AJ. Goals of obesity treatment. In: Fairburn CG, Brownell KD, eds. *Eating Disorders and Obesity: A Comprehensive Handbook,* 2nd ed. New York: The Guilford Press; 2002:507–511.

Buchwald H, Avidor Y, Braunwald E, et al. Bariatric surgery: A systematic review and meta-analysis. *JAMA* 2004;292:1724–1737.

Chanoine JP, Hampl S, Jensen C, et al. Effect of orlistat on weight and body composition in obese adolescents—a randomized controlled trial. *JAMA* 2005;293:2873–2883.

DeMaria EJ. Bariatric surgery for morbid obesity. *N Engl J Med* 2007;356:2176–2183.

Drent ML, van der Veen EA. Lipase inhibition: a novel concept in the treatment of obesity. *Int J Obes Relat Metab Disord* 1993;17:241–244.

Epstein LH, Myers MD, Raynor HA, et al. Treatment of pediatric obesity. *Pediatrics* 1998;101(Pt 2):554–570.

Epstein LH, Valoski A, Wing RR, et al. Ten-year outcomes of behavioral family-based treatment for childhood obesity. *Health Psychol* 1994;13:373–383.

Expert Committee Recommendations on the Assessment, Prevention, and Treatment of Child and Adolescent Overweight and Obesity: Summary Report. Barlow SE and the Expert Committee. *Pediatrics* 2007;120:S164–S192.

Flegal KM, Graubard BI, Williamson DF, et al. Cause-specific excess deaths associated with underweight, overweight, and obesity. *JAMA* 2007;298:2028–2037.

Gill TM, DiPietro L, Krumholz HM. Role of exercise stress testing and safety monitoring for older persons starting an exercise program. *JAMA* 2000;284:342–349.

Jelalian E, Saelens BE. Intervention for pediatric obesity: treatments that work. *J Pediatr Psychol* 1999;24:223–248.

Klein S, Wadden T, Sugerman HJ. AGA technical review on obesity. *Gastroenterology* 2002;123:882–932.

Klein S. Clinical obesity issues from an internist's perspective. *Obes Res* 2002;10(Suppl 1):87S–88S.

Kringelbach L. Cortical systems involved in appetite and food consumption. In: Kirkham TC, Cooper SJ, eds. *Appetite and Body Weight*. Burlington, MA: Elsevier Academic Press; 2007:5–26.

Kushner RF, Noble CA. Long-term outcome of bariatric surgery: an interim analysis. *Mayo Clin Proc* 2006;81:S46–S51.

National Heart Lung and Blood Institute (NHLBI) Obesity Education Initiative. Clinical Guidelines on the Identification, Evaluation, and Treatment of Overweight and Obesity in Adults: The evidence report. NIH Publication No. 98-4083. September 1998. p. 24. Available online at: http://www.nhlbi.nih.gov/guidelines/obesity/ob_gdlns.pdf.

National Institutes of Health, National Heart Lung and Blood Institute (NHLBI), and North American Association for the Study of Obesity. The practical guide: identification, evaluation, and treatment of overweight and obesity in adults. NIH Publication No. 00-4084. October 2000. Available online at: http://www.nhlbi.nih.gov/guidelines/obesity/prctgd_c.pdf.

Ogden CL, Carroll MD, Curtin LR, et al. Prevalence of overweight and obesity in the United States, 1999–2004. *JAMA* 2006;295:1549–1555.

Perri MG, Corsica JA. Improving the maintenance of weight lost in behavioral treatment of obesity. In: Wadden TA, Stunkard AJ, eds. *Handbook of Obesity Treatment.* New York: Guilford Press; 2002:357–379.

Pories WJ, Swanson MS, MacDonald KG, et al. Who would have thought it? An operation proves to be the most effective therapy for adult-onset diabetes mellitus. *Ann Surg* 1995;222:339–350.

Puhl R, Brownell KD. Bias, discrimination, and obesity. *Obes Res* 2001;9:788–805.

Rankinen T, Zuberi A, Chagnon YC, et al. The human obesity gene map: The 2005 update. *Obesity* 2006;14:529–644.

Razak F, Anand SS, Shannon H, et al. Defining obesity cut points in a multiethnic population. *Circulation* 2007;115:2111–2118.

Sjörström L, Lindroos AK, Peltonen M, et al. Lifestyle, diabetes, and cardiovascular risk factors 10 years after bariatric surgery. *N Engl J Med* 2004;351:2683–2693.

The Human Obesity Gene Map. http://obesitygene.pbrc.edu (Accessed on 7-7-2007).

Tsai AG, Wadden TA, Womble LG, et al. Commercial and self-help programs for weight control. *Psychiatr Clin North Am* 2005;28:171–192.

Tsai WS, Inge TH, Burd RS. Bariatric surgery in adolescents—recent national trends in use and in-hospital outcome. *Arch Pediatr Adolesc Med* 2007;161:217–221.

United States Department of Health and Human Services. *Healthy People 2010*, 2nd ed. With Understanding and Improving Health and Objectives for Improving Health. 2 vols. ed. Washington, DC: U.S. Government Printing Office; 2000.

Villareal DT, Apovian CM, Kushner RF, et al. Obesity in older adults: technical review and position statement of the American Society for Nutrition and NAASO, The Obesity Society. *Am J Clin Nutr* 2005;82:923–934.

Virtual Health Care Team. Lifestyle management of adult obesity. University of Missouri—Columbia School of Health Professions. www.vhct.org.

Wadden TA, Berkowitz RI, Womble LG, et al. Randomized trial of lifestyle modification and pharmacotherapy for obesity. *N Engl J Med* 2005;353:2111–2120.

Wilfley DE, Stein RI, Saelens BE, et al. The efficacy of maintenance treatment approaches for Childhood Overweight. *JAMA* 2007;298:1661–1673.

Hypoglycemia

Benjamin Cooperberg

INTRODUCTION

Healthy individuals maintain their plasma glucose within a narrow range. In the postprandial state, insulin secretion by the beta cell rises and glucose use and energy storage by target tissues increases. In the postabsorptive (fasting) state, plasma glucose is maintained between approximately 70 and 100 mg/dL, although it can fall further without causing symptoms in some individuals, especially in young women. Hypoglycemia occurs when plasma glucose falls below 54 mg/dL (3.0 mmol/L) with symptoms. The first defense against hypoglycemia is reduced insulin secretion. As glucose levels fall further, increased secretion of counter-regulatory hormones (glucagon and epinephrine) further reduces glucose use by tissues, increases release of glucose from liver stores (glycogenolysis), and increases glucose production and release by the liver (gluconeogenesis), all of which serve to raise plasma glucose levels. Later, other counter-regulatory hormones (cortisol and growth hormone) defend against hypoglycemia. These counter-regulatory mechanisms are essential for survival because glucose is the principle metabolic fuel for the brain under physiologic conditions. (After a period of prolonged fasting, the brain can use ketone bodies as fuel.) Hypoglycemia may occur when there is excess insulin, excess glucose consumption or loss, decreased counter-regulatory hormones, impaired responsiveness of target tissues to counter-regulatory hormones, or a combination of these factors.

Hypoglycemia is classified as **reactive** or **fasting**, depending on whether it occurs primarily in the post-prandial or fasting state, respectively.

CAUSES

Fasting Hypoglycemia

The most common cause of hypoglycemia is **drugs**. Insulin, sulfonylureas, and alcohol account for 70% of cases. Hypoglycemia can also be accidental, malicious, or surreptitious; factitious hypoglycemia should also be considered in any patient with a history of psychiatric illness, or access to insulin or oral hypoglycemia agents (e.g., health care workers, friends and relatives of people with diabetes). Although hypoglycemic agents used in the treatment of diabetes are the drugs most often implicated in iatrogenic hypoglycemia, it is important to remember that many other medications—some of which are commonly used—can also lower blood sugar. Included in this list are salicylates, quinine, quinolone antibiotics (especially gatifloxacin), haloperidol, disopyramide, angiotensin-converting enzyme (ACE) inhibitors, β-blockers, pentamidine, trimethoprim-sulfamethoxazole, and propoxyphene. Ingestion of alcohol during prolonged fasting (i.e., an alcohol binge) may lead to hypoglycemia by inhibition of gluconeogenesis.

In **critically ill states** such as end-stage liver disease, renal failure, starvation, and sepsis, glucose use may exceed production, thereby causing hypoglycemia. Counter-regulatory hormone deficiencies (adrenal insufficiency, growth hormone deficiency) rarely cause hypoglycemia unless there is more than one hormone deficiency. Non–islet cell **malignancies**, including lymphomas, hepatomas, leukemias, and teratomas, may cause hypoglycemia by secretion of insulin-like growth factor 2 (IGF-2), which can increase glucose use and suppress production.

When hypoglycemia is diagnosed, the endocrinologist is often consulted to investigate whether the patient has an **insulinoma**, a rare but life-threatening condition characterized by dysregulated insulin secretion by a pancreatic beta-cell tumor. The incidence of insulinoma is 1 to 2 cases per million patient-years. The median age at presentation is 47, with an age range from 8 to 82 years. Female-to-male ratio is 1.4:1. In younger patients, insulinoma is frequently associated with multiple endocrine neoplasia 1 (MEN1). Malignant insulinomas—10% of all such tumors—are more common in older patients. The symptoms of insulinoma include those of hypoglycemia. Insulinomas associated with MEN may be multifocal or malignant and may secrete other hormones such as gastrin or adrenocorticotropic hormone (ACTH). Because of frequent hypoglycemic episodes, these patients are prone to develop hypoglycemia unawareness, which may delay diagnosis.

Reactive (Postprandial) Hypoglycemia

Reactive hypoglycemia by definition occurs after meals. A common referral to endocrinologists is a patient who experiences symptoms of tremulousness, fatigue, anxiety, lightheadedness, decreased cognitive function, and excessive hunger about 2 hours after a meal. Usually, biochemical hypoglycemia is not documented. Most "reactive" hypoglycemia is often inappropriately diagnosed on the basis of low blood sugars during an oral glucose tolerance test (OGTT). At least 10% of normal subjects have blood glucose concentrations less than 50 mg/dL during an OGTT, and can have plasma glucose levels as low as 30 mg/dL without symptoms. Therefore, the **OGTT is not useful in making the diagnosis of reactive hypoglycemia.** When symptomatic low blood sugars after a mixed meal occur in patients with a history of **gastric surgery,** it is known as **alimentary hypoglycemia.** It has been speculated that rapid gastric emptying and glucose absorption lead to inappropriately high insulin levels for given glucose levels. If reactive hypoglycemia is observed in a patient status-post bariatric surgery, the possibility of **hyperinsulinemic hypoglycemia** must be considered as partial pancreatectomy may resolve these symptoms. These patients fall into the category of **non-insulinoma pancreatogenous hypoglycemia,** which consists of biochemical evidence of inappropriate hyperinsulinemia, often after a negative 72-hour fast, and hypertrophic beta cells on pathologic evaluation. Although fasting hypoglycemia is most characteristic of insulinoma, hypoglycemia in the post-prandial setting may occur. A rare cause of hypoglycemia is the presence of **autoantibodies** against insulin causing reactive hypoglycemia, or against the insulin receptor causing fasting hypoglycemia.

PRESENTATION

The diagnosis of hypoglycemia is confirmed by **Whipple's triad:**

- Symptoms of hypoglycemia
- Low plasma glucose concentration
- Relief of symptoms on raising the glucose levels

The neurogenic symptoms of hypoglycemia result from activation of the sympathetic nervous system, and the neuroglycopenic symptoms result from inadequate delivery of glucose to the brain (Table 31-1).

Neurogenic and neuroglycopenic symptoms begin to occur at a glycemic threshold of approximately 50 to 55 mg/dL. Plasma glucose levels of ~40 to 50 mg/dL are associated

TABLE 31-1	SYMPTOMS OF HYPOGLYCEMIA
Neurogenic (autonomic)	**Neuroglycopenic (brain glucose deprivation)**
Palpitations	Confusion
Tremor	Fatigue
Anxiety	Seizure
Sweating	Loss of consciousness
Hunger	Focal neurologic deficit
Paresthesia	

with gross behavioral changes, and levels of ~30 mg/dL and lower may produce coma, convulsions, and death. In individuals who experience recurrent hypoglycemia, these glycemic thresholds shift to lower plasma glucose concentrations. This phenomenon is known **hypoglycemia-associated autonomic failure (HAAF)** and is a common complication of tight glycemic control in people with diabetes. In most cases, avoidance of hypoglycemia for 2 to 3 weeks can restore awareness. In patients with poorly controlled diabetes mellitus, glucose counter-regulation and symptoms of hypoglycemia may occur at higher glucose concentrations.

MANAGEMENT

Absent a relevant drug history, critical illness, hormonal deficiency or non–beta-cell tumor, management of hypoglycemia centers on the question of whether the patient has an insulinoma, or other surgically curable condition. First, one must determine whether the patient really had a hypoglycemic episode with symptoms and a **documented plasma glucose <54 mg/dL**. If the patient's apparent hypoglycemia was asymptomatic, it is important to consider artifacts caused by improper collection, storage, or error in analytic methods. Measured plasma glucose can drop 10 to 20 mg/dL/hour after the blood sample is drawn, so it is important for samples to be processed quickly. In addition, large numbers of blood cells, as in patients with leukemia, can consume plasma glucose, thereby artifactually lowering the measured value, even in the presence of glycolytic inhibitors.

A **detailed history** is essential and should include the following aspects: the circumstances of the episode and its temporal relationship to meals or exercise, associated symptoms, weight changes, recurrence of the episode, drug/alcohol history, medication history, history of gastric surgery, personal or family history of diabetes or of MEN1 or MEN-associated conditions, comorbid conditions, and symptoms of other hormone deficiencies.

There are no specific physical findings associated with insulinoma. Other causes of hypoglycemia may be revealed by a complete **physical examination**, including signs of chronic alcohol use, other hormone deficiencies, or MEN1. Laboratory evaluation should focus on **documentation of insulin and C-peptide levels during an episode of symptomatic hypoglycemia** (plasma glucose <54 mg/dL). If the C-peptide is low in the presence of high insulin, exogenous insulin is indicated as the etiology. With high insulin and high C-peptide, screening for sulfonylurea and non-sulfonylurea secretagogues (repaglinide and nateglinide) should be performed to rule out surreptitious or inadvertent drug use.

To elicit an episode of hypoglycemia for **biochemical evaluation**, the patient may be instructed to initiate a supervised fast. It may be necessary to admit the patient to the hospital for a supervised 72-hour fast. In most healthy individuals, even after 72 hours of fasting, the plasma glucose remains >50 mg/dL. However, the blood sugar of some healthy women may fall below this level without symptoms. The patient may be asked to engage in

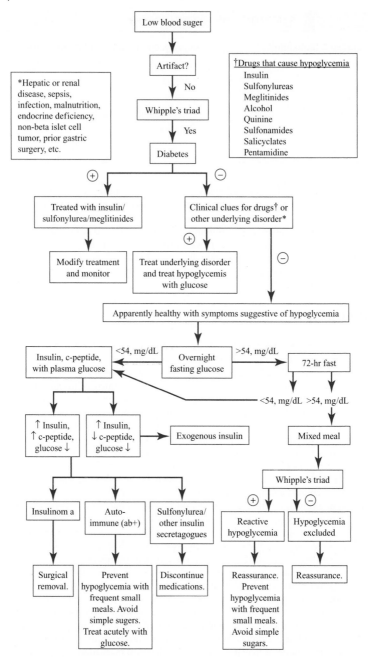

FIGURE 31-1. Algorithm for the differential diagnosis and management of hypoglycemia. (Adapted from Cryer PE. Glucose homeostasis and hypoglycemia. In: Larsen PR, et al., *Williams Textbook of Endocrinology*, 10th ed. Philadelphia: WB Saunders; 2003.)

moderate exercise to precipitate an episode of hypoglycemia. The fast is ended and the patient is treated for hypoglycemia with intravenous dextrose once symptomatic hypoglycemia is documented and appropriate samples are collected (diagnostic values in parentheses: glucose [<54 mg/dL], insulin [>3 μU/mL], C-peptide [>0.2 nmol/L], proinsulin [>5.0 pmol/L], β-hydroxybutyrate [<2.7 mmol/L]), and negative screens for insulin secretagogues are obtained. If Whipple's triad has been previously documented, the diagnostic fast can be concluded with an asymptomatic plasma glucose of <54 mg/dL. Alternatively, once symptomatic, the patient can receive 1 mg intravenous glucagon and a change in glucose of >25 mg/dL over 30 minutes is consistent with the diagnosis of insulinoma.

Immediate treatment of severe hypoglycemia includes intravenous dextrose (initial bolus of 1 ampule D50 (25 g) followed by infusion of glucose to maintain blood glucose >100 mg/dL) or 1 mg intramuscular or subcutaneous glucagon (in patients without ready intravenous access). Conscious patients may also be given readily absorbable carbohydrates (fruit juices, glucose tablets). However, to prevent recurrence, the underlying etiology must be corrected. Once a diagnosis of insulinoma is made biochemically, tumor localization is usually performed first by dual-phase thin-section multidetector computed tomography (CT) and endoscopic ultrasonography (this combination yields diagnostic sensitivity of nearly 100%). Intraoperative ultrasound may help precisely localize the tumor, especially when located in the head of the pancreas—the thickest aspect of the organ. The treatment of choice is surgical resection of the insulinoma, and this procedure is increasingly being performed laparoscopically. For solitary adenomas, surgery is curative. Multiple insulinomas associated with MEN1 are treated with an 80% subtotal pancreatectomy, although the recurrence rate is still 21% at 20 years. Medical therapy with diazoxide (notable side effects include edema and hirsutism), verapamil, or octreotide is reserved for patients who are not surgical candidates, who have recurrent disease and refuse reoperation, or who have inoperable disease. Frequent carbohydrate-rich meals may help prevent hypoglycemia.

An important role of the endocrinologist in the management of reactive hypoglycemia is reassurance of the patient and of the referring physician that the condition does not represent a life-threatening insulinoma. Treatment consists of frequent small feedings and avoidance of simple sugars. β-Blockers, anticholinergics, and intestinal α-glucosidase inhibitors may also have a role.

Patients should be educated about the symptoms of hypoglycemia and the appropriate corrective measures (including when to seek medical attention), and diabetic patients should be given a medical alert bracelet and a glucagon emergency kit.

One approach for the differential diagnosis and management of hypoglycemia is provided in Figure 31-1.

KEY POINTS TO REMEMBER

- Rule out artifact from collection, storage, or error in analytic methods.
- Confirm Whipple's triad for diagnosis.
- Healthy individuals can have low plasma glucose.
- The most common cause of hypoglycemia is drugs (especially insulin, sulfonylureas, and alcohol).
- Draw blood for diagnostic laboratory tests during the episode of hypoglycemia, and then immediately initiate treatment.
- The treatment of choice for insulinoma is surgical resection.
- OGTTs are not appropriate for diagnosis of reactive hypoglycemia.

REFERENCES AND SUGGESTED READINGS

Consoli A, Kennedy F, Miles J, et al. Determination of Krebs cycle metabolic carbon exchange in vivo and its use to estimate the individual contributions of gluconeogenesis and glycogenolysis to overall hepatic glucose output in man. *J Clin Invest* 1987; 80:1303–1310.

Cryer PE. Glucose homeostasis and hypoglycemia. In: Larsen PR, Kronenberg HM, Melmed S, et al., eds. *Williams Textbook of Endocrinology*, 10th ed. Philadelphia: WB Saunders; 2003:1604.

Cryer PE, Davis SN, Shamoon H. Hypoglycemia in diabetes. *Diabetes Care* 2003;26: 1902–1912.

Daughday W. The pathophysiology of IGF-II hypersecretion in non-islet cell tumor hypoglycemia. *Diabetes Rev* 1995;3:62–72.

Field J, Williams H. Artifactual hypoglycemia associated with leukemia. *N Engl J Med* 1961;265:946–948.

Lecavalier L, Bolli G, Cryer P, et al. Contributions of gluconeogenesis and glycogenolysis during glucose counterregulation in normal humans. *Am J Physiol* 1989;256(6 Pt 1): E844–E851.

Luyckx A, Lefebvre P. Plasma insulin in reactive hypoglycemia. *Diabetes* 1971;20: 435–442.

Marks V, Teale JD. Drug-induced hypoglycemia. *Endocrinol Metab Clin North Am* 1999;28:555–577.

Mitrakou A, Fanelli C, Veneman T, et al. Reversibility of unawareness of hypoglycemia in patients with insulinoma. *N Engl J Med* 1993;329:834–839.

Owen O, Morgan A, Kemp H, et al. Brain metabolism during fasting. *J Clin Invest* 1967; 46:1589–1595.

Seltzer H. Drug-induced hypoglycemia: a review of 1418 cases. *Endocrinol Metab Clin North Am* 1989;18:163–183.

Service GJ, Thompson GB, Service FJ. Hyperinsulinemic hypoglycemia with nesidioblastosis after gastric-bypass surgery. *N Engl J Med* 2005;353:249.

Service, FJ. Hypoglycemic disorders. *N Engl J Med* 1995;332:1144.

Tucker ON, Crotty PL, Conlon KC. The management of insulinoma. *Br J Surg* 2006; 93:264–275.

Diagnosis, Standards of Care, and Treatment for Hyperlipidemia

Anne C. Goldberg and Katherine E. Henderson

INTRODUCTION

Lipids are sparingly soluble molecules that include cholesterol, fatty acids, and their derivatives. Plasma lipids are transported by lipoprotein particles composed of proteins called **apolipoproteins**, and **phospholipids**, **cholesterol esters**, and **triglycerides**. Human plasma lipoproteins are separated into **five major classes** based on density: chylomicrons (least dense), very-low-density lipoproteins (VLDLs), intermediate-density lipoproteins (IDLs), low-density lipoproteins (LDLs), and high-density lipoproteins (HDLs). A sixth class, lipoprotein(a) [Lp(a)], resembles LDL in lipid composition and has a density that overlaps both LDL and HDL. Physical properties of plasma lipoproteins are summarized in Table 32-1.

LIPOPROTEIN METABOLISM

Exogenous Pathway

Dietary long-chain fatty acids and cholesterol are esterified and assembled into chylomicrons as triglycerides and cholesterol-esters, respectively. The predominant chylomicron apolipoprotein is apo B-48, but apo C-II and apo E mediate particle clearance. After entering the venous circulation from the thoracic duct, triglycerides are hydrolyzed to nonesterified fatty acids by the activity of lipoprotein lipase (LPL), with apo C-II serving as an enzyme cofactor. Triglyceride-depleted particles are called **chylomicron remnants** and are cleared by the hepatic chylomicron remnant receptor in an interaction mediated by apo E.

Endogenous Pathway

Hepatic triglycerides and cholesterol-esters are assembled into VLDL particles and secreted into the circulation. The main VLDL apolipoprotein is apo B-100 and it is a high-affinity ligand for the apo B/E (LDL) receptor. Triglycerides are hydrolyzed through the activity of LPL and apo C-II to create a triglyceride-depleted IDL particle. IDL may be cleared from the circulation by either the LDL receptor or the remnant receptor. It also may be further depleted of triglyceride by hepatic lipase to create a cholesterol-rich LDL particle. Circulating LDL enters the liver and extrahepatic tissues through interactions with the LDL receptor.

High-Density Lipoprotein Metabolism

Nascent HDL is secreted from the liver and small intestine as small apo A-I–containing discs. The discs acquire free cholesterol from peripheral tissues through the activity of the cholesterol efflux regulatory protein ABC1. The cholesterol is then esterified by the enzyme lecithin:cholesterol acyltransferase, with apo A-I serving as an enzyme cofactor. At

TABLE 32-1	PHYSICAL PROPERTIES OF PLASMA LIPOPROTEINS		
Lipoprotein	Lipid Composition[a]	Origin	Apolipoproteins
Chylomicrons	TG, 90%; chol, 3%	Intestine	B-48;C-I, C-II, C-III; E
VLDL	TG, 55%; chol, 20%	Liver	B-100; C-I, C-II, C-III; E
IDL	TG, 30%; chol, 35%	Metabolic product of VLDL	B-100; C-I, C-II, C-III; E
LDL	TG, 10%; chol, 50%	Metabolic product of IDL	B-100
HDL	TG, 5%; chol, 20%	Liver, intestine	A-I, A-II, A-IV; C-I, C-II, C-III; E
Lp(a)	TG, 10%; chol, 50%	Liver	B-100; apo (a)

chol, cholesterol; HDL, high-density lipoprotein; IDL, intermediate-density lipoprotein; LDL, low-density lipoprotein; Lp(a), lipoprotein(a); TG, triglyceride; VLDL, very-low-density lipoprotein.
[a]Balance of particle composition: protein and phospholipid.

this time, the particles are termed HDL_3. A larger HDL_2 particle is formed by acquisition of apolipoproteins and lipids released from delipidated chylomicrons and VLDL particles. HDL_2 is converted back to HDL_3 after removal of triglycerides by hepatic lipase or transfer of cholesterol esters to VLDL, IDL, or LDL particles. HDL transports cholesterol from peripheral tissues to the liver (reverse cholesterol transport) through transfer to apo B-100–containing lipoproteins or through clearance by the putative HDL catabolic receptor.

Atherosclerosis and Lipoproteins

Nearly 90% of patients with coronary heart disease (CHD) have some form of dyslipidemia. Increased levels of LDL, remnant lipoproteins, and Lp(a), as well as decreased levels of HDL, have all been associated with an increased risk of premature vascular disease.

Clinical Dyslipoproteinemias

Most dyslipidemias are multifactorial in etiology and reflect the effects of uncharacterized genetic influences coupled with diet, activity, smoking, alcohol use, and comorbid conditions such as obesity and diabetes mellitus. Differential diagnosis of the major lipid abnormalities is summarized in Table 32-2. The major genetic dyslipoproteinemias are reviewed in Table 32-3.

STANDARDS OF CARE FOR HYPERLIPIDEMIA

LDL cholesterol–lowering therapy, particularly with hydroxymethylglutaryl-coenzyme A (HMG-CoA) reductase inhibitors, lowers the risk of CHD-related death, morbidity, and revascularization procedures in hypercholesterolemic patients with (secondary prevention) or without (primary prevention) known CHD. Therefore, identification and management of high LDL cholesterol is the primary goal of the National Cholesterol Education Program's third expert report on cholesterol management in adults, or Adult Treatment Program III (ATP III).

The ATP III executive summary and full report can be viewed online at http://www.nhlbi.nih.gov/guidelines/cholesterol/.

TABLE 32-2	DIFFERENTIAL DIAGNOSIS OF MAJOR LIPID ABNORMALITIES

Lipid Abnormality	Primary Disorders	Secondary Disorders
Hypercholesterolemia	Polygenic, familial hypercholesterolemia, familial defective apo B-100	Hypothyroidism, nephrotic syndrome
Hypertriglyceridemia	Lipoprotein lipase deficiency, apo C-II deficiency, familial hypertriglyceridemia	Diabetes mellitus, obesity, metabolic syndrome, alcohol use, oral estrogen
Combined hyperlipidemia	Familial combined hyperlipidemia, type III hyperlipoproteinemia	Diabetes mellitus, obesity, metabolic syndrome, hypothyroidism, nephrotic syndrome
Low HDL	Familial alpha lipoproteinemia, Tangier's disease, familial HDL deficiency, lecithin:cholesterol acyltransferase deficiency	Diabetes mellitus, metabolic syndrome, hypertriglyceridemia, smoking

HDL, high-density lipoprotein.

Screening

Screening for hypercholesterolemia should begin **in all adults age 20 years or older**. Screening is best performed with a lipid profile (total cholesterol, LDL cholesterol, HDL cholesterol, and triglycerides) obtained after a 12-hour fast. If a fasting lipid panel cannot be obtained, total and HDL cholesterol should be measured. Measurement of fasting lipids is indicated if the total cholesterol is ≥ 200 mg/dL or HDL cholesterol is ≤ 40 mg/dL. If lipids are unremarkable and the patient has no major risk factors for CHD (Table 32-4), then screening can be performed every 5 years. Patients hospitalized for an acute coronary syndrome or coronary revascularization should have a lipid panel obtained within 24 hours of admission if lipid levels are unknown. Individuals with hyperlipidemia should be evaluated for potential **secondary causes**, including hypothyroidism; diabetes mellitus; obstructive liver disease; chronic renal insufficiency or nephrotic syndrome; or medications such as estrogens, progestins, anabolic steroids, and corticosteroids.

Risk Assessment

A major innovation of ATP III is a formal method of CHD risk assessment. ATP III now recognizes **five categories of CHD risk**—very high, high, moderately high, moderate, and lower risk. These CHD risk categories are defined in Table 32-5. Diabetes, noncoronary atherosclerosis (symptomatic cerebrovascular disease, peripheral artery disease, abdominal aortic aneurysm), or multiple risk factors conferring a 10-year CHD risk of more than 20% are considered CHD risk equivalents in ATP III. Risk assessment for patients without known CHD or CHD risk equivalents begins with consideration of five risk factors summarized in Table 32-4. A Framingham point score should be determined for any individual with two or more non–LDL cholesterol risk factors. (Framingham point score

TABLE 32-3 REVIEW OF MAJOR GENETIC DYSLIPOPROTEINEMIAS

Type of Genetic Dyslipidemia	Typical Lipid Profile	Type of Inheritance Pattern	Phenotypic Features	Other Information
Familial hypercholesterolemia (FH)	• Increased total (>300mg/dL) and LDL (>250 mg/dL) cholesterol • Homozygous form (rare) can have total cholesterol >600 mg/dL and LDL >550 mg/dL	Autosomal dominant	• Premature CAD • Tendon xanthomas • Xanthelasmata • Premature arcus corneae	Caused by mutations of the LDL receptor that lead to defective uptake and degradation of LDL
Familial combined hyperlipidemia (FCH)	• High levels of VLDL, LDL, or both • LDL apo B-100 level >130 mg/dL	Autosomal dominant	• Premature CAD • Patients do *not* develop tendon xanthomas	Genetic and metabolic defects are not established
Familial defective apolipoprotein B-100	• Similar to familial hypercholesterolemia		• Similar to familial hypercholesterolemia	Most all cases are caused by a glutamine for arginine mutation at amino acid 3500 of apo B-100
Type III hyperlipoproteinemia (familial dysbetalipoproteinemia)	• Symmetric elevations of cholesterol and triglycerides (300–500 mg/dL) • Elevated VLDL-to-triglyceride ratio >0.3)	Autosomal recessive	• Premature CAD • Tuberous or tuberoeruptive xanthomas • Planar xanthomas of the palmar creases are essentially pathognomonic	Many homozygotes are normolipidemic, and emergence of hyperlipidemia often requires a secondary metabolic factor such as diabetes mellitus, hypothyroidism, or obesity

Chylomicronemia syndrome	• Most patients have triglycerides in the range of 150–500 mg/dL • Clinical manifestations occur when triglycerides exceed 1500 mg/dL	Onset before puberty indicates deficiency of lipoprotein lipase or apo C-II, both autosomal recessive Familial hypertriglyceridemia is an autosomal-dominant disorder caused by overproduction of VLDL triglycerides and manifests in adults	• Eruptive xanthomas • Lipemia retinalis • Pancreatitis • Hepatosplenomegaly	Patients with familial hypertriglyceridemia or FCH may develop chylomicronemia syndrome in the presence of secondary factors such as obesity, alcohol use, or diabetes
Familial hypoalphalipoproteinemia	• HDL levels below the 10th percentile (<30 mg/dL for men and <40 mg/dL for premenopausal women)	Autosomal dominant	• Premature CAD • No characteristic findings on physical exam	

CAD, coronary artery disease; LDL, low-density lipoprotein; VLDL, very-low-density lipoprotein.

TABLE 32-4	MAJOR RISK FACTORS (EXCLUSIVE OF LOW-DENSITY LIPOPROTEIN [LDL] CHOLESTEROL) THAT MODIFY LDL GOALS[a]

Cigarette smoking

Hypertension (blood pressure ≥140/90 mm Hg or on antihypertensive medication)

Low high-density lipoprotein (HDL) cholesterol (<40 mg/dL)[b]

Family history of premature coronary heart disease (CHD) (CHD in male first-degree relative < age 55 years; CHD in female first-degree relative <65 years)

Age (men ≥45 years; women ≥55 years)

---

[a]In Adult Treatment Panel III, diabetes is regarded as a CHD risk equivalent.

[b]HDL cholesterol ≥60 mg/dL counts as a "negative" risk factor; its presence removes one risk factor from the total count.

From executive summary of the third report of the National Cholesterol Education Program (NCEP) expert panel on detection, evaluation, and treatment of high blood cholesterol in adults (Adult Treatment Panel III). *JAMA* 2001;285;2486, with permission.

algorithms for men and women are summarized in Table 32-6.) Patients with multiple non–LDL cholesterol CHD risk factors are then divided into those with a 10-year CHD risk >20%, 10% to 20%, or <10%. Presently, emerging risk factors (obesity; sedentary lifestyle; homocysteine, prothrombotic, and proinflammatory factors; and impaired fasting glucose) do not affect risk assessment, although they may influence clinical judgment when determining therapeutic options.

TABLE 32-5	ADULT TREATMENT PROGRAM III (ATP III) CATEGORIES OF CORONARY HEART DISEASE (CHD) RISK

Category	Definition
Very high risk	CHD and:
	Multiple risk factors (especially diabetes)
	Severe and poorly controlled risk factors (especially continued cigarette smoking)
	Multiple risk factors of the metabolic syndrome
	Acute coronary syndromes
High risk	CHD or CHD risk equivalent
Moderately high risk	2+ risk factors and 10-year CHD risk 10%–20%
Moderate risk	2+ risk factors and 10-year CHD risk <10%
Lower risk	0–1 risk factors

Adapted from Grundy SM, Cleeman C, Merz NB, et al. Implications of recent clinical trials for the National Cholesterol Education Program Adult Treatment Panel III Guidelines. *Circulation* 2004;110:227.

TABLE 32-6 · ESTIMATE OF 10-YEAR RISK (FRAMINGHAM POINT SCORES) FOR MEN AND WOMEN

Estimate of 10-year Risk for Men

Age (years)	Points
20–34	–9
35–39	–4
40–44	0
45–49	3
50–54	6
55–59	8
60–64	10
65–69	11
70–74	12
75–79	13

Total Cholesterol	Points Age 20–39	Age 40–49	Age 50–59	Age 60–69	Age 70–79
<160	0	0	0	0	0
160–199	4	3	2	1	0
200–239	7	5	3	1	0
240–279	9	6	4	2	1
≥280	11	8	5	3	1

	Points Age 20–39	Age 40–49	Age 50–59	Age 60–69	Age 70–79
Nonsmoker	0	0	0	0	0
Smoker	8	5	3	1	1

HDL (mg/dL)	Points	Systolic BP (mm Hg)	If Untreated	If Treated
≥60	–1	<120	0	0
50–59	0	120–129	0	1
40–49	1	130–139	1	2
<40	2	140–159	1	2
		≥160	2	3

Point Total	10-year Risk (%)	Point Total	10-year Risk (%)
<0	<1	9	5
0	1	10	6
1	1	11	8
2	1	12	10
3	1	13	12

(continued)

TABLE 32-6	ESTIMATE OF 10-YEAR RISK (FRAMINGHAM POINT SCORES) FOR MEN AND WOMEN *(Continued)*

Point Total	10-year Risk (%)	Point Total	10-year Risk (%)
4	1	14	16
5	2	15	20
6	2	16	25
7	3	≥17	≥30
8	4		

Estimate of 10-year Risk in Women

Age (years)	Points
20–34	−7
35–39	−3
40–44	0
45–49	3
50–54	6
55–59	8
60–64	10
65–69	12
70–74	14
75–79	16

Total Cholesterol	Points Age 20–39	Age 40–49	Age 50–59	Age 60–69	Age 70–79
<160	0	0	0	0	0
160–199	4	3	2	1	1
200–239	8	6	4	2	1
240–279	11	8	5	3	2
≥280	13	10	7	4	2

	Points Age 20–39	Age 40–49	Age 50–59	Age 60–69	Age 70–79
Nonsmoker	0	0	0	0	0
Smoker	9	7	4	2	1

HDL (mg/dL)	Points	Systolic BP (mm Hg)	If Untreated	If Treated
≥60	−1	<120	0	0
50–59	0	120–129	1	3
40–49	1	130–139	2	4
<40	2	140–159	3	5
		≥160	4	6

TABLE 32-6	ESTIMATE OF 10-YEAR RISK (FRAMINGHAM POINT SCORES) FOR MEN AND WOMEN (*Continued*)		
Point Total	10-year Risk (%)	Point Total	10-year Risk (%)
<9	<1	17	5
9	1	18	6
10	1	19	8
11	1	20	11
12	1	21	14
13	2	22	17
		23	22
14	2	24	27
15	3	≥25	≥30
16	4		

BP, blood pressure; HDL, high-density lipoprotein.

From Executive summary of the third report of the National Cholesterol Education Program (NCEP) expert panel on detection, evaluation, and treatment of high blood cholesterol in adults (Adult Treatment Panel III). *JAMA* 2001;285:2486.

Therapy for Hypercholesterolemia

ATP III thresholds for initiating cholesterol-lowering therapy with **therapeutic lifestyle change** (TLC; diet and exercise) and **hypolipidemic drugs** are summarized in Table 32-7. All patients requiring cholesterol-lowering therapy should implement a diet restricted in total and saturated fat intake in accordance with ATP III recommendations (Table 32-8). Moderate exercise and weight reduction is also recommended. A registered dietitian may be helpful to plan and start a fat-restricted and weight loss–promoting diet.

The ATP III LDL cholesterol treatment target for all high-risk patients is <100 mg/dL. For CHD patients in the **very-high-risk category**, an LDL cholesterol <70 mg/dL is a therapeutic option. An LDL cholesterol of ≥100 mg/dL is now identified as the threshold for simultaneous treatment with TLC and lipid-lowering agents. On the basis of outcomes in the Heart Protection Study (HPS), lipid-lowering drug therapy is also an option for patients with CHD and baseline LDL cholesterol <100 mg/dL. If a high-risk patient has hypertriglyceridemia or low HDL cholesterol, a fibrate or nicotinic acid (niacin) may be added to cholesterol-lowering therapy.

Patients with two or more non–LDL cholesterol risk factors and a Framingham point score predicting a 10-year CHD risk of 10% to 20% are considered at **moderately high risk** of CHD. Pharmacotherapy should be initiated if LDL cholesterol is ≥130 mg/dL. ATP III identifies an LDL cholesterol target <100 mg/dL as optional for this group, with drug therapy to be considered for patients with baseline LDL cholesterol 100 to 129 mg/dL. Patients with two or more risk factors and a 10-year risk <10% are candidates for drug therapy when LDL cholesterol remains ≥160 mg/dL despite TLC.

For **low-risk patients** (0–1 risk factors), cholesterol-lowering therapy should be considered if the LDL cholesterol is ≥190 mg/dL, especially for patients who have undergone a 3-month trial of TLC. Patients with very high LDL concentrations (≥190 mg/dL) often have a hereditary dyslipidemia and require treatment with multiple lipid-lowering agents.

TABLE 32-7	ADULT TREATMENT PROGRAM III (ATP III) LOW-DENSITY LIPOPROTEIN CHOLESTEROL (LDL-C) GOALS AND THRESHOLDS FOR THERAPEUTIC LIFESTYLE CHANGE (TLC) AND DRUG THERAPY		
Category	**LDL-C Goal**	**Start TLC**	**Start Drug Therapy**
Very high risk	<70 mg/dL	Any LDL-C	LDL-C ≥70 mg/dL
High risk	<100 mg/dL	≥100 mg/dL	≥100 mg/dL (consider if baseline LDL-C <100 mg/dL)
Moderately high risk	<130 mg/dL (<100 mg/dL optional)	≥130 mg/dL	≥130 mg/dL (optional if baseline LDL-C 100–129 mg/dL)
Moderate risk	<130 mg/dL	≥130 mg/dL	≥160 mg/dL
Lower risk	<160 mg/dL	≥160 mg/dL	≥190 mg/dL (optional if baseline LDL-C 160–189 mg/dL)

Adapted from Grundy SM, Cleeman C, Merz NB, et al. Implications of recent clinical trials for the National Cholesterol Education Program Adult Treatment Panel III Guidelines. *Circulation* 2004;110:227.

TABLE 32-8	NUTRIENT COMPOSITION OF THE THERAPEUTIC LIFESTYLE CHANGE (TLC) DIET
Nutrient	**Recommended Intake**
Saturated fat[a]	<7% of total calories
Polyunsaturated fat	Up to 10% of total calories
Monounsaturated fat	Up to 20% of total calories
Total fat	25%–35% of total calories
Carbohydrate[b]	50%–60% of total calories
Fiber	20–30 g/day
Protein	~15% of total calories
Cholesterol	<200 mg/day
Total calories (energy)[c]	Balance energy intake and expenditure to maintain desirable body weight/prevent weight gain

[a] Trans fatty acids are another low-density lipoprotein (LDL)–raising fat that should be kept at a low intake.
[b] Carbohydrate should be derived predominantly from foods rich in complex carbohydrates, including grains (especially whole grains), fruits, and vegetables.
[c] Daily energy expenditure should include at least moderate physical activity (contributing ~200 kcal/day).
From Executive summary of the third report of the National Cholesterol Education Program (NCEP) expert panel on detection, evaluation, and treatment of high blood cholesterol in adults (Adult Treatment Panel III). *JAMA* 2001;285:2486, with permission.

These patients should be referred to a lipid specialist, and family members should be screened with a fasting lipid battery. When LDL cholesterol is 160 to 189 mg/dL, drug therapy should be considered if the patient has a significant risk factor for cardiovascular disease, such as heavy tobacco use, poorly controlled hypertension, strong family history of early CHD, or low HDL cholesterol.

Response to therapy should be assessed after 6 weeks and the dose of medication titrated if the LDL cholesterol treatment target is not achieved. The initial dose of a cholesterol-lowering drug should be sufficient to achieve a 30% to 40% reduction in LDL cholesterol. If target LDL cholesterol has not been reached after 12 weeks, current therapy should be intensified by further dose titration, adding another lipid-lowering agent, or referral to a lipid specialist. Patients at goal should be monitored every 4 to 6 months.

Metabolic Syndrome

The constellation of abdominal obesity, hypertension, glucose intolerance, and an atherogenic lipid profile (hypertriglyceridemia; low HDL cholesterol; and small, dense LDL cholesterol) characterizes a condition called the **metabolic syndrome**. ATP III diagnostic criteria for the metabolic syndrome are summarized in Table 32-9. Approximately 22% of Americans qualify for a diagnosis of the metabolic syndrome by ATP III criteria. Prevalence is increased in older individuals, women, Hispanic Americans, and African Americans. Two large epidemiologic studies have demonstrated elevated all-cause and coronary mortality among men with the metabolic syndrome.

ATP III recognizes the metabolic syndrome as a **secondary treatment target** after LDL cholesterol is controlled. The report recommends treating the underlying causes of metabolic syndrome (overweight/obesity, physical inactivity) by implementing weight loss and aerobic exercise and managing cardiovascular risks, such as hypertension, that may persist despite lifestyle changes.

Hypertriglyceridemia

Recent analyses suggest that hypertriglyceridemia is an **independent cardiovascular risk factor**. Hypertriglyceridemia is often observed in the metabolic syndrome, and there are many potential etiologies for hypertriglyceridemia, including obesity, diabetes mellitus,

TABLE 32-9	ADULT TREATMENT PROGRAM III (ATP III) DIAGNOSTIC CRITERIA FOR THE METABOLIC SYNDROME
	ATP III[a]
Carbohydrate metabolism	Fasting glucose ≥110 mg/dL (>100 mg/dL in 2005 update)
Abdominal obesity[b]	Men, waist >40 in; women, waist >35 in
Dyslipidemia	Triglycerides ≥150 mg/dL; men, HDL cholesterol <40 mg/dL; women, HDL cholesterol <50 mg/dL
Hypertension	BP ≥130/85 mm Hg

BMI, body mass index; BP, blood pressure; HDL, high-density lipoprotein.
[a]To qualify for the diagnosis of metabolic syndrome by ATP III criteria, a patient must meet at least three of the five criteria (hyperglycemia, abdominal obesity, high triglycerides, low HDL cholesterol, high blood pressure).
[b]Waist circumferences in Asian and south Asian patients may require different cutpoints.

Category	LDL-C Target (mg/dL)	Non–HDL-C Target (mg/dL)
Very high risk	<70	<100
High risk	<100	<130
Moderately high risk	<130	<160
Moderate risk	<130	<160
Low risk	<160	<190

Adapted from Grundy SM, Cleeman C, Merz NB, et al. Implications of recent clinical trials for the National Cholesterol Education Program Adult Treatment Panel III Guidelines. *Circulation* 2004;110:227.

renal insufficiency, genetic dyslipidemias, and therapy with oral estrogen, glucocorticoids, or β-blockers. The ATP III classification of serum triglyceride levels is as follows:

- Normal: <150 mg/dL
- Borderline-high: 150 to 199 mg/dL
- High: 200 to 499 mg/dL
- Very high: ≥500 mg/dL

Treatment of hypertriglyceridemia depends on the degree of severity. For patients with very high triglyceride levels, triglyceride reduction through a very low fat diet (≤15% of calories), exercise, weight loss, and drugs (fibrates, niacin) is the primary goal of therapy to prevent acute pancreatitis. When patients have a lesser degree of hypertriglyceridemia, control of LDL cholesterol is the primary aim of initial therapy. TLC is emphasized as the initial intervention to lower triglycerides. Non–HDL cholesterol is a secondary treatment target. A patient's non–HDL cholesterol is calculated by subtracting HDL cholesterol from total cholesterol. Target non–HDL cholesterol level is 30 mg/dL higher than the LDL cholesterol target. LDL and non–HDL cholesterol treatment targets for various degrees of cardiovascular risk are summarized in Table 32-10.

Low High-Density Lipoprotein Cholesterol

Modifications from ATP II includes redefining low HDL cholesterol as <40 mg/dL. Low HDL cholesterol is an **independent CHD risk factor** that is identified as a non–LDL cholesterol risk and included as a component of the Framingham scoring algorithm. Etiologies for low HDL cholesterol include physical inactivity, obesity, insulin resistance, diabetes mellitus, hypertriglyceridemia, cigarette smoking, high (>60% calories) carbohydrate diets, and certain medications (β-blockers, anabolic steroids, progestins). Because therapeutic interventions for low HDL cholesterol are of limited efficacy, ATP III identifies LDL cholesterol as the primary target of therapy for patients with low HDL cholesterol. Low HDL cholesterol often occurs in the setting of hypertriglyceridemia and metabolic syndrome. Management of these conditions may result in improvement of HDL cholesterol. Aerobic exercise, weight loss, smoking cessation, menopausal estrogen replacement, and treatment with niacin or fibrates may elevate low HDL cholesterol.

Lipid-Lowering Therapy and Age

The risk of a fatal or nonfatal cardiovascular event increases with age, and most cardiovascular events occur in patients age 65 years and older. Secondary prevention trials with the

HMG-CoA reductase inhibitors have demonstrated significant clinical benefit for patients age 65 to 75 years. The Heart Protection Study failed to show an age threshold for primary or secondary prevention with simvastatin. Patients who are 75 to 80 years of age at study entry experienced a nearly 30% reduction in major vascular events. The Prospective Study of Pravastatin in the Elderly (PROSPER) trial found a significant reduction in major coronary events among patients age 70–82 years with vascular disease or CHD risks treated with pravastatin. **ATP III does not place age restrictions** on treatment of hypercholesterolemia in elderly adults.

ATP III recommends TLC for young adults (men age 20–35 years; women age 20–45 years) with an LDL level ≥130 mg/dL. Drug therapy should be considered in the following high-risk groups: (a) men who both smoke and have elevated LDL levels (160–189 mg/dL), (b) all young adults with an LDL ≥190 mg/dL, and (c) those with an inherited dyslipidemia.

TREATMENT OF HYPERLIPIDEMIA

Treatment of Elevated Low-Density Lipoprotein Cholesterol

Hydroxymethylglutaryl-Coenzyme A Reductase Inhibitors (Statins)
Statins are the treatment of choice for elevated LDL cholesterol. Available statins are summarized in Table 32-11.

The lipid-lowering effect of statins appears within the first week of use and becomes stable after approximately 4 weeks of use. Common side effects (5%–10% of patients) include gastrointestinal upset (abdominal pain, diarrhea, bloating, constipation), and muscle pain or weakness (which can occur without creatinine kinase elevations). Other potential side effects include malaise, fatigue, headache, and rash.

Elevations of liver transaminases 2 to 3 times the upper limit of normal are dose dependent and reversible with discontinuation of the drug. Liver enzymes should be measured before initiating therapy, at 8 to 12 weeks after dose initiation or titration, and then every 6 months. The medication should be discontinued if liver transaminases elevate to >3 times the upper limit of normal.

Because some of the statins undergo metabolism by the cytochrome P-450 enzyme system, taking them in combination with other drugs metabolized by this enzyme system increases the risk of **rhabdomyolysis**. Among these drugs are: fibrates (greater risk with gemfibrozil), itraconazole, ketoconazole, erythromycin, clarithromycin, cyclosporine,

TABLE 32-11	**CURRENTLY AVAILABLE STATINS**					
Name	Atorvastatin (Lipitor)	Fluvastatin (Lescol)	Lovastatin (Mevacor)	Pravastatin (Pravachol)	Rosuvastatin (Crestor)	Simvastatin (Zocor)
Dose range (mg/day p.o.)	10–80	20–80	10–80	10–80	5–40	10–80
Triglyceride effect (%)	13–32 ↓	5–35 ↓	2–13 ↓	3–15 ↓	10–35 ↓	12–36 ↓
LDL effect (%)	38–54 ↓	17–36 ↓	29–48 ↓	19–34 ↓	41–65 ↓	28–46 ↓
HDL effect (%)	4.8–5.5 ↑	0.9–12 ↑	4.6–8 ↑	3–9.9 ↑	10–14 ↑	5.2–10 ↑

HDL, high-density lipoprotein; LDL, low-density lipoprotein; ↑, increased; ↓, decreased.

nefazodone, and protease inhibitors. Statins may also interact with large quantities of grapefruit juice to increase the risk of myopathy, although the precise mechanism of this interaction is unclear. Simvastatin (Zocor) can increase levels of warfarin (Coumadin) and digoxin. Rosuvastatin (Crestor) may also increase warfarin levels.

Bile Acid Sequestrant Resins

Currently available bile acid sequestrant resins include:

- Cholestyramine (Questran): 4 to 24 g/day orally in divided doses before meals
- Colestipol (Colestid): tablets, 2 to 16 g/day orally; granules, 5 to 30 g/day orally in divided doses before meals
- Colesevelam (Welchol): 625-mg tablets; three tablets orally twice a day or six tablets orally daily with food (maximum, seven tablets per day)

Bile acid sequestrants typically lower LDL levels by 15% to 30%. These agents should not be used as monotherapy in patients with triglyceride levels >250 mg/dL because they can raise triglyceride levels. They may be combined with nicotinic acid or statins.

Common side effects of resins include constipation, abdominal pain, bloating, nausea, and flatulence. Bile acid sequestrants may decrease oral absorption of many other drugs, including warfarin, digoxin, thyroid hormone, thiazide diuretics, amiodarone, glipizide (Glucotrol), and statins. Colesevelam interacts with fewer drugs than the older resins. Other medications should be given 1 hour before or 4 hours after resins.

Nicotinic Acid (Niacin)

Niacin can lower LDL levels by ≥15%, lower triglyceride levels 20%–50%, and raise HDL levels by up to 35%. Crystalline niacin is given 1 to 3 g/day orally in 2–3 divided doses with meals. Extended-release niacin (Niaspan) is dosed at night. The starting dose is 500 mg orally, and the dose may be titrated monthly in 500-mg increments to a maximum of 2000 mg orally (administer dose with milk or crackers).

Common side effects of niacin include flushing, pruritus, headache, nausea, and bloating. Other potential side effects include elevation of liver transaminases, hyperuricemia, and hyperglycemia. Flushing may be decreased with use of aspirin 30 minutes before the first few doses. Hepatoxicity associated with niacin is partially dose dependent and appears to be more prevalent with over-the-counter time-released preparations.

Avoid use of niacin in patients with gout, liver disease, active peptic ulcer disease, and uncontrolled diabetes mellitus. Niacin can be used with care in patients with well-controlled diabetes (HgbA1c ≤7%). Serum transaminases, glucose, and uric acid levels should be monitored every 6 to 8 weeks during dose titration, and then every 4 months.

Cholesterol Absorption Inhibitors

Ezetimibe (Zetia) is currently the only available agent in this category. Ezetimibe appears to act at the brush border of the small intestine and inhibits cholesterol absorption. The recommended dosing is 10 mg orally, once daily. No dose adjustment is required for renal insufficiency, mild hepatic impairment, or in elderly patients. Ezetimibe may provide an additional 25% mean reduction in LDL when combined with a statin, and it provides an ~18% decrease in LDL when used as monotherapy. It is not recommended for use in patients with moderate to severe hepatic impairment.

There appear to be few side effects associated with ezetimibe. In clinical trials, there was no excess of rhabdomyolysis or myopathy when compared with statin or placebo alone. There is a low incidence of diarrhea and abdominal pain compared to placebo. Liver function monitoring is not required with monotherapy because there appears to be no significant impact on liver enzymes when this drug is used alone. Liver enzymes should be monitored when used in conjunction with a statin, as there appears to be a slight increased incidence of enzyme elevations with combination therapy.

Treatment of Hypertriglyceridemia

Nonpharmacologic Treatment

Nonpharmacologic treatments are important in the therapy of hypertriglyceridemia. Non-pharmacologic approaches include:

- Changing oral estrogen replacement to transdermal estrogen
- Decreasing alcohol intake
- Encouraging weight loss and exercise
- Controlling hyperglycemia in patients with diabetes mellitus
- Avoiding simple sugars and very high carbohydrate diets

Pharmacologic Treatment

Pharmacologic treatment of isolated hypertriglyceridemia consists of a fibric acid deriv-ative or niacin. Statins may be effective for patients with mild to moderate hyper-triglyceridemia and concomitant LDL elevation. (See the sections Nicotinic Acid [Niacin] and Hydroxymethylglutaryl-Coenzyme A Reductase Inhibitors [Statins] for dosing details.)

Currently available fibric acid derivatives include:

- Gemfibrozil (Lopid): 600 mg orally twice daily before meals
- Fenofibrate (multiple brands and doses available): typically 48 to 145 mg/day orally

Fibrates generally lower triglyceride levels 30% to 50% and increase HDL levels 10% to 35%. They can lower LDL levels by 5% to 25% in patients with normal triglyceride lev-els, but may actually increase LDL levels in patients with elevated triglyceride levels. Common side effects include dyspepsia, abdominal pain, cholelithiasis, rash, and pruritus. Fibrates may potentiate the effects of warfarin. Fibrates (particularly gemfibrozil) given in conjunction with statins may increase the risk of rhabdomyolysis.

Omega-3 Fatty Acids. Omega-3 fatty acids from fish oil can lower triglycerides when taken in high doses. The active ingredients are eiscosapentaenoic acid (EPA) and docosahexaenoic acid (DHA). To lower triglyceride levels, 1 to 6 g of EPA plus DHA is needed daily. Main side effects are burping, bloating, and diarrhea. A prescription form of omega-3 acid fatty acids is available and is indicated for triglycerides levels greater than 500 mg/dL; four tablets contain about 3.6 g of omega-3 acid ethyl esters and can lower triglycerides by 30%. In practice, omega-3 fatty acids are being used as an adjunct to statin or other drugs in patients with moderately elevated triglyceride levels. The combi-nation of omega-3 fatty acids plus statin has the advantage of avoiding the risk of myopa-thy seen in the statin-fibrate combination.

Treatment of Low High-Density Lipoprotein Cholesterol

Nonpharmacologic therapies are the mainstay of treatment, including smoking cessation, exercise, and weight loss. In addition, medications known to lower HDL levels should be avoided such as β-blockers, progestins, and androgenic compounds.

- Niacin is the most effective pharmacologic agent for increasing HDL levels. (See the section Nicotinic Acid [Niacin] in this chapter for dosing details.)

KEY POINTS TO REMEMBER

- Lowering total and LDL cholesterol reduces the risk of coronary death, myocardial infarction, stroke, and the need for coronary revascularization.
- All adults should be screened for hyperlipidemia and treated on the basis of risk assessment. All high-risk patients should be treated to an LDL cholesterol <100 mg/dL, and very-high-risk patients should be treated to an LDL cholesterol <70 mg/dL.
- All patients with elevated lipids should implement TLC.
- Statins are the treatment of choice for lowering LDL cholesterol. Other options for patients who cannot tolerate a statin include bile acid sequestrant resins, nicotinic acid, and ezetimibe.
- The response to therapy should be assessed every 6 weeks until the target LDL level is achieved.
- Nonpharmacologic treatments (e.g., diet and exercise) are very important in the therapy of hypertriglyceridemia.

REFERENCES AND SUGGESTED READINGS

Alberti KG, Zimmet PZ. Definition, diagnosis, and classification of diabetes mellitus and its complications. Part 1: diagnosis and classification of diabetes mellitus provisional report of a WHO consultation. *Diabet Med* 1998;15:539.

Ballantyne CM, Olsson AG, Cook TJ, et al. Influence of low high-density lipoprotein cholesterol and elevated triglycerides on coronary heart disease and response to simvastatin therapy in 4S. *Circulation* 2001;104:3046.

Cannon CP, Braunwald E, McCabe CH, et al. for the Pravastatin or Atorvastatin Evaluation and Infection Therapy-Thrombolysis in Myocardial Infarction 22 (PROVE IT-TIMI22) Investigators. Intensive versus moderate lipid lowering with statins after acute coronary syndromes. *N Engl J Med* 2004;350:1495.

Castelli WP, Garrison RJ, Wilson PW, et al. Incidence of coronary heart disease and lipoprotein cholesterol levels: the Framingham Study. *JAMA* 1986;256:2835.

Chong PH. Lack of therapeutic interchangeability of HMG-CoA reductase inhibitors. *Ann Pharmacother* 2002;36:1907–1917.

Downs JR, Clearfield M, Weis S, et al. for the AFCAPS/TexCAPS Research Group. Primary prevention of acute coronary events with lovastatin in men and women with average cholesterol levels: results of AFCAPS/TexCAPS. *JAMA* 1998;279:1615.

Executive summary of the third report of the National Cholesterol Education Program (NCEP) expert panel on detection, evaluation, and treatment of high blood cholesterol in adults (Adult Treatment Panel III). *JAMA* 2001;285:2486.

Feussner G, Wagner A, Kohl B, et al. Clinical features of type III hyperlipoproteinemia: analysis of 64 patients. *Clin Invest* 1993;71:362.

Ford ES, Giles WH, Dietz WH. Prevalence of metabolic syndrome among US adults: findings from the Third National Health and Nutrition Examination Survey. *JAMA* 2002;287:356.

Genest JJ, Martin-Munley SS, McNamara JR, et al. Familial lipoprotein disorders in patients with premature coronary artery disease. *J Am Coll Cardiol* 1992;19:792.

Grundy SM, Chait A, Brunzell JD. Familial combined hyperlipidemia workshop. *Arteriosclerosis* 1987;7:203.

Grundy SM, Cleeman JI, Merz NB, et al. Implications of recent clinical trials for the National Cholesterol Education Program Adult Treatment Program III Guidelines. *Circulation* 2004;110:227.

Innerarity TL, Mahley RW, Weisgraber KH, et al. Familial defective apolipoprotein B-100: a mutation of apolipoprotein B that causes hypercholesterolemia. *J Lipid Res* 1990;31:1337.

Knopp RH. Drug treatment of lipid disorders. *N Engl J Med* 1999;341:498.

Krauss RM, Lingren RT, Williams PT, et al. Intermediate-density lipoproteins and progression of coronary artery disease in hypercholesterolemic men. *Lancet* 1987;2:62.

Kugiyama K, Doi H, Motoyama T, et al. Association of remnant lipoprotein levels with impairment of endothelium-dependent vasomotor function in human coronary arteries. *Circulation* 1998;97:2519.

Lakka HM, Laaksonen DE, Lakka TA, et al. The metabolic syndrome and total and cardiovascular disease mortality in middle aged men. *JAMA* 2002;288:2709.

MRC/BHF Heart Protection Study of cholesterol lowering with simvastatin in 20,536 high-risk individuals: a randomized placebo-controlled trial. *Lancet* 2002;360:7–22.

Package insert. Crestor (Rosuvastatin). Wilmington, DE: AstraZenica Pharmaceuticals; November 2007.

Package insert. Lescol (fluvastatin sodium). East Hanover, NJ: Novartis Pharmaceuticals Corporation; October 2006.

Package insert. Lipitor (atorvastatin calcium tablets). Morris Plains, NJ: Parke-Davis Pharmaceutical Research; November 2007.

Package insert. Mevacor (lovastatin). West Point, PA: Merck and Co, Inc.; May 2007.

Package insert. Pravachol (pravastatin sodium). Princeton, NJ: Bristol-Myers Squibb Company; March 2007.

Package insert. Zetia (ezetimibe). North Wales, NJ: Merck/Schering-Plough Pharmaceuticals; September 2007.

Package insert. Zocor (simvastatin). West Point, PA: Merck and Co, Inc.; May 2007.

Pasternak RC, Smith JC Jr, Bairey-Merz CN, et al. (2002) ACC/AHA/NHLBI Clinical Advisory on the Use and Safety of Statins. *Circulation* 2002;106:1024–1028.

Sachs FM, Pfeffer MA, Moye LA, et al. The effect of pravastatin on coronary events after myocardial infarction in patients with average cholesterol levels. *N Engl J Med* 1996; 335:1001.

Scandinavian Simvastatin Survival Study Group. Scandinavian Simvastatin survival study. *Lancet* 1994;344:1383.

Shepherd J, Blauw GJ, Murphy MB, et al. Pravastatin in elderly individuals at risk of vascular disease (PROSPER): a randomized controlled trial. PROspective Study of Pravastatin in the Elderly at Risk. *Lancet* 2002;360:1623.

Shepherd J, Cobbe SM, Ford I, et al. Prevention of coronary heart disease with pravastatin in men with hypercholesterolemia. *N Engl J Med* 1995;333:1301.

Steinberg D, Gotto AM. Preventing coronary artery disease by lowering cholesterol levels: fifty years from bench to bedside. *JAMA* 1999;282:2043.

Stone NJ, Levy RI, Fredrickson DS, et al. Coronary artery disease in 116 kindred with familial type II hyperlipoproteinemia. *Circulation* 1974;49:476.

Tall AR. Plasma high density lipoproteins. Metabolism and relationship to atherogenesis. *J Clin Invest* 1990;86:379.

The Long-Term Intervention with pravastatin In Ischemic Disease (LIPID) study group. Prevention of cardiovascular events and death with pravastatin in patients with coronary heart disease and a broad range of initial cholesterol levels. *N Engl J Med* 1998;339:1349.

Third Report of the Expert Panel on detection, evaluation, and treatment of high blood cholesterol in adults (Adult Treatment Panel III). http://www.nhlbi.nih.gov/guidelines/cholesterol/index.htm.

Note: Two supplements of the *American Journal of Cardiology* have lipid drug safety reports from the National Lipid Association. April 17, 2006 Volume 97 (8) and March 19, 2007 Volume 99 (6). There are extremely useful articles about all of the drugs and their side effects as well as clinical trial information.

Multiple Endocrine Neoplasia Syndromes

33

Manu V. Chakravarthy

INTRODUCTION

Multiple endocrine neoplasia (MEN) syndromes are sporadic or hereditary neoplastic disorders of more than one endocrine organ. Broadly, there are two distinct syndromes: MEN1 and MEN2. Each of these syndromes is characterized by complete penetrance but variable expressivity. The main subtypes of MEN2 are MEN2A, with its variant, familial medullary thyroid cancer (FMTC), and MEN2B. The identification of the genetic and molecular basis of these syndromes has enhanced our understanding of their pathogenesis, and thereby improved our ability to diagnose and treat these conditions more effectively. Both MEN syndromes have an autosomal-dominant pattern of inheritance and provide examples of different genetic mechanisms of tumorigenesis. MEN1 is caused by loss of function or inactivation of a tumor suppressor gene. On the other hand, MEN2 is caused by gain of function or activation of a proto-oncogene.

CAUSES

(See Table 33-1.)

Multiple Endocrine Neoplasia 1

MEN1 is inherited as an autosomal dominant trait with an incidence of 2 to 20 per 100,000 in the general population. The gene for MEN1 has been identified and is located on the long arm of chromosome 11 (11q13). The *MEN1* gene functions as a tumor suppressor gene and encodes a 610 amino acid nuclear protein called menin. The complete function of menin is not yet fully known, although studies suggest it might have a role in transcriptional regulation. Although ~10% of *MEN1* mutations arise *de novo*, more than 400 different germline mutations have been identified. However, there is no correlation between the genotype and phenotype in MEN1, making genetic screening and rational therapeutic intervention difficult.

Multiple Endocrine Neoplasia 2

MEN2 is also a rare autosomal-dominant syndrome with an estimated incidence of 1 to 10 per 100,000 in the general population. It has been identified in 500 to 1000 kindred worldwide. Two main subtypes are recognized: MEN2A and MEN2B. A variant of the MEN2A syndrome is familial medullary thyroid carcinoma (FMTC). Among these syndromes, MEN2A accounts for 80% of cases, FMTC for 15%, and MEN2B for 5%. Nearly all patients with the MEN2 syndrome will develop medullary thyroid carcinoma (MTC), which is derived from the cells of the neural crest rather than from thyroid follicular cells. Approximately 25% of patients with MTC have one of the MEN2 variants. Pheochro-

TABLE 33-1	GENERAL FEATURES OF MEN1 AND MEN2 SYNDROMES	
	MEN1	**MEN2**
Incidence	2–20 per 100,000	1–10 per 100,000
Inheritance	Autosomal dominant	Autosomal dominant
Gene	*MEN1* gene	*RET* gene
Gene product	Menin (nuclear protein)	RET (transmembrane tyrosine kinase–linked protein)
Location	Chromosome 11 (11q13)	Chromosome 10 (10q11-2)
Function	Tumor suppresser gene	Proto-oncogene
Type of mutation in tumors	Inactivation	Activation
Genotype–phenotype correlation	No	Yes
Genetic testing guides intervention to prevent and cure cancer	No	Yes

Adapted from Brandi ML, et al. Guidelines for diagnosis and therapy of MEN type 1 and type 2. *J Clin Endocrinol Metab* 2001;86:5658–5671.

mocytoma is the second most common tumor in MEN2, and is present in ~50% of patients.

The gene for MEN2 has been identified and its function well characterized. MEN2 is caused by specific mutations in the *RET* proto-oncogene, located on chromosome 10 (10q11-2) containing 21 exons, and encodes a membrane-bound tyrosine kinase receptor. In contrast to MEN1, there is a high degree of correlation between a specific *RET* mutation and clinical phenotype. Eighty percent to 98% of cases of MEN2A and FMTC are caused by mutations involving exon 10 or exon 11 that lead to ligand-independent homodimerization of the receptor with constitutive activation and downstream signaling of the mitogen-activated protein (MAP) kinase pathway. On the other hand, more than 95% of MEN2B cases exhibit a mutation at exon 16 that leads to autophosphorylation and alteration of substrate specificity. Therefore, these are the exons that are routinely screened for *RET* mutations, and because of the tight genotype–phenotype correlation, both genetic screening as well as curative therapeutic interventions are feasible.

PRESENTATION

(See Table 33-2.)

Multiple Endocrine Neoplasia 1

Although the presentation can be variable, the three most common features of the MEN1 syndrome are parathyroid, enteropancreatic, and pituitary tumors. Thus clinically, a patient with primary hyperparathyroidism and either a pituitary adenoma or an islet cell tumor is considered to have MEN1.

TABLE 33-2   CLINICAL MANIFESTATIONS OF MEN1, MEN2A, AND MEN2B

MEN1	MEN2A	MEN2B
Hyperparathyroidism (~95%)	**Medullary thyroid cancer (~100%)**	**Medullary thyroid cancer (~100%)**
Enteropancreatic tumors (30%–80%)	**Pheochromocytoma (~50%)**	**Pheochromocytoma (~50%)**
• Gastrinoma (50%)	**Hyperparathyroidism (~30%)**	**Other**
• Insulinoma (10%)	**Other**	• Mucosal neuroma (95%)
• Glucagonoma	• Cutaneous lichen amyloidosis	• Intestinal ganglioneuromatosis (40%)
• VIPoma	• Hirschsprung's disease	• Marfanoid habitus (75%)
• Non-hormone secreting		
Pituitary tumors (15%–90%)		
• Prolactinoma (60%)		
• GH-secreting (acromegaly) (25%)		
• ACTH-secreting (Cushing's disease) (6%)		
• Non-hormone secreting		
Other tumors		
• Facial angiofibromas and collagenomas (70%–88%)		
• Multiple lipomas (30%)		
• Adrenocortical tumors (5%–40%)		
• Carcinoid tumors (3%)		

GH, growth hormone; VIP, vasoactive-intestinal polypeptide.

Adapted from Brandi ML, et al. Guidelines for diagnosis and therapy of MEN type 1 and type 2. *J Clin Endocrinol Metab* 2001;86:5658–5671; Lakhani VT, et al. The multiple endocrine neoplasia syndromes. *Ann Rev Med* 2007;58:253–265.

Parathyroid Tumors

The most common and earliest manifestation of MEN1 is primary hyperparathyroidism, which occurs in nearly 95% of patients by the age of 50 years. Hyperparathyroidism in MEN1, compared to its sporadic counterpart typically presents around at age 20 to 25 years (vs. 55–60 years), with an equal male-to-female ratio (compared to 1M:3F ratio), and involves all four glands (rather than a single adenoma). Although most patients are asymptomatic, they may present with typical symptoms and signs of hypercalcemia (polyuria, myalgias, fatigue, renal stones).

Enteropancreatic Tumors

Enteropancreatic tumors are the second most common tumors, and occur in 30% to 80% of MEN1-affected individuals. They can be functional or nonfunctional. Symptoms of hormone excess usually occur by age 40, although with biochemical testing and imaging, asymptomatic tumors in carriers can be identified much earlier.

Gastrinoma is the most common enteropancreatic tumor, presenting in ~50% of MEN1 patients. An initial diagnosis of gastrinoma should suggest MEN1, because 25% to 30% of all gastrinoma patients have MEN1. The tumor causes hypergastrinemia with increased gastric acid output (Zollinger-Ellison syndrome). It is usually multicentric and has malignant potential. More than half of the gastrinomas in MEN1 have already metastasized before diagnosis, although the metastatic tumors in MEN1 are usually less aggressive than sporadic gastrinoma tumors. These tumors account for the major morbidity and mortality associated with MEN1. They are often located in the duodenum and may be associated with pancreatic tumors. Patients may present with peptic ulcer disease, diarrhea, cachexia, and abdominal pain.

Insulinoma is the second most common enteropancreatic tumor, occurring in ~10% of patients with MEN1 syndrome. Most insulinomas arise spontaneously because <5% of patients with insulinoma have MEN1 syndrome. Patients typically present with fasting hypoglycemia. The finding of inappropriately elevated plasma levels of insulin, C-peptide, and proinsulin in a hypoglycemic patient is highly suggestive of insulinoma. The tumors are usually too small to be identified by computed tomography (CT) or magnetic resonance imaging (MRI); however, intraoperative ultrasound usually identifies the tumor within the pancreas. For further details, see Chapter 31, Hypoglycemia.

Pituitary Tumors

Anterior pituitary adenomas are seen in 15%–90% of patients with MEN1, and are the initial presenting tumors in 10% to 25% of cases. Two-thirds are microadenomas, which are usually functional and commonly secrete prolactin, resulting in the expected symptoms of prolactin excess (amenorrhea and galactorrhea in women; impotence in men). Nearly one-fourth of these pituitary tumors secrete growth hormone resulting in acromegaly, and a smaller percentage secrete adrenocorticotropic hormone (ACTH) resulting in Cushing's disease. The presentation, diagnosis, and management are similar to those of sporadic pituitary adenomas (see Chapter 1, Pituitary Adenomas.)

Other Tumors

Patients with MEN1 syndrome can also present with multiple lipomas, facial angiofibromas, and collagenomas. Adrenocortical tumors, both functional and nonfunctional, occur in 5% to 40% of patients with MEN1. Hypercortisolism can be ACTH-dependent (pituitary adenoma or ectopic ACTH syndrome) or ACTH-independent (adrenal adenoma). Although statistically most cases are caused by pituitary adenomas, it is nevertheless important to differentiate between the various causes by biochemical testing (see Chapter 14, Cushing's Syndrome).

Carcinoid tumors are present in ~3% of MEN1 patients. Nearly all carcinoid tumors in MEN1 originate in tissues arising from the embryologic foregut. Thymic carcinoids are predominantly seen in males, can be asymptomatic until a late stage, and tend to be more aggressive than in sporadic tumors. Bronchial carcinoids, by contrast, tend to occur mainly in females, can secrete ACTH, and may present with Cushing's syndrome. Gastric enterochromaffin-like cell carcinoids have been found incidentally during gastric endoscopy for gastrinoma in MEN1. Carcinoid syndrome generally does not occur unless the tumor has metastasized to the liver (see Chapter 34, Carcinoid Syndrome).

Multiple Endocrine Neoplasia 2

The presenting features of MEN2 are largely dependent on the subtype (see Table 33.2). However, the common underlying feature in virtually all patients with MEN2A, MEN2B, and FMTC is the development of MTC, and is the most common cause of morbidity and death in patients with the MEN2 syndrome.

Medullary Thyroid Cancer

MTC is the first clinical manifestation in MEN2 kindreds because of its earlier and higher penetrance, occurring in nearly all patients with MEN2. MTC is preceded by C-cell hyperplasia (CCH), with resultant secretion of calcitonin, which serves as an excellent plasma tumor marker. CCH progresses to microscopic MTC, followed by local disease (usually multicentric), and eventually by metastatic disease (commonly to lymph nodes, lung, liver, and bones). MTC usually presents as a thyroid nodule and/or increased serum calcitonin.

The severity of MTC depends on the MEN2 subtype. It tends to be more aggressive in MEN2B, presenting usually before 5 years of age. By contrast, MTC is the only manifestation of FMTC (a variant of MEN2A), and has an indolent clinical course. FMTC presents later in life, with a peak incidence in the fourth and fifth decades. It tends to be less aggressive than the other subtypes of MEN2. However, the criteria to characterize kindred as having FMTC include MTC in more than 10 carriers in the kindred, multiple carriers or affected members older than age 50, and an adequate history to rule out pheochromocytoma or hyperparathyroidism. Such strict diagnostic criteria are necessary because some MEN2A patients may manifest only MTC and thus be incorrectly designated as FMTC, with the resulting danger of missing a diagnosis of pheochromocytoma.

Pheochromocytoma

Almost one-half of the patients with MEN2A and MEN2B have pheochromocytoma. Compared to sporadic cases, pheochromocytoma in MEN2 is almost always benign, bilateral, confined to the adrenal glands, and presents earlier in life. If unrecognized, it can present as hypertensive crisis during surgery for MTC early in childhood. The clinical presentation, diagnosis, and management are similar to that seen in sporadic cases (see Chapter 15, Pheochromocytoma).

Hyperparathyroidism

Primary hyperparathyroidism is seen in about one-third of the patients with MEN2A, but it is rarely seen in MEN2B. It is usually caused by four-gland hyperplasia, although it is less aggressive than in MEN1. The clinical presentation, diagnosis, and management are similar to those in MEN1 and that seen in sporadic cases (see Chapter 22, Hyperparathyroidism). It is important to evaluate the parathyroid glands during thyroidectomy for patients with MEN2A because they may be enlarged even though the preoperative calcium level is normal.

Other Features Assioicated with MEN2B

In addition to MTC and pheochromocytoma, patients with MEN2B also manifest a characteristic marfanoid habitus, but do not have lens subluxation or aortic disease. Ganglioneuromas occur in 95% of MEN2B patients, which can present at the lips, eyelids, and tongue, giving these patients a characteristic phenotype that can be apparent at birth. Intestinal ganglioneuromatosis can occur as early as infancy with gastrointestinal motility disorders.

MANAGEMENT

MEN1

To diagnose MEN1 syndrome in an individual, the patient must have two of the three main MEN1-related tumors: parathyroid, pituitary, and enteropancreatic. Familial MEN1 is defined as at least one case of MEN1 plus a first-degree relative with one of the three tumors.

Treatment

Patients with MEN1 are not treated until there is clinical or biochemical evidence of a characteristic disease because there is no genotype–phenotype correlation, and, consequently, there is no rationale for prophylactic intervention in an attempt to prevent the disease. However, a patient with a known *MEN1* mutation should be followed closely for evidence of the tumors that are characteristically associated with this syndrome.

Parathyroid Tumors. The most common surgical approach is either a four-gland parathyroidectomy with autotransplantation, or a 3.5-gland parathyroidectomy. Minimally invasive parathyroidectomy is not recommended, as the hyperparathyroidism in MEN1 patients is invariably due to hyperplasia of all four glands. A decrease in PTH >50% from baseline indicates adequate resection of parathyroid tissue. There is a high incidence of recurrence. In one series, 10 years after parathyroidectomy, 50% of the MEN1 patients had recurrent hyperparathyroidism. Because calcimimetics have proved effective in the treatment of patients with hypercalcemia from other causes, they might also have a role in treating persistent or recurrent hypercalcemia following surgery in MEN1 patients.

Enteropancreatic Tumors. Proton pump inhibitors are the treatment of choice to effectively control hypergastrinemia, but they are administered at double the usual dose (e.g., omeprazole 40 mg orally daily; pantoprazole 80 mg orally daily). The role of surgery in management of gastrinoma in MEN1 is still controversial. It is usually reserved for patients who are (a) refractory to or intolerant of medical therapy, (b) have gastrinomas >2 cm, or (c) at increased risk of metastasis. Outcomes of surgery are also relatively poor in MEN1 patients (only 16% disease-free survival), compared to those with sporadic gastrinomas (45% disease-free survival). Patients with persistent or recurrent gastrinomas after surgery could undergo repeat surgery, or medical therapy with 5-fluorouracil, octreotide, or interferon.

Surgery is the treatment of choice for insulinoma and is usually curative. For other islet cell tumors, surgery is still a first-line indication, since medical therapy alone is unsatisfactory. Tumor recurrence is treated symptomatically with agents such as octreotide.

Pituitary and Other Tumors. The treatment for MEN1 patients with these tumors as well as those with carcinoid or adrenocortical tumors is similar to that for patients who develop these tumors sporadically. After medical or surgical treatment, patients should be followed for recurrence or persistent disease, as is usually done.

Screening

Once an index case of MEN1 is identified, genetic counseling and testing should be considered for all family members. The age to start screening is still controversial. Direct DNA analysis for mutations in the *MEN1* gene identifies patients who have inherited a mutated allele and are destined to develop MEN1. Once an individual is identified as high risk for MEN1 (positive gene test or family history), periodic biochemical screening to detect symptoms related to hormone excess associated with the tumors characteristic of MEN1 should be carried out. However, as mentioned previously, because of a lack of genotype–phenotype correlation, prophylactic treatments have no beneficial role in patients with MEN1.

On the basis of current consensus guidelines, a proposed screening scheme for tumor expression in a carrier of *MEN1* mutation is as follows:

Parathyroid Tumors
- Serum ionized calcium and PTH annually, starting at age 8 years. A sestamibi scan to be considered if biochemical tests are positive.

Enteropancreatic Tumors
- Fasting gastrin and secretin-stimulated gastrin annually, starting at age 20 years. An octreotide scan to be considered if biochemical tests are positive.

- Fasting glucose with or without insulin annually, starting at age 5–20 years. Selective measurement of pancreas vein insulin during arterial calcium infusion may also be considered based on the clinical picture.
- Chromogranin A and glucagon annually, starting at age 20 years for other enteropancreatic tumors as indicated, followed up with octreotide scan, CT, or MRI if biochemical tests are positive.

Pituitary Tumors
- Prolactin and insulin-like growth factor 1 (IGF-1) annually, starting at age 5 years. MRI if biochemical tests are positive.

MEN2

Genetic Testing

The MEN2 syndrome is a great example of a genetic disorder in which genetic testing allows for early diagnosis and effective prophylactic surgical intervention. In patients who present with a suspicious thyroid nodule, fine-needle aspiration biopsy may establish the diagnosis of MTC. Once an index case is identified (any patient with MTC), the individual should be tested for *RET* oncogene mutations by direct DNA sequence analysis in exons 10, 11, 13, 14, and 15 for MEN2A and FMTC, and exon 16 for MEN2B. This molecular genetic test has a sensitivity of 95%.

Only if the patient tests positive for a mutation in one of these exons, should *RET* molecular genetic analysis be extended to the patient's first-degree relatives (parents and children). If either parent tests positive, all the at-risk family members should be tested for that mutation. Therefore, the main indications for molecular genetic testing include:

- Confirmation of diagnosis of MEN2A, FMTC, and MEN2B
- Presymptomatic screening of family members at risk
- Identification of germline mutations to distinguish sporadic from familial MTC

Given a relatively low false-negative rate (2%–5%), if an individual tests negative for the *RET* mutation, he or she is not likely to be at risk for development of the MEN2 syndrome. In such cases, the patient could have a sporadic MTC or pheochromocytoma. Less likely is the possibility of a highly unusual or new *RET* mutation. Although entirely replaced by *RET* mutation analysis for carrier diagnosis, the calcitonin test can be used in such situations in which the MEN2 carrier ascertainment with DNA testing is not helpful or no *RET* mutation is detected. It is important to note that *RET* genetic testing does not obviate the need for biochemical studies to detect pheochromocytoma or hyperparathyroidism in MEN2 patients. In addition, *RET* genetic testing before symptoms develop cannot identify spontaneous mutations that have not yet occurred.

Screening and Treatment

Medullary Thyroid Carcinoma. A key issue is to distinguish individuals who have MEN2 from those with sporadic MTC. This is particularly relevant for individuals who present with multifocal MTC with a negative family history. Because MTC is the first clinical manifestation and is the major cause of morbidity and mortality in patients with MEN2A, MEN2B, and FMTC, total thyroidectomy with regional lymphadenectomy is the treatment of choice for MTC whether patients have hereditary or sporadic disease. In fact, all patients thought to have sporadic MTC should undergo *RET* mutation analysis as ~10% of putative sporadic cases have been shown to harbor germline *RET* mutations. Mutations in codons 768, 804, and 891 of the *RET* oncogene are specific for FMTC, as kindreds with these mutations only develop MTC and are not at risk for pheochromocytoma or hyperparathyroidism.

The decision to perform thyroidectomy in MEN2 patients should be based on the results of *RET* mutation testing, rather than on biochemical (calcitonin) testing. This recommendation is derived from the fact that there is not only a clear relationship between the particular *RET* codon mutation and aggressiveness of the MTC, but that early detection and intervention can significantly alter the clinical course of MTC. Therefore, the timing of prophylactic thyroidectomy is dependent on the risk-group stratification based on the *RET* codon mutation:

- Mutation in codon 918 associated with MEN2B is considered to have the "highest" risk for development of MTC, and, hence, total thyroidectomy is recommended by 6 months of age.
- Mutations in codons 611, 618, 620, and 634 associated with MEN2A are deemed of "higher" risk; total thyroidectomy is recommended by 5 years of age.
- Mutations in codon 768 and 804 associated with FMTC are considered "high" risk; total thyroidectomy is recommended by 5 to 10 years of age.

After thyroidectomy, patients are screened with serial calcitonin measurements, as it is often the first index of persistent or recurrent MTC. Local disease can be surgically resected, whereas widespread metastases are difficult to cure, since conventional chemotherapy or radiotherapy is not very effective.

Pheochromocytoma. Screening for pheochromocytoma with annual plasma and/or urinary fractionated metanephrine measurements is done in all MEN2 patients. The age at which to begin the screening also depends on specific codon mutations. Screening should start between 5 and 7 years of age in families with high-risk mutations (codons 611, 618, 634, and 918), and between 10 and 15 years of age in those with mutations in less high-risk codons (codon 768). An abnormal biochemical test should be followed by CT or MRI to localize tumors. Some advocate routine imaging every 3 to 5 years, even in the presence of normal biochemical tests.

Approximately one-fourth of patients with no known family history of pheochromocytoma may have an inherited disease caused by a mutation other than *RET*, including mutations in the genes for von Hipple-Lindau (*VHL*), neurofibromatosis type 1 (*NF1*), and genes encoding the B and D subunits of mitochondrial succinate dehydrogenase (*SDHB* and *SDHD*). Therefore, any patient with presumably sporadic pheochromocytoma in the following clinical settings should be screened for mutations in these genes using a stepwise approach:

- Bilateral adrenal pheochromocytoma without MTC: first screen for mutations in *VHL*; if negative, then screen for mutations in *RET*.
- Age <20 years with sporadic unilateral adrenal pheochromocytoma: first screen for mutations in *VHL*; if negative, then screen for mutations in *RET*; if negative, then screen for mutations in *SDHB*.
- Age >20 years with sporadic unilateral adrenal pheochromocytoma: first screen for mutations in *SDHB*; if negative, then screen for mutations in *SDHD*.

Treatment of pheochromocytoma in MEN2 is similar to that in sporadic cases (see Chapter 15, Pheochromocytoma). If a pheochromocytoma is detected at the same time as MTC, adrenalectomy should be performed before thyroidectomy with appropriate adrenergic blockade to avoid intraoperative catecholamine crisis. Laparoscopic adrenalectomy is the recommended surgical approach. Those patients with evidence of unilateral disease should have unilateral adrenalectomy followed by annual biochemical testing to detect recurrence. If the adrenal lesion by pathology is a pheochromocytoma and unilateral adrenalectomy is performed, then ~50% will develop a contralateral pheochromocytoma over 10 years. Those with evidence of bilateral disease must undergo bilateral adrenalectomy. When bilateral adrenalectomy is required, appropriate pre- and intraoperative stress-dose glucocorticoid coverage should be given, followed by both glucocorticoid and mineralocorticoid replacement for life.

Hyperparathyroidism. Those at risk for hyperparathyroidism (with mutations in codons 611, 618, 620, and 634) should be screened annually with ionized calcium and intact PTH, starting at the age of 15 years. Hyperparathyroidism is managed with subtotal parathyroidectomy or total parathyroidectomy with autotransplantation. If parathyroid hyperplasia is found at the time of thyroidectomy, this should be considered as hyperparathyroidism even in the absence of biochemical evidence of disease.

KEY POINTS TO REMEMBER

- MEN syndromes are rare, autosomal-dominant disorders.
- The three main features of the MEN1 syndrome are hyperparathyroidism, enteropancreatic tumors, and anterior pituitary tumors. The syndrome is associated with both hormone excess (PTH, prolactin, gastrin) and malignant tumors (gastrinoma, carcinoid).
- Surgery is the treatment of choice for hyperparathyroidism and insulinoma, whereas medical treatment is preferred for gastrinoma in MEN1 patients.
- Although the *MEN1* germline mutation test is recommended for MEN1-carrier detection, this is mainly for information purposes as there is no role for prophylactic medical or surgical intervention given the lack of genotype–phenotype correlation. This is in stark contrast to patients with the MEN2 syndrome.
- MEN2 has two main subtypes: MEN2A and MEN2B. FMTC is a mild variant of MEN2A, and hence is diagnosed only from rigorous criteria to avoid missing a diagnosis of MEN2A with its risk of pheochromocytoma.
- MTC and pheochromocytoma are the main tumors associated with MEN2A and MEN2B.
- The main morbidity from MEN2 is MTC, with the aggressiveness of MTC being highest in MEN2B, followed by MEN2A and FMTC.
- Hyperparathyroidism is present mainly in MEN2A, whereas MEN2B is associated with ganglioneuromas and marfanoid habitus.
- Genetic testing is critical in the MEN2 syndrome because such testing allows for early diagnosis and effective prophylactic surgical intervention. MEN2-carrier detection by *RET* germline mutation testing is the basis for recommending thyroidectomy to prevent or cure MTC.

REFERENCES AND SUGGESTED READINGS

Brandi ML, Gagel RF, Angeli A, et al. Guidelines for diagnosis and therapy of MEN type 1 and type 2. *J Clin Endocrinol Metab* 2001;86:5658–5671.

Burgess JR, Greenaway TM, Shepherd JJ. Expression of the MEN-1 gene in a large kindred with multiple endocrine neoplasia type 1. *J Intern Med* 1998;243:465–470.

Chandrasekharappa SC, Guru SC, Manickam P, et al. Positional cloning of the gene for multiple endocrine neoplasia type 1. *Science* 1997;276:404–407.

de Groot JWB, Links TP, Plukker JT, et al. RET as a diagnostic and therapeutic target in sporadic and hereditary endocrine tumors. *Endocr Rev* 2006;27:535–560.

Doherty GM, Olson JA, Frisella MM, et al. Lethality of multiple endocrine neoplasia type 1. *World J Surg* 1998;22:581–585.

Eng C, Clayton D, Schuffenecker I, et al. The relationship between specific RET proto-oncogene mutations and disease phenotype in multiple endocrine neoplasia type 2. *JAMA* 1996;276:1575–1579.

Gagel RF, Marx SJ. Multiple endocrine neoplasia. In: Larsen PR, et al., eds. *Williams Textbook of Endocrinology*, 10th ed. Philadelphia: WB Saunders; 2003:1717–1762.

Krause DS, Van Etten RA. Tyrosine kinases as targets for cancer therapy. *N Engl J Med* 2005;353:172–187.

Lakhani VT, You YN, Wells SA. The multiple endocrine neoplasia syndromes. *Annu Rev Med* 2007;58:253–265.

Machens A, Niccoli-Sire P, Hoegel J, et al. Early malignant progression of hereditary medullary thyroid cancer. *N Engl J Med* 2003;349:1517–1525.

Mulligan LM, Kwok JB, Healey CS, et al. Germ-line mutations of the RET proto-oncogene in multiple endocrine neoplasia type 2A. *Nature* 1993;363:458.

Mulligan LM, Ponder BA. Genetic basis of endocrine disease: multiple endocrine neoplasia type 2. *J Clin Endocrinol Metab* 1995;80:1989–1995.

Skinner MA, Moley JA, Dilley WG, et al. Prophylactic thyroidectomy in multiple endocrine neoplasia type 2A. *N Engl J Med* 2005;353:1105–1113.

Thakker RV. Multiple endocrine neoplasia type 1. *Endocrinol Metab Clin North Am* 2000;29:541–562.

Tramp D, Farren B, Wooding C, et al. Clinical studies of multiple endocrine neoplasia type 1 (MEN1). *QJM* 1996;89:653–669.

Wells SA, Chi DD, Toshima K, et al. Predictive DNA testing and prophylactic thyroidectomy in patients at risk for multiple endocrine neoplasia type 2A. *Ann Surg* 1994;220:237–247.

Wells SA, Skinner MA. Prophylactic thyroidectomy, based on direct genetic testing in patients at risk for multiple endocrine neoplasia type 2 syndromes. *Exp Clin Endocrinol Diabetes* 1998;106:29–34.

Wiench M, Wygoda Z, Gubala E, et al. Estimation of risk of inherited medullary thyroid carcinoma in apparent sporadic patients. *J Clin Oncol* 2001;19:1374–1380.

Carcinoid Syndrome

Manu V. Chakravarthy

INTRODUCTION

Carcinoid syndrome refers to the cluster of symptoms mediated by the systemic release of vasoactive compounds and hormones produced by carcinoid tumors. The term *karzinoide* was first introduced by Oberndorffer in 1907 to describe intestinal tumors that histologically resembled carcinomas but did not behave in their aggressive manner. Carcinoid tumors are rare, slow-growing neuroendocrine tumors arising from enterochromaffin cells, which are frequently identified in the mucosa of the intestine and bronchus. The overall prevalence of carcinoid tumors in the United States is estimated to be 1 to 2 cases per 100,000 persons. Because of their indolent nature, these tumors are often considered only after the onset of the carcinoid syndrome, which in turn, does not typically occur until the tumor has metastasized to the lungs or liver.

Carcinoid tumors contain neurosecretory granules that synthesize, store, and release substances, such as serotonin, histamine, prostaglandins, kallikrein, bradykinins, substance P, gastrin, corticotropin, and neuron-specific enolase. The most prominent of these substances is serotonin (5-hydroxytryptamine), the degradation of which results in 5-hydroxyindoleacetic acid (5-HIAA), which is excreted in the urine. When released into the systemic circulation, serotonin can result in the symptoms of carcinoid syndrome: flushing (purplish or red), diarrhea (watery and explosive), tachycardia, hypotension, bronchoconstriction, telangiectasia, and right-sided heart disease or failure. Symptoms can be exacerbated by consuming foods rich in tyramine, such as blue cheese, chocolate, and red wine.

Carcinoid tumors are classified according to their embryologic site of origin into carcinoids of the **foregut** (10%; bronchi, stomach), **midgut** (75%; small intestine, appendix, proximal large bowel), and **hindgut** (15%; distal colon, rectum). Recently, the World Health Organization (WHO) presented new classifications based on their malignant potential: *well-differentiated endocrine tumor* (proliferation index [PI] <2%); *well-differentiated endocrine carcinoma* (PI >2% but <15%); *poorly differentiated endocrine carcinoma* (PI >15%); *mixed exocrine—endocrine tumors;* and *tumor-like lesions.* More than 75% of carcinoid tumors are located in the gastrointestinal tract, ~25% are in the lung, and <1% are in the kidneys and ovaries. Within the gastrointestinal tract, carcinoids of the small intestine are the most common (29%), followed by tumors of the rectum (14%), stomach (5%), and appendix (5%). "Typical" carcinoids have a characteristic histologic appearance of monotonous sheets of small round cells with uniform nuclei and cytoplasm without pleomorphism or mitoses. "Atypical" carcinoids have features associated with more aggressive behavior, such as greater nuclear atypia, higher mitotic rates, and/or necrosis.

CAUSES

The molecular pathogenesis of carcinoid tumors is incompletely understood. Sporadic foregut carcinoids, as well as those associated with multiple endocrine neoplasia 1 (MEN1) (primary hypergastrinemia [Zollinger-Ellison syndrome]), display allelic losses at chromosome 11q13. Somatic *MEN1* gene mutations have also been reported in one-third of sporadic foregut tumors. Duodenal carcinoid tumors (localized in or close to the ampulla of Vater) producing somatostatin are associated with neurofibromatosis-1. For midgut carcinoids, the major areas of chromosomal loss are 18q (54%), 9p (15%), 11q (13%), and 16q (12%). Bronchial carcinoids are associated with mutations of the *p53* tumor suppressor gene and abnormal expression of proteins involved in apoptosis, including Bcl-2 and Bax. The expression of various growth factors (basic fibroblast growth factor, vascular endothelial growth factor, transforming growth factor α and β, trefoil peptides, and platelet-derived growth factor) and some of their receptors has also been reported in carcinoid tumors.

Although the precise cause for the flushing seen in carcinoid syndrome is uncertain, the other manifestations of the syndrome, especially diarrhea and bronchospasm, appear to be largely attributable to the excessive serotonin. Right-sided valvular heart disease is also caused by high serum levels of serotonin and is a later complication of this syndrome resulting in endocardial fibrosis and thickening of the heart valves, with resultant pulmonic stenosis and tricuspid insufficiency. Mitral valves are usually less affected because of the metabolism of serotonin in the lungs. Other potential causes for these findings must also be considered in the differential diagnosis (Table 34-1).

TABLE 34-1   **DIFFERENTIAL DIAGNOSIS OF CARCINOID SYNDROME**

Flushing

Physiologic

- Menopause, hot drinks, anxiety disorder, benign cutaneous flushing

Medications

- Diltiazem, amyl nitrate, nicotinic acid, levodopa, bromocriptine, alcohol plus disulfram

Diseases

- Systemic mastocytosis, basophilic chronic granulocytic leukemia, VIPoma, pheochromocytoma, medullary carcinoma of the thyroid, renal cell carcinoma, diencephalic seizures

Diarrhea

- Gastroenteritis, inflammatory bowel disease, infectious colitis, VIPoma, laxative abuse

Bronchospasm

- Asthma, anaphylaxis, pulmonary edema, bronchial foreign body

Valvular heart disease

- Rheumatic heart disease, subacute bacterial endocarditis, dilated cardiomyopathy, ischemic heart disease with papillary muscle dysfunction

---

Adapted from Robertson RG, et al. Carcinoid tumors. *Am Fam Physician* 2006;74:429–434; Sitaraman SV, Goldfinger SE. The carcinoid syndrome. In: Rose BD, ed. *UpToDate,* Waltham, MA: UpToDate; 2007.

PRESENTATION

Symptoms of the carcinoid syndrome vary in intensity and timing. They are also usually vague, nonspecific, and organ-related, causing relatively long delays in diagnosis. The average time from symptom onset to diagnosis is more than 9 years. At presentation, 40% to 60% of patients are asymptomatic. Many carcinoid tumors are found incidentally during surgery for other reasons, usually at appendectomy (1 of 300 appendectomies) or surgery for acute pancreatitis, or surgery for bowel obstruction or diseases of the female reproductive tract. Symptoms from the tumor itself can range from mild abdominal discomfort to intermittent intestinal obstruction. Occasionally a carcinoid tumor can be the lead point for an intermittent intestinal intussusception. Carcinoid tumors characteristically present at age 50 to 60, have a higher incidence in African Americans, and are slightly more frequent in women (55%).

A majority of the patients with small bowel carcinoid tumors present with metastases to lymph nodes and/or liver. The lungs and liver metabolize many of the substances secreted by carcinoid tumors, thereby preventing their release into the systemic circulation until metastases develop. This may explain why patients who have carcinoid tumors have the syndrome only if they have hepatic metastases. However, if the syndrome is present, it does not necessarily mean there is metastatic disease, as the liver may not have immediately cleared the bioactive products. Carcinoid syndrome occurs in only 10% of all patients with carcinoid tumors, and it is most often associated with midgut tumors, whereas bronchial and other extraintestinal carcinoids rarely cause the syndrome.

Symptoms and Signs

Flushing
Flushing is usually dry without diaphoresis and occurs in 85% of patients with carcinoid syndrome. In midgut carcinoid, flushing is usually of faint pink to red color and involves the face and upper trunk down to the nipples. Flushing is initially provoked by alcohol and food containing tyramines (blue cheese, chocolate, red wine). With time, flushing may occur spontaneously. It typically lasts for 1 to 5 minutes and may occur many times per day. Flushing associated with foregut tumors is more intense, lasts for hours, is frequently followed by telangiectasias, and involves the upper trunk and the limbs.

Diarrhea
Diarrhea is usually secretory (watery, nonbloody) and persists with fasting. Stools may vary from a few to >30/day and can be explosive. If accompanied by severe abdominal cramping, diarrhea could be due to mesenteric fibrosis. Diarrhea is usually not temporally related to flushing episodes.

Bronchospasm
Ten percent to 20% of patients with carcinoid syndrome have wheezing and dyspnea, often during flushing episodes.

Carcinoid Heart Disease
Carcinoid heart disease can be seen in 60% to 70% of patients with metastatic carcinoid tumors. It is characterized by fibrous thickening of the endocardium, valve leaflets, atria, and ventricles. Valvular heart disease is the most common pathologic feature, with tricuspid valve regurgitation and pulmonary valve stenosis seen in 97% and 88% of patients, respectively. Clinical manifestations are those of right-sided valvular heart disease and include peripheral edema, ascites, and pulsatile hepatomegaly.

Carcinoid Crisis
Carcinoid crisis is a life-threatening form of carcinoid syndrome that is triggered by specific events such as anesthesia, surgery, or chemotherapy, which presumably stimulates the

release of an overwhelming amount of vasoactive compounds. Symptoms include flushing with extreme changes in blood pressure, and may also include arrhythmias, bronchospasm, and altered mental status.

Other Manifestations
Pellagra dermatosis (hyperkeratosis and pigmentation), Peyronie's disease of the penis, occlusion of the mesenteric arteries and veins, and intraabdominal/retroperitoneal fibrosis leading to intestinal and/or urethral obstruction may also be present. Rarely, carcinoid tumors of foregut or of hindgut origin can cause bone metastases. These tumors can secrete corticotropin-releasing hormone (CRH) and adrenocorticotropic hormone (ACTH) (resulting in ectopic Cushing's syndrome), or growth hormone (resulting in acromegaly). Gastric carcinoids are associated with MEN1.

MANAGEMENT

Diagnosis
Carcinoid tumors pose a diagnostic challenge because they often are asymptomatic and indolent. Given the various other conditions apart from the carcinoid syndrome that result in diarrhea or flushing (see Table 34-1), the evaluation is primarily directed to address two key issues: (a) verify that the presenting symptoms are due to an actively secreting carcinoid tumor, and (b) localize the tumor.

Biochemical Testing
The most useful initial diagnostic test for carcinoid syndrome is to measure **24-hour urinary excretion of 5-HIAA,** which is the end product of serotonin metabolism. This test has a sensitivity of 75% and specificity of nearly 100%. The normal range of 5-HIAA excretion is <6 mg/day (Barnes-Jewish Hospital ref range). Most patients with the carcinoid syndrome have urinary 5-HIAA levels >100 mg/day; in one study the range was from 99 to 2070 mg/day. However, in other patients with the carcinoid syndrome, only modest elevations (up to 30 mg/day) are seen, comparable to that observed in patients with celiac sprue, Whipple's disease, or after the ingestion of high tryptophan-containing foods. Therefore, before ordering the measurement of urinary 5-HIAA, it is critical to note those factors that lead to either false-positive or false-negative test results (Table 34-2). 5-HIAA levels also appear to correlate well with tumor mass, and can be used as a marker for the extent of disease.

Although urinary 5-HIAA excretion is useful in patients with midgut carcinoid tumors, this test may not be useful in patients with suspected foregut carcinoids because they often lack aromatic amino acid decarboxylase, the enzyme that converts 5-hydroxytryptophan to serotonin. Consequently, foregut carcinoids will have high levels of 5-hydroxytryptophan instead. However, this metabolite cannot be accurately measured in clinical laboratories within the United States currently, and, therefore, other studies need to be performed to localize the tumor directly.

Another biochemical test that can be used is **chromogranin A,** a glycoprotein that is secreted with other hormones by neuroendocrine tumors. Although chromogranin A levels appear to be a sensitive marker of carcinoid tumors, this test has poor specificity because chromogranin levels are also increased in other conditions unrelated to neoplastic processes, such as decreased renal and liver function, inflammatory bowel disease, physical stress and trauma, and hypergastrinemia caused by achlorhydria (e.g., chronic use of proton pump inhibitors, atrophic gastritis, or retained gastric antrum). Therefore, chromogranin A measurements are not generally used for the diagnosis of the carcinoid syndrome. Nevertheless, it can be used as a marker of tumor progression or regression, since changes in its level precede the radiographic detection of the tumor. An increased chromogranin A

TABLE 34-2	FACTORS THAT FALSELY INCREASE OR DECREASE URINARY 5-HIAA CONCENTRATION

False-Positive

Foods

- Avocados, pineapples, bananas, kiwi fruit, plums, eggplant, walnuts, pecans

Drugs

- Nicotine, caffeine, acetaminophen, guafenesin, phenobarbital, reserpine, ephedrine, phentolamine, fluorouracil, melphalan

False-Negative

Drugs

- Ethanol, aspirin, isoniazid, heparin, monoamine oxidase inhibitors, corticotropin, imipramine, levodopa, methyldopa, phenothiazines

level has been shown to be an independent predictor of poor overall survival, and correlates with tumor burden (except in gastrinoma).

According to some recent reports, determination of **whole blood serotonin** concentration may be more sensitive than urinary 5-HIAA levels, and may be useful in cases when the latter results are equivocal. For example, in patients with the carcinoid syndrome, the fasting whole blood serotonin concentration ranged from 790 to 4500 ng/mL, in contrast to healthy subjects who had a range of 71 to 310 ng/mL. However, the specificity of this test is undetermined. In addition, several factors can affect total blood serotonin levels: Selective serotonin reuptake inhibitor (SSRI) antidepressant medications reduce blood serotonin concentrations, whereas paragangliomas such as extra-adrenal pheochromocytomas can increase serotonin levels.

If the preceding biochemical tests are normal or only marginally elevated in a patient who describes obvious flushing and other features of the carcinoid syndrome, **provocative testing** with epinephrine (starting at 2 mcg intravenous boluses up to a maximum of 10 mcg) or intravenous pentagastrin (0.06 mg/kg body weight) might be considered, both of which have nearly 100% sensitivity. The test is considered positive if the patient has flushing, hypotension, and tachycardia that appears between 45 and 120 seconds after an injection and lasts for at least 1 minute. The test is stopped after the first positive response. The advantage of the pentagastrin provocation test over the epinephrine test is that it induces flushing in patients with either foregut or midgut tumors.

Imaging

Once the biochemical diagnosis of carcinoid syndrome is confirmed, the tumor must be localized. Abdominal CT scanning is the diagnostic procedure of choice for tumor staging, as it identifies the primary tumor, mesenteric lymph node enlargement, and liver metastases. Carcinoids that have infiltrated have a characteristic CT appearance that is spiculated with a stellate pattern. The presence of somatostatin receptors in carcinoid tumors has allowed the use of indium-111 octreotide scintigraphy for tumor imaging. This test has nearly 90% sensitivity in patients with carcinoid syndrome. Therefore, both abdominal CT and octreotide scintigraphy have complementary roles in localization procedures, with the added advantage of octreoscan in predicting responses to octreotide therapy.

Other modalities such as MRI (sensitive for detecting extrahepatic disease), endoscopic ultrasound/intraoperative ultrasound, and video capsule endoscopy are usually reserved for those patients with suspected carcinoid tumors that have not been localized by CT or the octreoscan. Chest CT scan can be used to localize bronchial carcinoid tumors, and echocardiography can help in establishing the severity of carcinoid heart disease.

Treatment

The key management issues in patients with carcinoid tumors include removal of the tumor (if metastases have not occurred) and control of symptoms.

The treatment of choice for a patient who has a localized carcinoid tumor is surgery. Tumors <2 cm in the appendix can be treated with appendectomy. Larger appendiceal carcinoids require right hemicolectomy. Carcinoids of the small intestine are generally removed by segmental resection with mesenteric lymph node excision. Radical excision of the rectum is recommended for rectal carcinoids and radical colectomy for colonic carcinoids. Bronchial carcinoids are usually removed surgically. The efficacy of various therapies may be evaluated by the magnitude of their biochemical response (e.g., >50% reduction in urinary 5-HIAA levels) or tumor response rate (e.g., reduction in tumor size on imaging studies).

Because more than 90% of patients with the carcinoid syndrome have metastatic disease (except bronchial and ovarian tumors, which may cause symptoms without metastasis), surgery plays a limited role in the treatment of such patients. However, potentially curative surgery can be offered to the rare patient with resectable hepatic or isolated brain metastasis, or to patients with bronchial and ovarian carcinoids. Patients with carcinoid syndrome may need to be pretreated with octreotide to reduce the incidence of carcinoid crisis, which can be precipitated during induction of anesthesia or surgical manipulation of tumors.

Specific treatment for the various symptoms of the carcinoid syndrome is also necessary. Several drugs have shown efficacy for patients with flushing and severe diarrhea, such as octreotide, prednisone, phenoxybenzamine, and chlorpromazine. Selective bronchodilators can be used to control symptoms of wheezing. However, in patients with severe symptoms, the only drug that is likely to be effective with acceptable toxicity is octreotide. Flushing and diarrhea resolve in 75% to 80% of patients treated with 50 mcg of subcutaneous octreotide 3 times per day.

Side effects of octreotide include anorexia, nausea and vomiting, which can be minimized by gradual titration of the dose (maximum 1500 mcg/day in divided doses). However, long-acting preparations of octreotide (lanreotide SR) are also available for more convenient dosing of once every 10 days, and studies have shown equal efficacy with both lanreotide SR and octreotide. Another common complication includes the development of asymptomatic cholesterol gallstones or gallbladder sludge in ~25% of patients during the first 18 months of therapy, as octreotide reduces postprandial gallbladder contractility and emptying. Prophylactic treatment with ursodeoxycholic acid may help reduce this complication.

The role of surgery in advanced disease is unclear. When resection is not possible, other treatment options for patients with metastatic carcinoid disease include the use of radiofrequency ablation and cryoablation, either alone or in conjunction with surgical debulking. In uncontrolled trials, hepatic artery embolization resulted in marked symptomatic improvement in up to 75% of patients with hepatic metastases from carcinoid with reductions in flushing and diarrhea. The addition of interferon-alfa has also been effective in controlling symptoms in patients whose disease is resistant to therapy with octreotide alone. Cytotoxic chemotherapy (streptozocin, cyclophosphamide, fluorouracil, doxorubicin) has had limited success in the treatment of metastatic carcinoid tumors.

Prognosis

Carcinoid tumors are slow-growing, and even with metastases survival is measured in terms of years rather than months. The prognosis is based on the location, size, invasiveness, and histology of the primary tumor. The best survival rates are for appendiceal tumors (~85%), followed by bronchopulmonary (~75%) and rectal (~70%) tumors. The presence of functional abnormalities of the tricuspid valve and the carcinoid syndrome portends a poorer median survival. Data from the U.S. National Carcinoid Register showed an overall median 5-year survival for all patients of 82%. Median survival in patients with localized tumors was 94%, those with regional lymph node metastases 64%, and those with metastatic tumors 0% to 27%.

KEY POINTS TO REMEMBER

- Carcinoid tumors are rare, slow-growing neuroendocrine tumors. The systemic release of serotonin and other vasoactive peptides from carcinoid tumors results in the carcinoid syndrome.
- The principal features of carcinoid syndrome include flushing, diarrhea, sweating, wheezing, abdominal pain, and cardiac fibrosis.
- Carcinoid syndrome occurs in only 10% of patients with carcinoid tumors, and particularly in the presence of hepatic metastases. However, bronchial and ovarian carcinoids can result in the syndrome, even in the absence of metastatic disease.
- The most useful initial diagnostic test for carcinoid syndrome is measurement of 24-hour urinary excretion of 5-HIAA.
- The treatment of choice for a patient with a localized carcinoid tumor is surgery.
- Medical treatment of metastatic carcinoid tumors includes the use of octreotide.

REFERENCES AND SUGGESTED READINGS

Fink G, Krelbaum T, Yellin A, et al. Pulmonary carcinoid: presentation, diagnosis, and outcome in 142 cases in Israel and review of 640 cases from the literature. *Chest* 2001;119:1647–1651.

Janson ET, Holmberg L, Stridsberg M, et al. Carcinoid tumors: analysis of prognostic factors and survival in 301 patients from a referral center. *Ann Oncol* 1997;8:685–690.

Kulke M, Mayer R. Carcinoid tumors. *N Engl J Med* 1999;340:858–868.

Kvols LK, Moertel CG, O'Connell MJ, et al. Treatment of malignant carcinoid syndrome: evaluation of a long-acting somatostatin analogue. *N Engl J Med* 1986;315:663–666.

Modlin IM, Sandor A. An analysis of 8305 cases of carcinoid tumors. *Cancer* 1997; 79:813–829.

Öberg KE. Carcinoid tumors, carcinoid syndrome, and related disorders. In: Larsen PR, Kronenberg HM, Melmed S, et al., eds. *Williams Textbook of Endocrinology*, 10th ed. Philadelphia: WB Saunders; 2003:1857–1876.

Richter G, Stöckmann F, Conlon JM, et al. Serotonin release into blood after food and pentagastrin. Studies in healthy subjects and in patients with metastatic carcinoid tumors. *Gastroenterology* 1986;91:912–918.

Robertson RG, Geiger WJ, Davis NB. Carcinoid tumors. *Am Fam Physician* 2006; 74:429–434.

Sitaraman SV, Goldfinger SE. The carcinoid syndrome. In: Rose BD, ed. *UpToDate*. Waltham, MA: UpToDate; 2007.

Vinik AI. Carcinoid tumors. In: DeGroot L, Jameson JL, eds. *Endocrinology*, 4th ed. Philadelphia: WB Saunders; 2001:2533–2546.

Autoimmune Polyendocrine Syndromes

35

Matteo Levisetti

INTRODUCTION

The autoimmune polyendocrine syndromes comprise a heterogeneous group of disorders that are characterized by the autoimmune destruction of endocrine glands and other self tissues. Autoimmune polyendocrine syndrome type I (APS-I) is diagnosed when at least two of the three defining conditions are present: mucocutaneous candidiasis, hypoparathyroidism, and adrenal insufficiency. The initial manifestation of APS-I typically occurs in infancy and presents with persistent candidal infections of the skin and mucous membranes. The subsequent development of hypocalcemia, due to hypoparathyroidism, is the feature that usually leads to the diagnosis of APS-1 in affected children. Adrenal insufficiency typically develops after the hypoparathyroidism, with both glucocorticoid and mineralocorticoid deficiency. Autoimmune polyendocrine syndrome type II (APS-II) is more common than APS-I, and is generally diagnosed in adulthood. APS-II is generally defined by the presence in an individual of two or more of the following diseases: primary adrenal insufficiency, type 1A diabetes mellitus, Graves' disease, autoimmune hypothyroidism, celiac disease, pernicious anemia, or primary hypogonadism (Table 35-1).

CAUSES

APS-I, also known as autoimmune polyendocrinopathy-candidiasis-ectodermal dystrophy, APECED, is caused by mutations in the autoimmune regulator (*AIRE*) gene found on chromosome 21. The pattern of inheritance of APS-I is autosomal recessive. The AIRE protein, a transcription factor, is expressed in the medullary epithelial cells of the thymus and mediates the expression of peripheral tissue antigens, a function that is required for the deletion of autoreactive T cells and the establishment of self-tolerance. Mutations in this gene presumably lead to incomplete negative selection and escape to the periphery of self-reactive T cells, which in turn, initiate the destruction of various endocrine glands and self tissues.

APS-II is genetically complex and has no clear pattern of inheritance. Many of the diseases of APS-II are associated with certain human leukocyte antigen (HLA) alleles: HLA-DQ2/DQ8 and type 1A diabetes, for example. The exact mechanisms that lead from HLA class II–associated susceptibility to organ-specific autoimmune disease are unknown.

PRESENTATION

History

A complete and thorough history is essential for the proper evaluation and management of patients with the autoimmune polyendocrine syndromes. Detailed information with regard to the timing and presentation of known autoimmune and endocrine diagnoses

TABLE 35-1	AUTOIMMUNE POLYGLANDULAR SYNDROMES	
	APS-I	**APS-II**
Prevalence	Rare	Common
Genetics	*AIRE* mutations, autosomal recessive	Polygenic, HLA association
Common phenotype	Mucocutaneous candidiasis	Adrenal insufficiency
	Hypoparathyroidism	Type 1A diabetes
	Adrenal insufficiency	Thyroiditis
	Ungual dystrophy, enamel hypoplasia	
Associated conditions	Hypogonadism	Hypogonadism
	Alopecia	Alopecia
	Vitiligo	Vitiligo
	Celiac disease	Pernicious anemia
	Type 1A diabetes	Myasthenia gravis
	Pernicious anemia	Celiac disease
	Thyroiditis	Rheumatoid arthritis
	Chronic active hepatitis	Sjögren's syndrome

APS, autoimmune polyglandular syndrome; *AIRE*, autoimmune regulator gene, chromosome 21.

should be documented. The history should include careful inquiry about any signs or symptoms that would be consistent with any of the endocrine disorders that make up the autoimmune polyendocrine syndromes. Special attention should be addressed to symptoms of potentially life-threatening conditions: fatigue and weight loss in adrenal insufficiency, or polyuria and polydipsia in type 1A diabetes mellitus. The family history is important, since APS-I has an autosomal-recessive pattern of inheritance. APS-II occurs more frequently within families but without a clear Mendelian pattern of inheritance.

Physical Examination

The examination should include full evaluation for any of the findings that accompany the individual disorders that make up the syndromes. Chronic hyperpigmentation and orthostatic hypotension are signs of adrenal insufficiency. Patients with type 1A diabetes mellitus may be tachycardic and volume depleted. Slow relaxation phases of deep tendon reflexes and periorbital edema are signs of hypothyroidism. Pernicious anemia may cause pallor, impaired vibratory sensation, and ataxia. The skin, hair, nails, teeth, and oral mucosa should be examined carefully for any abnormalities. Vitiligo and alopecia are common components of both APS-I and II. Patients with APS-I may have characteristic dental enamel hypoplasia, mucocutaneous candidiasis, and nail dystrophy.

MANAGEMENT

Diagnostic Evaluation

Many of the autoimmune disorders that make up the autoimmune polyendocrine syndromes have long prodromal phases during which time tissue-specific autoantibodies appear in the serum. The repertoire of autoantibodies present in a given individual serves as a guide to diseases that may develop, as the risk for a given disease tends to increase as the number and quantity of autoantibodies targeting that tissue increases. For example, the 5-year risk of developing type 1A diabetes in first-degree relatives of affected individuals is >50% if multiple anti-beta cell autoantibodies are present.

Laboratory Evaluation

The major laboratory approaches to the diagnosis of the autoimmune polyendocrine syndromes are **serologic tests for autoantibodies** against involved glands and tissues, and **evaluation of end-organ function and hormone secretion.** Evaluation for the presence of adrenal (21-hydroxylase), thyroid (peroxidase and thyroglobulin), islet cell (insulin, glutamic acid decarboxylase, and ICA512), and parietal cell (H+/K+-ATPase) autoantibodies (Table 35-2) may assist in confirming clinical suspicion of tissue autoimmunity or in assessing risk for future endocrinopathy. However, routine serologic testing should not replace careful clinical assessment of endocrine sufficiency. Endocrine organ function should be evaluated by laboratory measurement of the **appropriate hormones:** adrenal (cosyntropin-stimulation testing, serum electrolytes, aldosterone, and renin), thyroid (thyroid-stimulating hormone and free levothyroxine), pancreatic islet (fasting glucose or glucose tolerance testing), parathyroid (ionized serum calcium and intact parathyroid hormone), and gonads (estrogen or testosterone, follicle-stimulating hormone, and luteinizing hormone). **Serum vitamin B_{12} levels** and **complete blood counts** with differentials may be done to evaluate for pernicious anemia, and patients with **tissue transglutaminase autoantibodies** may require endoscopy with small bowel biopsy to document celiac disease. **Genetic testing** for known mutations in the *AIRE* **gene** is available for patients and their families if APS-I is suspected.

Treatment

At the present time there are no safe and effective therapies targeting the generalized autoimmunity that underlies the pathogenesis of the autoimmune polyendocrine syndromes. Patients with APS-I/II require close monitoring, and the clinician should maintain a high index of suspicion for the development of additional autoimmune diseases in these individuals. Therapies for the individual components of the syndromes are discussed in other chapters and the management of each disease is essentially the same in the patient with APS. A few points deserve special consideration:

- Patients with APS-I and chronic oral candidiasis should be treated aggressively with antifungal medication (fluconazole) and closely monitored given the elevated risk of oral cancers in these individuals.
- The development of additional endocrine disorders in a patient may complicate the clinical picture of the known disease, and certain examples deserve special consideration. Symptomatic hypotension or hypoglycemia leading to a decrease in insulin dosing in a patient with type 1A diabetes may be manifestations of adrenal insufficiency.

TABLE 35-2	ORGAN-SPECIFIC AUTOANTIBODIES
Type 1A diabetes: insulin, glutamic acid decarboxylase, ICA512
Thyroiditis: thyroid peroxidase, TSH receptor, thyroglobulin
Adrenal insufficiency: 17-α-hydroxylase and 21-α-hydroxylase
Pernicious anemia: parietal cell H+/K+-ATPase
Celiac disease: tissue transglutaminase
Hypoparathyroidism: calcium-sensing receptor
Hepatitis: cytochrome P-450, mitochondrial, nuclear, and smooth muscle antigen

- Thyroid hormone replacement in a patient with hypothyroidism may precipitate life-threatening addisonian crisis if concomitant adrenal insufficiency is present. It is wise to evaluate adrenal function by dynamic testing in patients with multiple autoimmune endocrinopathies prior to starting levothyroxine therapy.
- Pernicious anemia is treated by intramuscular injections of cyanocobalamin. Celiac disease generally responds to a gluten-free diet; however, mineral and vitamin supplementation may be required if significant malabsorption persists.
- In a patient with autoimmune hypothyroidism and APS-II, the unexplained requirement for increased thyroid hormone dosing to maintain euthyroidism may reflect malabsorption of drug due to the onset of celiac disease.

KEY POINTS TO REMEMBER

- Patients with APS-I or APS-II require careful observation and management given the high risk of developing additional autoimmune disorders and endocrine deficiencies.
- Special attention to the potential development of conditions that can be life-threatening, such as adrenal insufficiency or type 1A diabetes, is essential. Patients should be educated about signs and symptoms of disorders for which they are at risk, so that early diagnosis and treatment may limit the morbidity and mortality caused by these conditions.
- When a rare disorder, such as autoimmune hypoparathyroidism, occurs spontaneously, the probability that other autoimmune disorders are present or will develop is high, and there is greater clinical utility in screening for other hormone deficiencies and/or for the presence of autoantibodies. When a common autoimmune disease is present in isolation, such as hypothyroidism, the development of additional autoimmune endocrine disorders is much less common, and further endocrine and serologic testing should be guided by clinical suspicion.

REFERENCES AND SUGGESTED READINGS

Ahonen P, Myllarniemi S, Sipila I, et al. Clinical variation of autoimmune polyendocrinopathy-candidiasis-ectodermal dystrophy (APECED) in a series of 68 patients. *N Engl J Med* 1990;322:1829–1836.

Aaltonen J, Björses P, Perheentupa J, et al. An autoimmune disease, APECED, caused by mutations in a novel gene featuring two PHD-type zinc-finger domains. *Nat Genet* 1997;17:399–403.

Anderson MS, Venanzi ES, Klein L, et al. Projection of an immunological self shadow within the thymus by the AIRE protein. *Science* 2002;298:1395–1401.

Chen QY, Kukreja A, Maclaren NK. The autoimmune polyglandular syndromes. In DeGroot LJ, Jameson JL, eds. *Endocrinology*, 4th ed. Philadelphia: WB Saunders; 2001:587–599.

Eisenbarth GS, Gottlieb, PA. Autoimmune polyendocrine syndromes. *N Eng J Med* 2004; 350:2068–2079.

Neufeld M, Maclaren NK, Blizzard RM. Two types of autoimmune Addison's disease associated with different polyglandular autoimmune (PGA) syndromes. *Medicine (Baltimore)* 1981;60:355–362.

Perheentupa J. APS-I/APECED: the clinical disease and therapy. *Endocrinol Metab Clin North Am* 2002;31:295–320.

Schatz DA, Winter WE. Autoimmune polyglandular syndrome. II. Clinical syndrome and treatment. *Endocrinol Metab Clin North Am* 2002;31:339–352.

Villasenor J, Benoist C, Mathis D. AIRE and APECED: molecular insights into an autoimmune disease. *Immunol Rev* 2005;204:156–164.

Endocrine Disorders in HIV/AIDS

36

Paul Hruz and Kevin Yarasheski

INTRODUCTION

Human immunodeficiency virus (HIV) causes the acquired immunodeficiency syndrome (AIDS). In 2006, approximately 40 million people worldwide were living with HIV/AIDS, including ~18 million women and 2.3 million children. HIV is transmitted by exchange of blood, semen, or vaginal secretions through mucosal membranes. HIV can be transmitted during homosexual and heterosexual contact, during childbirth (mother-to-child transmission) and breast feeding, by blood transfusion, and by needles shared during intravenous drug use. HIV targets $CD4^+$ T lymphocytes, where it integrates into the host DNA, replicates, and produces new virions that infect and reduce T-cell number. This weakens host immunity and renders the host susceptible to common pathogens. Currently, there is no vaccine or cure for HIV.

There are many antiretroviral medications that effectively inhibit HIV replication by acting at different steps in the HIV life cycle (Table 36-1). When prescribed in proper combinations, highly active antiretroviral therapy (HAART) has reduced HIV-related morbidity and mortality rates so effectively that HIV infection is considered a chronic manageable infection that can be controlled for many years. Life expectancy for HIV-infected people is much longer than it was 10 years ago. From 1995 to 2001, mortality from HIV decreased by ~70%. **Now HIV-positive people die more frequently from injury, cancer, heart disease, or drug abuse than from AIDS.**

New anti-HIV medication classes are currently being tested that target other steps in the HIV life cycle, including maturation inhibitors and integrase inhibitors (raltegravir [Isentress]). Newer HIV medications and regimens are always needed to reduce pill burden, drug resistance, and toxicities.

Existing medication regimens have toxicities and they contribute to undesirable endocrine, metabolic, and body composition alterations. The pathogenesis of these disorders is multifactorial, and can also result directly from HIV infection per se, the medications used to treat HIV and HIV-related opportunistic infections, and indirectly from other chronic viral infections (e.g., hepatitis B virus [HBV], hepatitis C virus [HCV]), rapid immune reconstitution associated with HAART, advancing age, underlying genetic predisposition, poor lifestyle habits (diet, inactivity, tobacco, alcohol, recreational drug use), and drug–drug interactions. HIV infection and anti-HIV medications have been associated with several endocrine, metabolic, and anthropomorphic complications including: insulin resistance, hyperglycemia, adrenal insufficiency, hyperparathyroidism, hypogonadism, dyslipidemia, central adiposity, peripheral adipose wasting (lipoatrophy), muscle wasting, and osteopenia. Chronic inflammation associated with HIV infection, insulin resistance, dyslipidemia, and abdominal obesity are all pro-atherogenic processes. Therefore, cardiometabolic disease risk may be elevated in HIV-infected individuals treated with HAART. Its detection and treatment should be considered and integrated into current treatment paradigms for HIV-infected patients.

TABLE 36-1 ANTIRETROVIRAL CLASSES AND DRUG NAMES

Entry (CCR5–CXCR4) Inhibitors	Fusion Inhibitors	Nonnucleoside Reverse Transcriptase Inhibitors (NNRTI)	Nucleotide Reverse Transcriptase Inhibitors (NtRTI)	Nucleoside Reverse Transcriptase Inhibitors (NRTI)	Aspartyl Protease Inhibitors (PI)	Combination Drug Tablets
Selzentry	Fuzeon	Viramune	Viread	Emtriva	Agenerase[a]	Atripla: Efavirenz + Emtriva + Viread
		Rescriptor		Epivir	Aptivus[a]	Combivir: Epivir + Retrovir
		Efavirenz		Hivid	Crixivan[a]	
		Etravirine– (TMC125)		Retrovir	Invirase[a]	Epzicom: Ziagen + Epivir
				Videx	Kaletra[a]	
				Zerit	Lexiva[a]	Trizivir: Ziagen + Epivir + Retrovir
				Ziagen	Norvir	Truvada: Viread + Emtriva
					Prezista[a]	
					Reyataz[a]	
					Viracept	

[a]Often combined with Norvir.

Optimal care for HIV-infected people includes a high index of suspicion for endocrinopathies; physical and laboratory assessment of potential metabolic abnormalities; consideration of HBV, HCV and other sexually transmitted diseases (STDs); counseling on smoking cessation, recreational drug use, and weight management; careful consideration and implementation of treatment regimens that minimize risk; and initiation of specific therapies for endocrine abnormalities once they manifest (including therapeutic lifestyle changes in diet and exercise, lipid-lowering agents, insulin sensitizers/secretagogues, and anti-hypertensives).

PRESENTATION

Risk Factors

All patients with HIV infection are at risk for the development of endocrine disorders. In patients not receiving antiretroviral therapy, inflammatory cytokine production due to active disease, AIDS wasting, and the presence of opportunistic infections can all contribute to this risk. With the initiation of treatment, immune reconstitution can precipitate autoimmune diseases such as hyperthyroidism. Antiretroviral medications (particularly Crixivan, Norvir, and Zerit) can directly or indirectly increase the risk of metabolic abnormalities such as insulin resistance and dyslipidemia. It is important to remember that a patient's underlying genetic risk and environmental factors (such as overnutrition and sedentary lifestyle) can combine with disease-related risk factors to lead to overt manifestation of latent endocrine disease. For instance, reduced bone mineral density, which is associated with HIV infection and initiation of antiretroviral therapy, can also result from traditional risk factors for osteopenia (smoking and alcohol intake, use of corticosteroids, advanced age, low body weight, inadequate calcium intake and/or vitamin D deficiency).

History

A family history of early myocardial infarction, type 2 diabetes, or autoimmune disease can contribute to a patient's background risk and should be evaluated. Because it is common for patients to switch treatment regimens because of issues of compliance, viral resistance, and drug toxicities, detailed questioning on both prior and current antiretroviral therapies should be undertaken. Specific assessment of a patient's diet and physical activity level should be made. Many of the physical manifestations of endocrine disease may be subclinical or subtle, or may evolve slowly over months to years. A careful review of systems with specific attention to complaints that may reflect endocrine dysfunction is essential. Patients are often most aware of and concerned about facial lipoatrophy, visceral adiposity, and other features of lipodystrophy (altered/disproportionate body fat distribution), and in most cases these concerns can be validated by objective measures of fat distribution. Direct questioning may uncover evidence of diabetes mellitus (polyuria, polydipsia, nocturia), hypogonadism (decreased libido, erectile dysfunction, weakness, depressed mood), thyroid disease (thermal intolerance, unintentional weight change, altered bowel function), or adrenal insufficiency (weight loss, nausea, dizziness, abdominal pain, fatigue).

Physical Examination

Together with a patient's own report, the physician's subjective observation of changes in fat content and/or distribution can be used as a simple screen for lipodystrophy. **Lipoatrophy** can be seen as a loss of fat in the face and extremities. **Lipohypertrophy** is frequently observed as increased abdominal girth, the presence of a dorsocervical fat pad ("Buffalo hump"), and/or increased breast size in women. Objective changes in body fat composition (peripheral lipoatrophy and/or increased visceral adiposity) can be quantified by measurement of skin fold thickness, limb and abdominal circumference, and calculation of the waist-to-hip ratio. **Visceral adiposity** can be considered significantly elevated if the waist-to-hip ratio is greater than 0.90 in men and 0.80 in women. The use of an abdominal circumferences >102 cm in men and >88 cm in women may also reflect abnormal abdominal fat accumulation. Although computed tomography (CT) and magnetic resonance imaging (MRI) scans are more sensitive and accurate for identifying lipodystrophy; these tests are expensive, not practical for use in routine screening, and are generally used as research tools. Male patients with **hypogonadism** may exhibit testicular atrophy, changes in hair growth and/or gynecomastia. The clinical signs of **thyroid disease,** if present, are similar to those observed in the general population.

Laboratory Evaluation

Glucose Homeostasis

Screening for abnormal glucose homeostasis in HIV-infected patients can be performed in the same manner as in HIV-negative patients at risk for the development of type 2 diabetes mellitus (see Chapter 29, Diabetes Mellitus Type 2). The simplest and most cost-effective method is the determination of fasting blood sugar levels. Patients with insulin resistance will have normal fasting blood sugars as long as pancreatic beta-cell function is preserved. Oral glucose tolerance testing may be more sensitive in detecting early glucose intolerance, providing a better indication of peripheral glucose disposal than fasting glucose levels, which primarily reflect hepatic insulin sensitivity.

Dyslipidemia

A fasting lipid profile should be obtained in all HIV-infected patients prior to the initiation of antiretroviral therapy and within 3 to 6 months after starting a new treatment regimen. If no abnormalities are detected with these initial screens, repeat testing should be done at least annually. Hypertriglyceridemia and low high-density lipoprotein (HDL) cholesterol levels are the most commonly observed lipid changes in HIV-infected patients. Mild to moderate elevations in low-density lipoprotein (LDL) cholesterol levels can also be observed in patients, particularly with the restoration to health following initiation of effective antiretroviral therapy. Markedly elevated LDL cholesterol levels should prompt the investigation of an underlying genetic dyslipidemia and/or attention to the dietary consumption of saturated fat. The Infectious Diseases Society of America (IDSA) has issued comprehensive guidelines for the treatment of dyslipidemia in HIV-infected persons, and adherence to National Cholesterol Education Program (NCEP) recommendations with the stratification of goals according to coronary heart disease (CHD) risk categories is advisable (see Chapter 32, Diagnosis, Standards of Care, and Treatment for Hyperlipidemia).

Thyroid Function

The prevalence of thyroid dysfunction in HIV-infected patients is low and only rarely caused by the direct manifestations of active disease (such as *Pneumocystis carinii*–induced thyroiditis). Therefore, routine screening in asymptomatic patients is not generally necessary. However, because of the background prevalence in the general population and the nonspecific clinical signs of thyroid dysfunction, patients with a clinical history suggestive of hyper- or hypothyroidism can be screened with standard thyroid studies (i.e., serum thyroid-stimulating hormone [TSH] alone or together with total or free thyroxine [T_4] levels). Although a TSH level will identify most patients with primary hypothyroidism, this test may fail to identify patients with secondary hypothyroidism owing to pituitary disease. In interpreting the results of such tests, it is important to recognize that changes indicative of nonthyroidal illness (normal or low TSH with low T_4 levels) may be present in seriously ill patients. Elevated total T_4 levels in patients with normal TSH levels may also reflect the increased thyroid-binding globulin levels that are frequently observed in early HIV infection. In such patients, free T_4 levels are generally normal.

Adrenal Function

Although HIV-infected patients only rarely exhibit overt clinical symptoms of adrenal dysfunction, subclinical changes in adrenal steroid levels can frequently be detected. This includes higher basal serum cortisol and lower dihydroepiandrosterone levels. The lipodystrophy observed in patients on HAART led to initial suspicion for Cushing's syndrome; however, HIV patients have been shown to have normal suppression of cortisol levels following dexamethasone administration. In patients with advanced disease, opportunistic infection of the adrenal gland (e.g., by cytomegalovirus [CMV]) or use of medications that interfere with normal steroid metabolism (e.g., ketoconazole) can lead to adrenal insufficiency. Megestrol acetate (Megace) is used in patients with HIV/AIDS to treat anorexia and wasting; this drug can be associated with secondary adrenal insufficiency owing to disruption of the hypothalamic–pituitary–adrenal axis and with worsening glucose intolerance due to potential glucocorticoid activity. Drug–drug interactions such as the concomitant use of inhaled fluticasone propionate and ritonavir (Norvir) can lead to clinically significant cortisol excess. Although routine screening for adrenal disease is not necessary, in patients who exhibit symptoms suggestive of adrenal insufficiency, a standard ACTH stimulation test can be performed (see Chapter 11, Adrenal Insufficiency). Cushing's syndrome can usually be distinguished clinically from HIV-associated lipodystrophy. However, if hypercortisolemia is suspected, a 24-hour urinary free cortisol measurement or a dexamethasone suppression test can be performed (see Chapter 14, Cushing's Syndrome).

Gonadal Function

Because of the diurnal variation in testosterone levels, it is preferable to screen for hypogonadism with an early morning serum collection. Sex-hormone binding globulin levels are often elevated in HIV-infected men; therefore, total testosterone levels may be normal despite low free testosterone levels. If testosterone levels are low, measurement of gonadotropin levels (luteinizing hormone [LH], follicle-stimulating hormone [FSH]) can distinguish between primary and secondary disease. In addition to adverse effects on adrenal function, Megace can also suppress the pituitary–gonadal axis. In patients with secondary hypogonadism, the assessment for other pituitary abnormalities should be considered, including the measurement of serum prolactin and MRI of the pituitary gland, particularly in patients with headache, visual changes, or evidence of other pituitary hormone deficiencies (see Chapter 19, Male Hypogonadism).

Bone and Mineral Metabolism

The identification of patients with osteopenia/osteoporosis can facilitate preventative measures directed toward reducing the risk of fractures in the aging HIV-infected patient population. Dual energy x-ray absorptiometry (DEXA) of the hip and lumbar spine provides the most reliable and quantifiable data. Assessment of calcium and vitamin D status (25-OH vitamin D level) can also be helpful. Vitamin D deficiency can be observed in HIV-infected individuals and may at least contribute partially to the hyperparathyroidism that has been occasionally reported. Although serum calcium levels may be low, this is most commonly due to low serum albumin levels. This can be distinguished from true hypocalcemia by the determination of ionized calcium levels.

MANAGEMENT

The successful management of HIV-infected patients with or at-risk for endocrinopathies requires an integrated approach that addresses predisposing factors, optimal antiretroviral therapies, management of comorbidities, and selective use of pharmacologic agents with awareness of potential drug–drug interactions. A summary of potential treatment options available for the metabolic, endocrinologic, and body composition abnormalities is provided

TABLE 36-2	POTENTIAL TREATMENT OPTIONS AVAILABLE FOR METABOLIC, ENDOCRINOLOGIC, AND BODY COMPOSITION ABNORMALITIES	
Problem	**Treatment Options/Interventions**	**Potential Risks/Specific Comments**
Osteopenia/ osteoporosis	Optimization of calcium intake, vitamin D levels	
	Bisphosphonates	Long–term benefit in reducing fracture risk is unclear
	Testosterone (if hypogonadism present)	
Dyslipidemia		
Increased triglycerides	Gemfibrozil, fenofibrate	
Low HDL	Increase physical activity	
Elevated LDL	HMG-CoA reductase inhibitors	Use with PIs may lead to toxicity
Insulin resistance	Lifestyle changes	
	Metformin	May precipitate lactic acidosis (risk possibly increased by use of NRTIs)
	Thiazolidinediones	Heart disease risk? Bone loss in women?
Lipoatrophy	Avoidance of thymidine analogs (particularly d4T)	Drug switching may affect viral suppression
	Uridine	Expensive, unproven
	Surgical implant of biodegradable or permanent fillers	
Visceral adiposity	Lifestyle changes (increased exercise)	May exacerbate lipoatrophy
	Growth hormone	Expensive, not FDA approved for this indication

in Table 36-2. For some of the endocrinopathies such as thyroid disease, hypogonadism, and adrenal insufficiency, treatment strategies can follow those established for the HIV-negative population. In others such as HIV-associated lipodystrophy, insulin resistance, and dyslipidemia, active etiologic and outcomes research remains in progress and it is likely that revisions to existing treatment guidelines and/or the development of novel therapies will evolve with time. This is particularly relevant to the management of HIV-associated lipodystrophy. Changes in antiretroviral therapy, particularly the switch from thymidine analogs (such as Zerit) to Viread- or Ziagen-containing regimens, have been shown to modestly increase limb fat. Limited data suggest that the use of select thiazolidinediones or uridine may also increase limb fat. Infusion of biodegradable or permanent fillers has been used to treat facial lipoatrophy. Visceral adiposity can be reduced with increased physical activity and dietary modification, but this does not improve lipoatrophy. Some preliminary data suggest that growth hormone and growth hormone secretagogues, although expensive and not approved by the Food and Drug Administration (FDA) for this purpose, may reduce visceral fat content in HIV-infected people.

In patients with insulin resistance and/or elevated lipids, switching to a nonprotease inhibitor (PI)-containing antiviral regimen, if possible, may be beneficial. In contrast to Crixivan and Norvir, newer PIs such Reyataz do not appear to impair insulin sensitivity and can be considered when continued PI use is desired. HMG-CoA reductase inhibitors ("statins") can be used cautiously to treat elevated LDL cholesterol levels. Drug interactions are possible with statins that are primarily metabolized by the same P-450 3A4 pathway as PIs. Therefore, simvastatin and lovastatin should be avoided. Pravastatin or atorvastatin can be used safely with careful titration to the minimum effective dose. Low-dose fluvastatin is a recommended alternative in PI-treated patients. Cerivastatin and rosuvastatin appear to be safe in PI-treated patients. With marked elevations in triglycerides (>1000 mg/dL), treatment with a fibrate (gemfibrozil or fenofibrate) is indicated due to the increased risk of pancreatitis. Niacin is less effective in patients on HAART and has been associated with worsening insulin resistance.

KEY POINTS TO REMEMBER

- HIV-infected patients are at increased risk for a number of endocrine, metabolic, and body composition changes.
- HIV infection itself, opportunistic infections, disease-related comorbidities, antiretroviral therapy, together with background genetic factors and modifiable lifestyle risk factors all contribute to the incidence of endocrine and metabolic disease.
- A high index of suspicion together with judicious screening and confirmatory laboratory testing is required to diagnose HIV-associated endocrinopathies.
- The complexity of antiretroviral drug regimens, limited experimental data on effective therapies, and significant potential for drug–drug interactions present numerous challenges to the treatment of HIV-associated endocrine, metabolic, and body composition disorders.

REFERENCES AND SUGGESTED READINGS

Carr A. Treatment strategies for HIV lipodystrophy. *Curr Opin HIV AIDS* 2007;2: 332–338.

Crum NF, et al. A review of hypogonadism and erectile dysfunction among HIV-infected men during the pre- and post-HAART eras: diagnosis, pathogenesis, and management. *AIDS Patient Care STDS* 2005;19:655–671.

Crum NF, et al. Graves' disease: an increasingly recognized immune reconstitution syndrome. *AIDS* 2006;20:466–469.

Dube MP, et al. Guidelines for the evaluation and management of dyslipidemia in human immunodeficiency virus (HIV)-infected adults receiving antiretroviral therapy: recommendations of the HIV Medical Association of the Infectious Diseases Society of America and the Adult AIDS Clinical Trials Group. *Clin Infect Dis* 2003;37:613–627.

Gavrila A, et al. Improvement in highly active antiretroviral therapy-induced metabolic syndrome by treatment with pioglitazone but not with fenofibrate: a 2 × 2 factorial, randomized, double-blinded, placebo-controlled trial. *Clin Infect Dis* 2005;40: 745–749.

Grinspoon S, Carr A. Cardiovascular risk and body-fat abnormalities in HIV-infected adults. *N Engl J Med* 2005;352:48–62.

Grundy SM, et al. Implications of recent clinical trials for the National Cholesterol Education Program Adult Treatment Panel III guidelines. *Circulation* 2004;110:227–239.

Grunfeld C, et al. Recombinant human growth hormone to treat HIV-associated adipose redistribution syndrome: 12-week induction and 24-week maintenance therapy. *J Acquir Immune Defic Syndr* 2007.

HIV Medicine. http://www.hivmedicine.com/index.htm (accessed May 2007).

Martinez E, et al. Management of dyslipidaemia in HIV-infected patients receiving antiretroviral therapy. *Antivir Ther* 2004;9:649–663.

McComsey GA, et al. Uridine supplementation in HIV lipoatrophy: pilot trial on safety and effect on mitochondrial indices. *Eur J Clin Nutr* 2007;1-7doi:10.1038/sj.ejcn.1602793.

Moyle GJ, et al. A randomized comparative trial of tenofovir DF or abacavir as replacement for a thymidine analogue in persons with lipoatrophy. *AIDS* 2006;20:2043–2050.

Schambelan M, et al. Management of metabolic complications associated with antiretroviral therapy for HIV-1 infection: recommendations of an International AIDS Society-USA panel. *J Acquir Immune Defic Syndr* 2002;31:257–275.

Tebas P, et al. Accelerated bone mineral loss in HIV-infected patients receiving potent antiretroviral therapy. *AIDS* 2000;14:F63–F67.

Third report of the National Cholesterol Education Program (NCEP) Expert Panel on Detection, Evaluation, and Treatment of High Blood Cholesterol in Adults (Adult Treatment Panel III) final report. *Circulation* 2002;106:3143–3421.

Yarasheski KE, Marin D, Claxton S, et al. Endocrine, metabolic and body composition disorders. In: Powderly WG, ed. *Manual of HIV Therapeutics,* 2nd ed. Philadelphia: Lippincott Williams & Wilkins; 2001:154–167.

Index

Page numbers followed by *f* refer to figures; page numbers followed by *t* refer to tables.